Abigail Woods · Michael Bresalier
Angela Cassidy · Rachel Mason Dentinger

Animals and the Shaping of Modern Medicine

One Health and its Histories

Abigail Woods
Department of History
Kings College London
London, UK

Angela Cassidy
Department of Politics
University of Exeter
Exeter, UK

Michael Bresalier
Department of History
Swansea University
Swansea, UK

Rachel Mason Dentinger
University of Utah
Salt Lake City, UT, USA

https://doi.org/10.1007/978-3-319-64337-3

To the animals (human and non-human) who brought us together.

Preface

It is not long since the question 'Where are the animals in medical history?' prompted yawning and shuffling of feet among scholars of that discipline. While in the wider world the health agenda known as 'One Medicine' or 'One Health' was gathering momentum by highlighting the deeply interconnected nature of human and animal health and the need for integrated approaches to it, with a few key exceptions, scholars in medical history continued to believe that the only animals important to medicine were human animals. Conference organizers asked if animals belonged on medical history programmes; conference delegates voted with their feet; and scholarly discussions proceeded largely in ignorance of how animals and animal health had shaped—and been shaped by—the history of human health, medicine and society.

This was the situation that inspired the programme of research on which this volume is based. Generously sponsored by the Wellcome Trust,[1] it set out to explore the zoological foundations of human medicine, to illuminate the history of animals in medicine, and to develop an empirically grounded history of the recent movement for One Health. Research began at Imperial College London in 2011 and terminated at King's College London in 2016. It was conducted by a team of four scholars—Abigail Woods (principal investigator), Michael Bresalier,

[1]Programme Grant reference 092719/Z/10/A.

Rachel Mason Dentinger and Angela Cassidy—who are the joint authors of this volume.

Combining first degrees in veterinary medicine and the life sciences, with scholarly careers that straddle the history and sociology of veterinary medicine, human medicine and biology, we formed an interdisciplinary team well equipped to study the history of medicine as an interdisciplinary, interspecies phenomenon. Each of us has worked on discrete research projects that address a different aspect of this issue. This volume presents findings from each project, in five sample chapters that bear the authors' names.

However, the work as a whole is a shared endeavour. It grew out of our many meetings, in which we reviewed existing historical accounts of animals and medicine, and worked together to develop a shared language, conceptual apparatus and approach to studying their interconnected histories. It aspires to greater cohesion and coherence than a standard edited volume. It was also more difficult to write—more difficult, even, than a standard monograph in which only a single author has to make decisions about arguments and narrative. We found few precedents to guide us: team working is relatively new to the discipline of history, and, judging by certain publishers' responses to the notion of a volume with four authors, it is equally unfamiliar to academic publishing. Consequently, we have had to develop our working, writing and publishing practices by trial and error. This has been a very time-consuming but ultimately fulfilling experience. The mutual support and advice of colleagues has pushed our scholarship to a higher level, and enabled us to work on a broader canvas than would have been possible otherwise.

We are very grateful to Palgrave for supporting our vision and helping us to realize it. We hope that our readers—whether medical historians, animal historians or participants in One Health today—will find this an interesting and a thought-provoking volume. We also hope that it will persuade our colleagues in medical history that without asking 'Where are the animals?' and 'What do they do?', we cannot truly understand what has constituted medicine in history or what it has become today.

Many people have contributed to the preparation of this volume. Collectively, we wish to thank the Wellcome Trust for funding our research, colleagues (especially Dr. Kathryn Schoefert) in the Centre for the History of Science, Technology and Medicine at King's College London for their ongoing support, and the various audiences, reviewers and expert advisors who have provided constructive feedback on our findings in the course of the research programme. Abigail Woods would also like to thank Department III at the Max Planck Institute for the History of Science, Berlin, for hosting her during the spring term of 2017, which was a crucial writing-up phase. Angela Cassidy would like to thank new colleagues at the University of Exeter for their support during writing up, and the scientists and veterinarians she interviewed as part of this research for their essential insights into One Health and disciplinary politics in the twenty-first century. Rachel Mason Dentinger would also like to thank new colleagues at the University of Utah for providing support during the completion of this book. Michael Bresalier would like to thank archivists at the Food and Agriculture Organization (Fabio Ciccarello) and the World Health Organization (Reynald Erard) for their support of the research for his chapter, his new colleagues at Swansea University for embracing his work, and Abigail Woods for her remarkable support in completing the job.

London, UK	Abigail Woods
Swansea, UK	Michael Bresalier
Exeter, UK	Angela Cassidy
Salt Lake City, USA	Rachel Mason Dentinger

Contents

List of Figures

List of Tables

CHAPTER 1

Introduction: Centring Animals Within Medical History

In a recent handbook on the history of medicine, authors Robert Kirk and Michael Worboys argued that 'In no body of scholarship is it more obvious, puzzling and true to say that "animals disappear."'[1] Literally, of course, this is not the case, for as Etienne Benson points out,

> to a limited but important extent, writing about human history is always—already writing about animals … Humans are a kind of animal that (like all kinds of animal) has been and continues to be profoundly reshaped by its interactions with other kinds of animals … All history is animal history, in a sense.

However, Benson acknowledges the difference between scholarship that incorporates the impact of animal life on humans but is essentially focused on humans, and that which aims 'to explore the history of nonhuman animals as subjects in their own right and for their own sakes'.[2] Nearly all medical history scholarship falls into the former category. While animals do feature in it, and to an increasing degree since the turn of the twenty-first century,[3] they are usually shadowy, marginal creatures, 'mere blank

[1] Kirk and Worboys (2011), p. 561.

[2] Benson (2011) p. 5.

[3] Recent reviews of this literature include: Rader (2007), Kirk and Worboys (2011), Woods (2016, 2017a, 2017b), Kirk (2017).

A. Woods et al., *Animals and the Shaping of Modern Medicine*,
Medicine and Biomedical Sciences in Modern History,
https://doi.org/10.1007/978-3-319-64337-3_1

pages onto which humans wrote meaning'.[4] They appear because of their implications for human health and medicine, or because of their capacity to illuminate wider developments in human history, such as the growth of government, colonialism and international trade.

This volume breaks new ground in applying Benson's second perspective to medical history: 'to explore the history of nonhuman animals as subjects in their own right and for their own sakes'.[5] Humans remain important, of course, for ultimately we can only know about animals from the records that humans have created, and which reflect human interests in animals. However, by taking animals seriously as historical subjects, it is possible to shed a different light on human history by revealing the myriad ways in which animals have influenced human actions and perceptions. Adopting this approach also illuminates animals as creatures with their own histories, which have been profoundly altered by their relationships with humans, and the roles that humans have decided they should perform. It results in a richer, less anthropocentric account of the medical past, which reveals how, in different times and places, animals have experienced medicine, how they have been produced by it and how they have changed it.

In widening the historical lens to incorporate animals and their fashioning into medical subjects and objects, this volume pursues three key goals. First, it seeks to make a programmatic contribution to the field of medical history by elucidating some of the largely unrecognized ways in which animals have informed the knowledges, practices and social formations of medicine. Through analysing key contexts in which animals have attracted medical attention and with what effects, it will expose a series of medical problems, concerns, personnel and practices that barely feature in existing scholarship. In addition, by studying the historical positioning of animals at the shifting boundaries between medicine, veterinary medicine and the life sciences, it will cast new light on the relationships between these fields. It will thereby demonstrate how, by attending to the more-than-human dimensions of medicine, we reach new understandings of its historical identity, participants and manner of pursuit.

Second, the volume seeks to enhance the burgeoning field of animal history by offering the first substantive account of animals in medicine.

[4] Fudge (2006).

[5] Benson (2011) p. 5.

Expanding beyond much-studied laboratory contexts to explore the medical history of animals in zoos, on farms, in hospitals, post-mortem rooms and international policy arenas, it illuminates the diverse species that have participated in medicine, the many roles they have played in it, and how their bodies and habits have both shaped and been shaped by its ideas, practices and institutions. Crucially, the volume highlights how these diverse species forged multispecies networks, thereby extending animal history's typical focus on the dyadic relationships between humans and another species of animal.

The third objective of this volume is to speak to the twenty-first-century initiative known as One Health (OH). Featuring prominently in medical, veterinary and scientific publications, and in national and international health policy and position statements, OH pursues an expansive vision of improving health and wellbeing through the multidisciplinary study of problems at the interface of humans, animals and their environments. For its proponents, OH represents a necessary response to a host of shared threats to human and animal health, such as emerging diseases that transmit between animals and humans, antimicrobial resistance, food insecurity, food safety and climate change. They argue that such issues cannot be tackled effectively within the traditional disciplinary compartments of human medicine, veterinary medicine and the life sciences. Rather, integrated, coordinated approaches are required, in which the health of animals is considered in relation to the health of humans and the environment.[6] This volume situates OH within a longer historical context by illuminating certain precedents to this way of working. It also offers a critical, empirically grounded perspective on its operation today by exploring the circumstances that gave rise to its emergence as a self-conscious movement, and how its proponents conceptualize the roles of animals within it.

In addressing these three objectives, the volume also addresses three distinct audiences: historians of animals, historians of science and medicine, and health professionals concerned with OH today. The remainder of this chapter introduces the history of animals as a field of enquiry, and situates this study in relation to it. While historians of animals will be familiar with its discussion of the methodological and conceptual issues

[6]For example: Gibbs (2014), American Veterinary Association, Centers for Disease Control and Prevention, One Health Initiative.

that are important to the writing of animal histories, we present them here for the benefit of medical historians who may not be familiar with them. We also provide an important overview of how we approach the history of animals in medicine, and conclude by elaborating on the volume's objectives, outlining its research questions and introducing the case studies that follow.

1.1 Why Animals?

The ways in which non-human animals have shaped human history is a pressing and important issue for historians today. Recent years have witnessed increasing engagement with the subject, manifesting in a burgeoning body of literature that draws on perspectives from material culture studies, science and technology studies, zoology, performance studies, and environmental, social and cultural history. Directing their attention to a variety of animal species, authors have addressed the lives and experiences of animals, their categorization and manipulation by humans, their relationships with humans and environments, and their representations within art and literature.[7] The eclectic methods of animal history, and the many differences between its animal subjects (some of which had more historical similarities with humans than with each other) have led some historians to ask whether it can be said to constitute a coherent field of enquiry, or whether it primarily offers an approach to animals which can be applied to all existing types of history.[8] Insofar as animal history is a field, this volume is intended to be a contribution to that body of work, but it also draws on animal history ideas and approaches in order to develop new perspectives on medical history.

Animal historians acknowledge that the significance of animals to war, agriculture, science, colonialism, sport and the environment means that they have long featured in scholarly histories, but usually as supporting

[7] Seminal works include: Ritvo (1987), Kete (1994), Anderson (2004). Valuable edited collections include: Henninger-Voss (2002), Rothfels (2002), Kalof and Resl (2007), Brantz (2010), Shaw (2013a, 2013b), Nance (2015). An even larger scholarship addresses the contemporary dimensions of human–animal relationships, drawing on disciplines such as philosophy, anthropology, geography, English literature and cultural studies. For an introductory overview, see Marvin and McHugh (2014). Key authors who have set the framework for thinking about these issues include: Agamben (2002), Derrida (2002), Wolfe (2003), Haraway (2008).

[8] Swart (2007), Andrews (n.d.).

actors in the drama of human history. Their stated intention is to bring animals in from the margins and position them at the centre of historical analysis in order to explore the intertwining of human and animal lives, and the development of human ideas about, and relationships with, animals.[9] Conceptualizing animals as creatures with their own histories and the unintentional capacity to effect historical change, authors seek to trace 'the many ways in which humans construct and are constructed by animals in the past'.[10] The purpose of these analyses is not simply to fill a gap in the writing of human history but to rethink conventional historiographies. This volume follows their lead in acknowledging animals as shapers of medicine in history, and also as shapers of the ways in which we, as scholars, perceive and write about medical history.[11]

Developments beyond the academy have helped to precipitate this 'animal turn'. Since the later twentieth-century, animal-related causes, from opposition to factory farming and animal experimentation, to the wider improvement of animal welfare, have gained increasing public support and political traction. Portrayed variously as victims of, or contributors to, environmental degradation, animals have also become a key aspect of wider concerns about human interactions with the natural world. Meanwhile, the impacts of diseases such as bovine spongiform encephalopathy (BSE) and avian influenza, which emerged in animals and spread to people, have made the health connections between humans and animals more visible and threatening. These developments have prompted much reflection on human responsibilities for non-human others, and how to live sustainably with them.[12] They have also encouraged animal scientists such as ethologists, vets and ecologists, to study the sentience and subjectivities of animals, and their relationships with their environments.[13]

Enhanced concern for animals and human–animal relations in the present has helped to draw attention to their pasts within different domains of historical scholarship. Situating animals within nature as constituents

[9] Ritvo (2002), Fudge (2002), Kean (2012), Sivasundaram (2015).

[10] Fudge (2006).

[11] We thank Tamar Novick of the Max Planck Institute for the History of Science, Berlin, for making this observation.

[12] Ritvo (2002), Shaw (2013a, 2013b), Vandersommers (2016).

[13] For example: Bekoff (2002), Grandin and Johnson (2005).

of environments and ecosystems, environmental historians have explored the interplay between 'nature' and 'culture' in the shaping of human pasts.[14] Challenging the very notion of a nature–culture dichotomy and the priority it awards to human 'culture' over animal 'nature', post-humanist scholars have sought to understand how human and animal differences, essences and linkages have been constructed through historically specific encounters.[15] By contrast, for social and cultural historians, the fact that 'humans are always, and have always been, enmeshed in social relations with animals'[16] calls for a social historical approach to animal histories. Their work has established animals as the latest beneficiaries of 'history from below', a genre that originated in the 1970s with E.P. Thompson's history of the working classes, and expanded subsequently to incorporate other neglected historical subjects such as women, colonized peoples, marginalized ethnic groups and the mentally ill.[17] The animals studied tend to be celebrity animals, charismatic wildlife and those domesticated species that have entered into close relationships with humans. Other, more marginal creatures have been neglected. This volume offers a partial corrective by examining the medical histories of some uncharismatic and historically overlooked animals, such as tapeworms and farmed livestock.

As with the other groups targeted by 'history from below', there is an explicit political dimension to much animal history writing. Some scholars, who locate themselves within the field of critical animal studies, aim to improve animal lives in the present by uncovering and criticizing the ways in which humans have exploited them in the past.[18] For other animal historians, these narratives of animal domination and oppression are too simplistic. They, too, are often keen to effect present-day changes in attitudes to animals by revealing their treatment in the past. Consequently, they remain alert to the power dynamics that have informed past human–animal relationships.[19] However, they also emphasize the complexity and historical specificity of those relationships,

[14] McNeill (2000), Nash (2005), Cronon (1990).

[15] Lorimer (2009), Cole (2011).

[16] Philo and Wilbert (2000) p. 2. See also Swart (2007) p. 276, Eitler (2014) p. 262.

[17] Ritvo (2002), Kean (2012). For a history of animals as workers, see Hribal (2007).

[18] Taylor and Twine (2014), Institute for Critical Animal Studies.

[19] Fudge (2012).

and the 'resistance, compliance and compromise' that variously characterized them.[20] This volume follows their lead in believing that historians have a moral obligation to document how human actions have impacted animal lives. It seeks to develop a nuanced understanding of the human–animal relationships that were forged through medical research and practice, and to analyse the implications of those relationships for humans, animals and medicine.

1.2 Writing Animal Histories

There are particular challenges associated with writing the history of animals. Some scholars have questioned whether it is even possible. Pearson and Weismantel state that the challenges are at once ontological ('a question of imagining animal being'), epistemological (because our communications with animals are non-verbal) and methodological (how can we write authentic animal histories when the only records that survive of them were created by humans?). They suggest that these difficulties are linked: if animals have no voices, they cannot leave records from which historians can write their pasts; without language, consciousness or intentionality they are unable to participate in history except as subjects of biological evolution. For some commentators, it follows that the study of animals belongs within the natural sciences not the humanities—which are by definition concerned with human society and culture.[21] This stance has roots in Christian theology, which asserts human dominion over animals, and in Enlightenment thinking, which posits fundamental distinctions between humans and animals, nature and culture.[22]

These dichotomies and the exceptional status they award to humans have been challenged by post-modern and post-humanist scholarship, and by studies of developments within technoscience, food production and climate science, which provide concrete examples of the impossibility of separating nature from society.[23] Historical analyses lend support to these challenges. By illuminating circumstances in which particular

[20] Pooley-Ebert (2015) p. 165.

[21] Pearson and Weismantel (2010).

[22] Thomas (1983).

[23] Latour (1993), Mitchell (2002), Schrepfer and Scranton (2003), Agamben (2002), Lorimer (2009).

humans (notably women, the mentally ill and certain ethnic groups) were invested with animal characteristics, and certain animals (notably horses, dogs and primates) were awarded privileged, quasi-human status, it reveals that human–animal boundaries are not fixed in nature but shaped by human society and culture. Therefore animals and animality are not distinct from, but constitutive of the human, in ways that change over time and place.[24]

If the human–animal boundary is blurred, then where does this leave assertions that without cognition or conscious thought, animals cannot be active historical subjects? Scholars have tackled this question by considering whether the ability to act on history can exist separately from the intention to do so, and whether animals can be historical subjects without necessarily possessing subjectivity. They suggest that while animals do not understand or care about human knowledge, politics and cultures, nevertheless they can make a difference to them. Therefore, in principle, animals do possess agency—where agency constitutes the ability to act.[25] For animal historians, the nature of that agency is an empirical question. It is not a natural, permanent attribute; rather, it emerges and is performed through social relationships, which vary by time, space and species.[26]

In locating animal agency within human–non-human encounters, many scholars draw on ideas associated with Actor Network Theory (ANT). Developed within the field of science studies by Bruno Latour, Michel Callon and John Law in the 1980s, ANT sought to remove distinctions between nature and society. It represented a critical response to prevailing understandings of scientific knowledge and technical innovation as either realist or sociological.[27] It has since been adopted and developed by scholars in many other disciplines. ANT has many variants but it essentially proposes a relational way of understanding the world. In widening the traditional analytical lens to incorporate interacting human and non-human entities, it opens up a space for animals as historical actors. ANT presents agency, and actors, as products of the unstable web

---

[24] Ritvo (1995), Fudge (2002), Ritvo (2007), Hochadel (2010), Bourke (2011), Davis (2014).

[25] Fudge (2006), Law and Mol (2008), McFarland and Hediger (2009).

[26] Philo and Wilbert (2000), Eitler (2014), Pooley-Ebert (2015).

[27] Callon and Law (1986), Latour (1988, 2005).

of relations (or networks) in which all are embedded. The configuration of these networks affects how the capacity to act is distributed among and deployed by its members. Their actions reshape ideas and practices, bodies and materials, experiences and social relations, and, by extension, the network itself. In this formulation, it is not only the animal's capacity to effect historical change but also the animal itself which is constantly being reconfigured through its embeddedness in multiple interactive, ever-changing relationships.[28]

Animal studies scholars frequently cite ANT when reflecting on the agency of animals. However, their recognition that pre-existing power differentials, social contexts and species differences have an important bearing on network formation, the relationships of its participants, and consequently on the animal's ability to act, seems to support criticisms of ANT's 'flat ontology'—its refusal to acknowledge any differences between actors other than those created through networks.[29] While we agree with such criticisms, we, too, find ANT to be a useful heuristic device because of the significance it awards to relationships. It suggests that through scrutinizing 'the entire lived experience of quotidian and extraordinary interactions—embodied and imaginary, material and symbolic—that occur within space and in particular locations, and involve humans and animals in multiple forms of engagement and exchange',[30] we can work out how animals have changed medicine and have, in turn, been changed by it.[31] Moreover, by privileging relationships, as ANT exhorts us to, we are able to identify the interconnections between multiple species.[32]

Thinking about animals in history has also been profoundly influenced by Donna Haraway's writing. While acknowledging the uneven distribution of pain and suffering between human and animals, she perceives their relationships to be characterized by mutual adaptation rather than exploitation, and seeks to determine how, in historically and culturally specific circumstances, humans and animals come together in 'material-semiotic nodes or knots in which diverse bodies and meanings coshape

---

[28] Pearson (2013) pp. 128–45, Eitler (2014).

[29] Barron (2003), McLean and Hassard (2004).

[30] Pearson and Weismantel (2010).

[31] Kean (2012).

[32] Pettit et al. (2015).

one another'.[33] As Law and Mol point out, this does not mean that animals have the capacity to control history, just that by entering into relationships with human and other non-human actors they are able to make a difference to it. Their analysis of Cumbrian sheep during the British 2001 foot-and-mouth disease epidemic offers some concrete examples. The variable bodily responses of sheep to encounters with the foot-and-mouth disease virus affected whether the vets that inspected them were able to detect and respond to it. The hill sheep's ability to know its place or 'heft' on the hills fashioned the landscape in ways that were valued by humans, and which led ultimately to their exemption from the government's contiguous culling policy. These outcomes were not necessarily predictable: they resulted from the unstable, indeterminate webs of practices that drew together and were created by sheep and their co-actors. Law and Mol conclude that the important question is not *whether* but *how* animals act.[34]

We will address this question by analysing the roles that animals have performed within medical research and practice. Some of these roles will be familiar to medical historians. In laboratories, animals were fashioned into experimental subjects and manipulated to cast light on health and disease. Animals that fell sick performed roles as disease victims, and were sometimes transformed into patients. Alternatively, or additionally, they were regarded as hosts and potential transmitters of infection. Animals have also performed other, less well-documented roles in medicine: as pathological specimens, points of comparison with other species, commercial products, shapers and victims of food systems and natural environments, and vehicles for personal and professional advancement. They have often performed several roles simultaneously or sequentially throughout their lives and afterlives. Roles have reshaped animals, physically and conceptually, and therefore impacted on their histories. Roles also had their own histories that were influenced partly by human–animal relationships and their disruption by disease, and also by prevailing ideas of disease and the tools available to conceptualize, investigate and manage it. While it was humans who awarded roles to animals, animals were not passive recipients. Their bodies, behaviours and relationships with humans have invited the awarding of particular roles

---

[33] Haraway (2008) p. 4.

[34] Law and Mol (2008) p. 74.

and influenced their performance within them. Different roles have provided animals with different opportunities to shape medicine, with ramifications for the health of both humans and animals. The concept of the animal role therefore offers a useful tool for illuminating the historical co-constitution of humans, animals and medicine.

1.3 Animals in Medical History

Inspired by Haraway's thinking, in 2011, Kirk and Worboys called for the history of medicine to be rewritten as a history of interspecies interactions.[35] However, to date, few scholars have adopted this approach. There are only a handful of key works that foreground the relationships between humans and animals, and these focus narrowly on experimental settings.[36] Studies of the co-constitution of animals and medicine are also few in number and derive more from the history of the life sciences than medical history.[37] For the most part, animals fade into the background of medical history writing.[38] Scholars influenced by the 'animal turn' have not been drawn to study the history of medicine, while historians of medicine have remained largely unaware of the 'animal turn'.

This situation has not arisen because animals were unimportant to medicine. On the contrary, as this volume and its extended bibliography demonstrate, they have been integral to its history. Medical scientists employed animals to develop new knowledge of bodies, minds and diseases; to generate biological products, and to test the safety and efficacy of drugs. Animals supplied nutrition to humans and transmitted diseases to them. The state of animal health powerfully influenced—and was influenced by—their environments. Animals were treated as patients, fashioned into pathological specimens, and their diseases compared across species. So far, however, these animal roles have been studied from a largely human perspective. Their capacity to shape medicine has attracted little attention, and they have been rarely studied as medical subjects 'in their own right and for their own sakes'—not even within the field of

[35] Kirk and Worboys (2011).

[36] Rupke (1990), Todes (1997), Dror (1999), Guerrini (2003), Schlich and Schlünder (2009), Kirk (2014).

[37] Clarke and Fujimura (1992), Clause (1993), Kohler (1994), Rader (2007).

[38] Woods (2017b).

veterinary history, which is ostensibly focused on the health of animals as a problem in its own right.[39]

We can offer only tentative explanations for why animal histories of medicine have yet to be written. It may be because of the dominance of cultural studies' perspectives within animal and human–animal history, which have tended to foreground animals' cultural and symbolic roles in society rather than delving into the content and material practices of animal science and medicine. It may also result from a preference for writing the histories of individual animals that are visible in today's society and with which humans develop empathetic bonds: pet animals, zoo animals and charismatic wildlife species. Farm animals, which have wielded considerable influence over human health, are comparatively neglected. Such explanations do not apply to historians of medicine. The field's long-lasting engagement with ANT,[40] its preoccupation with the histories of bodies and material practices, the scientific training of many of its scholars, and their expertise—generated through writing patient histories—in thinking about medical history 'from below', means that the tools for writing animal-centred histories of medicine are already in circulation.[41] The failure to apply them may be due to the anthropocentrism that characterized most fields of history writing until relatively recently. However, we believe that disciplinary traditions may also be to blame.

It is now more than 20 years since the late Roy Porter asserted that, 'in the academic world, it is automatically assumed that a "historian of medicine" is a person who works on the history of human medicine'.[42] He attributed this assumption to modernist notions of human difference from, and primacy over, animals. While in the intervening years these notions have come increasingly under attack, scholars have not significantly revised their perceptions of what constitutes medical history. There remains an implicit assumption that human health and medicine lie at the heart of this field. Sick animals whose health had no direct consequence for humans are relegated to the small subfield of veterinary

[39] Benson (2011) p. 5. Susan Jones is one of the few veterinary historians to foreground animals and their relationships with humans. A good example is Jones (1997). See also Degeling (2009).

[40] Latour (1988).

[41] Porter (1985), Beier (1987), Warner (1999), Gillis (2006), Cooter (2010), Crozier (2010), Hurren (2012).

[42] Porter (1993) p. 19.

history, while other aspects of animal life are studied by historians of biology. We hold that this compartmentalization is artificial and unhelpful. It does not reflect the historical positioning of animals within these fields, and it produces a narrowly anthropocentric framing of 'medicine' which is frequently at odds with its historical identity.

This volume challenges such conceptions by revealing that modern medicine, as developed in the West over the last two centuries, was a more-than-human endeavour, whose boundaries with veterinary medicine and biology were porous and in a constant state of flux. In certain historical contexts, animals contributed to the compartmentalization of these domains. In others, they helped to break down the barriers between them, particularly through their investigation within boundary-crossing fields such as parasitology, zoology, comparative medicine, nutrition and agriculture.[43] Animals contributed to the formation of these fields, and were, in turn, formed by them. By elucidating these processes, this volume not only sheds light on the history of animals. In identifying the ideas, methods, problems, places and people who engaged with their health, it also develops a new perspective on medicine itself—and therefore on what constitutes the field of medical history.

In developing this animal-centred medical history, we have had to engage with the tricky issue of how to write the histories of non-verbal creatures when the only records that survive of them were created by humans. Some scholars have attempted to overcome this problem by using modern scientific understandings of animals to retrospectively interpret their behaviours and experiences.[44] As historians of science and medicine, we find this approach deeply problematic, because in granting a timeless universality to scientific interpretations that are in fact products of specific historical circumstances, it reifies the nature–culture divide.[45] Other scholars have argued that the problem cannot be overcome; that it is impossible to truly 'know' the authentic historical animal because surviving records are mere cultural representations of them.[46] Swart has challenged this view. Questioning the very notion of authenticity, she points out that the 'facts' about animals are always

[43] Woods (2017c).

[44] For example: Pearson (2013), Foote and Gunnels (2015), Pooley-Ebert (2015).

[45] Latour (1993).

[46] Fudge (2002) p. 6.

human interpretations, not 'real' accounts of them.[47] Benson goes further by arguing that because animals have informed the human production of records of them, such records—or traces—are more than cultural representations; they comprise 'material-semiotic remnants' of animals, a nexus of language and materiality that offer 'unintentional indexes of a now-absent presence'.[48]

Inspired by Benson's thinking around animal traces, we approach medical historical records of animals as evidence of their interactions with humans, whose analysis reveals how animals made a difference to, and were changed by, medicine. We perceive multiple layers of animal traces which gained meaning in reference to each other. There are the immediate material remains of diseased animal bodies such as taxidermy and museum specimens. Then there are the narratives, statistics and images that humans have created from these materials and from other long-dead animals whose remains were not preserved. Finally, there are the knowledge-practices and social relationships that were fashioned by and from these creations. In studying these traces, we ask not only what they reveal about the health of animals in history and the roles that animals played in medicine. By reflecting on why this 'animal archive' was created in the first place, we also learn about the animal's capacity to attract human attention, and the relationships that bound them.[49]

1.4 One Health and its Histories

One of the inspirations and intended audiences for this work is the contemporary movement for OH, whose features and early twenty-first-century emergence are explored in Chapter 6. OH is underpinned by the belief that some of the most important health threats faced today are not species specific, and consequently can only be tackled by interdisciplinary working across the domains of human medicine, veterinary medicine and the life sciences. Its integrated approach to human and animal health implies that medicine cannot achieve its goals through a purely anthropocentric approach. Just as other contemporary agendas have prompted historians to study animal pasts, so has the push for OH drawn our attention to the roles played by animals in the history of medicine.

[47] Swart (2015).

[48] Benson (2011) p. 3.

[49] Tortorici (2015).

While the term OH is new, the concept is not. This is well recognized by OH advocates, who use historical observations of human–animal health connections in attempts to legitimize their agenda, and win momentum and funding for it.[50] They locate the roots of OH in an earlier agenda known as One Medicine (OM), which developed in the 1960s and 1970s with the aim of bringing human and veterinary medicine into closer alignment.[51] OM was, in turn, presaged by work dating back to the nineteenth century in the fields of comparative medicine and veterinary public health, where human and animal health problems were considered in tandem.[52] OH advocates offer a single, highly selective interpretation of this history. They highlight the work of key high-profile figures whose work crossed the human–animal divide and had a lasting impact on medicine: Louis Pasteur, Robert Koch, William Osler, Theobald Smith, John McFadyean and Rudolph Virchow (who is frequently quoted, in the absence of any identifiable source material, as stating that 'between human and animal medicine there is no dividing line').[53] Extracting these individuals from their historical contexts, OH advocates present them as far-sighted geniuses who recognized the merits of a OH approach. There is little understanding of what, within the context of the time, these men thought they were doing and why; whether their work was typical or unusual; and how animals might have shaped, or been shaped, by it.

One of the goals of this volume is to develop a more critical, evidence-based, animal-centred history of OH by documenting and explaining the circumstances in which animals and their diseases became important to human medical agendas. By identifying what motivated their investigation by a range of lesser-known individuals, how these investigations were pursued in policy and practice, and with what implications for human and animal health, the book will illuminate precedents to OH today, and draw insights of relevance to its future operation. It will also offer an explanation for the emergence of OH as a self-conscious twenty-first-century agenda and unpack the place of animals within it.

---

[50] Woods and Bresalier (2014).

[51] Schwabe (1984), Zinsstag et al. (2011).

[52] Bresalier et al. (2015).

[53] Schwabe (1984), Michell (2000) pp. 101–6, Day (2008) pp. 151–3.

We do not attempt a complete account of the history of animals in medicine: the subject is too vast and too neglected.[54] Instead, we aim to set a new research agenda and to illustrate where it might lead through a series of case studies that are drawn from the authors' individual research programmes. These studies explore animal histories of medicine, and histories of animals in medicine, on scales ranging from the local to the global, from the 1830s to the present day. They are designed to be read separately as standalone examples of the contexts in which animals became important to medicine and the difference they made to it. Read collectively, they illuminate the diverse species, spaces, methods, people, problems and contexts of enquiry that were involved in constructing animal health as a medical problem. In tracing how that construction changed over time, they also trace the shifting place of animals within medicine, and how animals moulded its relationships with veterinary medicine and the life sciences.

Cross-cutting questions include: What circumstances attracted human attention to animals and their diseases, and what networks developed around them? How can we account for the attention paid to animals by members of the medical profession, which is generally assumed to be exclusively concerned with the health of humans? How and where were investigations and interventions performed on animals, and what roles did animals play within them? While our human protagonists' affective relationships with animals are generally impossible to discern, the concept of the animal role permits analysis of the multiple values that humans assigned to animals. We also ask: What difference did animals make to medicine—to its ideas, practices, the health of its human and animal subjects, and its interpersonal and interdisciplinary relationships? What difference did medicine make to animals—to their bodies and experiences in life, the manner and timing of their deaths, and to their afterlives?

In selecting which aspects of the history of animals in medicine to study, we made a deliberate decision not to focus on the laboratory-based subjects of experimental medicine. This is partly because these animals, notably rodents and dogs, already feature in the handful of existing animal-centred accounts of medical history. It is also because

[54] For a chronological overview, see Bresalier et al. (2015).

experimental medicine is already overrepresented within medical history scholarship. The widely held perception that the pursuit of knowledge through experiments is one of the defining features of modern medicine, means that scholars have dedicated considerable attention to its history, starting with the growth of experimental physiology around 1800, and progressing to the emergence of other experimental sciences: bacteriology in the 1860s and 1870s, pharmacology, endocrinology, nutrition science and immunology in the decades around 1900, and biomedicine in the post-Second World War era.[55] The attention lavished on the topic is such that many scholars seem to assume by default that the history of animals in medicine is a history of experimental animals, or 'animal models' of disease, that were manipulated in laboratories for the benefit of human health.

This volume seeks to dislodge that perception through a series of case studies that decentre not only humans but also laboratory-based experimentation from the history of modern medicine. The studies address a series of other important medical contexts whose histories have been obscured by the historiographical focus on the laboratory: natural history, zoology, parasitology, comparative anatomy, ecology, nutrition and agriculture. Lying at the borderlands of human medicine, veterinary medicine and the life sciences, and shedding light on their shifting points of intersection, analysis of these contexts shifts the historical focus away from laboratory rodents and dogs towards a wide array of other species that hardly ever feature in accounts of medical history: zoo animals, Scottish sheep, cows of the developing world, and the tapeworm, *Echinococcus granulosus*. These animals performed various roles, including, but not confined to, those of disease victims, patients, experimental material, shapers and products of their environments, hosts and transmitters of infection, tools for thinking comparatively across species, spontaneous (as opposed to experimentally designed) models of disease, and sources of human nutrition. Their investigation relied not only on experimental practices but also on observation, categorization, comparison, statistical analysis and clinical trials. These methods were applied far beyond the laboratory, in animal houses, post-mortem rooms, hospitals, farms, field stations and slaughterhouses. By drawing our attention to these historically neglected aspects of medicine, the animals studied in this volume also expand and

---

[55] Guerrini (2003), Lowy (2003), Rader (2007), Schlich et al. (2009), Löwy (2011), Franco (2013).

alter received conceptions of what constituted medicine in history, and who were its key actors.

The first case study, presented in Chapter 2, is situated in Britain's mid-nineteenth-century zoological gardens, particularly those located in London and Dublin. It documents the diseases and deaths that beset their diverse animal inhabitants, and argues that as a consequence, the zoos became important sites of medical research and practice. It shows how medical men who helped to run the zoos, and medical visitors who hoped to make their names within them, used their knowledge and practice of human medicine and comparative anatomy to advance the health of zoo animals, and devise comparative pathological understandings of their diseases. These men awarded animals the roles of patients, victims of their environments, pathological specimens and points of interspecies comparison. They manipulated animal bodies, surroundings and management in ways that were shaped by animal biologies and behaviours. Through these activities, the zoo became medical, and medicine zoological. An array of vertebrate species fell under the medical gaze, and helped to generate new knowledge of health and disease that found applications in human medicine.

In Chapter 3 the focus shifts to diseased and dying sheep on farms in and around Scotland at the turn of the twentieth century. It reveals how these animals came to be regarded as victims of their environment, and positioned at the hub of a research network containing farmers, doctors, vets, natural historians and zoologists. It examines the investigations performed by this network, and how sheep fashioned and were fashioned by them. It then describes and explains key changes to the network, which shifted the location of investigations from farms to laboratories, and distanced doctors and practical farmers from the scientific study of sheep. Awarded new roles as hosts and transmitters of infection, sheep lost influence over investigators' activities. Meanwhile, veterinarians sought to capture sick sheep for themselves by claiming superior knowledge that derived from their unique relationships with them. In these ways, sheep first integrated, and then contributed to widening divisions between the various experts in their diseases.

Chapter 4 is concerned with diseased and undernourished dairy cattle, and how they came to be perceived not simply as threats to farming profits but as contributors to world hunger and ill health. Moving from interwar Britain and its empire, to the post-war international stage, it explores how developments in nutritional science and veterinary medicine, combined with economic depression, food shortages and the effects of war, drew attention to the undernourished, unhealthy bodies of both humans and cows, and suggested connections between them. By the early 1950s, under the United Nations and its agencies, cows had become key participants in the campaign against human hunger in the developing world. Their unproductive bodies inspired the formation of new health structures that brought together experts in human health, nutrition, veterinary medicine and agricultural science to create new types of cow that would prove more capable of supporting human health and nutrition.

Chapter 5 continues to cross borders between nations and disciplines in its study of the tapeworm, *Echinococcus granulosus*, and the ideas and investigations it inspired. It is particularly concerned with the work of parasitologist Calvin Schwabe, who is better known as a progenitor of the recent movement for OH. For Schwabe, *Echinococcus* was an animal in its own right, an active, opportunistic participant in both human and non-human ecological and cultural interactions. In following Schwabe as he followed *Echinococcus*, from the laboratory into human communities and multispecies ecosystems, and from Beirut to Kenya to California, this chapter reveals that the roots of his commitment to unifying human and veterinary medicine lay in his deep-seated engagement with the parasite. His investigations into its body and behaviour led him to view distinctions between human and non-human species as culturally contingent rather than fundamentally biological. This fed his conviction that human and veterinary medicine could only function truly effectively when practised in tandem.

Chapter 6 takes forward the story of OH by exploring its emergence as a self-conscious movement, dedicated to the integrated study of problems at the interface between human health, animal health and the environment. It explores how Schwabe's work influenced, and was reconfigured by, this movement, and locates its early development in several research and policy networks, which produced not one but several different forms of OH. The chapter also examines how human–animal health relationships have inspired and shaped OH, and how they are represented—in sometimes contradictory ways—in the texts and images produced by its researchers and advocates. It argues that in privileging the roles of animals as transmitters of diseases to humans, and experimental models of human diseases, OH rebrands longstanding research agendas that are far more concerned with the health of humans than that of animals.

Chapter 7 concludes by summarizing what these chapters have revealed about the medical history of animals and the animal history of medicine. It reflects on the implications of these findings for how historians think about and study the history of medicine, and for how OH advocates conceptualize and pursue their integrating agenda. The volume ends with an annotated bibliography of animals in the history of medicine, which offers an entry point for scholars who are new to the field and is organized around some of the key animal roles that are explored in the chapters.

Bibliography

Agamben, Giorgio. *The Open: Man and Animal*. Stanford: Stanford University Press, 2002.

American Veterinary Association. "One Health – It's All Connected." Accessed February 19, 2017. https://www.avma.org/onehealth.

Anderson, V. *Creatures of Empire: How Domestic Animals Transformed Early America*. Oxford: Oxford University Press, 2004.

Andrews, Thomas. "Review of Nance, S. (ed.) The Historical Animal." Accessed February 19, 2017. https://networks.h-net.org/node/19397/reviews/148458/andrews-nance-historical-animal.

Barron, Colin. "A Strong Distinction between Humans and Non-Humans is No Longer Required for Research Purposes: A Debate between Bruno Latour and Steve Fuller." *History of the Human Sciences* 16 (2003): 77–99.

Beier, L.M. *Sufferers and Healers: The Experience of Illness in Seventeenth Century England*. London: Routledge, 1987.

Bekoff, M. *Minding Animals: Awareness, Emotion and Heart*. Oxford: Oxford University Press, 2002.

Benson, E. "Animal Writes: Historiography, Disciplinarity, and the Animal Trace." In *Making Animal Meaning*, edited by L. Kalof and G.M. Montgomery, 3–16. East Lansing: Michigan State University Press, 2011.

Bourke, Joanna. *What it Means to be Human: Reflections from 1791 to the Present*. London: Virago, 2011.

Brantz, D. (ed.) *Beastly Natures: Animals, Humans and the Study of History*. London: University of Virginia Press, 2010.

Bresalier, M., A. Cassidy and A. Woods. "One Health in History." In *One Health: The Theory and Practice of Integrated Health Approaches*, edited by J. Zinsstag, E. Schelling, D. Waltner-Toews, M. Whittaker and M. Tanner, 1–15. Wallingford: CABI, 2015.

Callon, Michel and John Law. "Some Elements of a Sociology of Translation: Domestication of the Scallops and the Fishermen of St Brieuc Bay." In *Power, Action and Belief: A New Sociology of Knowledge*, edited by John Law, 196–223. London: Routledge, 1986.

Cassidy, Angela, Rachel Mason Dentinger, Kathryn Schoefert and Abigail Woods. "Animal Roles and Traces in the History of Medicine.' In Animal Agents: The Non-Human in the History of Science, edited by Amanda Rees. *BJHS Themes* 2 (2017): 11–33.

Centres for Disease Control and Prevention. "One Health." Accessed February 19, 2017. https://www.cdc.gov/onehealth.

Clarke, Adele and Joan Fujimura (eds.). *The Right Tools for the Job: At Work in Twentieth-Century Life Sciences.* Princeton: Princeton University Press, 1992.

Clause, Bonnie. "The Wistar Rat as a Right Choice: Establishing Mammalian Standards and the Ideal of a Standardized Mammal." *Journal of the History of Biology* 26 (1993): 329–49.

Cole, Lucinda. "Introduction: Human–Animal Studies and the Eighteenth Century." *The Eighteenth Century* 52 (2011): 1–10.

Cooter, Roger. "The Turn of the Body: History and the Politics of the Corporeal." *Arbor Ciencia, Pensamiento y Cultura* 186 (2010): 393–405.

Cronon, William. "Modes of Prophecy and Production: Placing Nature in History," *Journal of American History* 76 (1990): 1122–31.

Crozier, Ivan. "Bodies in History – The Task of the Historian." In *The Cultural History of the Human Body, vol. 6 1920-present*, edited by I. Crozier, 1–20. London: Bloomsbury, 2010.

Davis, David Brion. *The Problem of Slavery in the Age of Emancipation.* New York: Knopf, 2014.

Day, Michael. "One Health and the Legacy of John McFadyean." *Journal of Comparative Pathology* 139 (2008): 151–3.

Degeling, Chris. "Picturing the Pain of Animal Others: Rationalising Form, Function and Suffering in Veterinary Orthopaedics." *History and Philosophy of the Life Sciences* 31 (2009): 377–403.

Derrida, J. "The Animal That Therefore I Am (More to Follow)." *Critical Inquiry* 28 (2002): 369–418.

Dror, O.E. "The Affect of Experiment. The Turn to Emotions in Anglo-American Physiology, 1900-1940." *Isis* 90 (1999): 205–37.

Eitler, Pascal. "Animal History as Body History: Four Suggestions from a Genealogical Perspective." *Body Politics* 2 (2014): 259–74.

Foote, N. and C. Gunnels. "Exploring Early Human-Animal Encounters in the Galapagos Islands Using a Historical Zoology Approach." In *The Historical Animal*, edited by Susan Nance, 203–20. New York: Syracuse University Press, 2015.

Franco, Nuno Henrique. "Animal Experiments in Biomedical Research: A Historical Perspective." *Animals* 3 (2013): 238–73.

Fudge, Erica. *Perceiving Animals: Humans and Beasts in Early Modern English Culture.* Urbana: University of Illinois Press, 2002.

Fudge, Erica. "A Left-Handed Blow: Writing the History of Animals." In *Representing Animals*, edited by N. Rothfels, 3–18. Bloomington: Indiana University Press, 2002.

Fudge, Erica. "Ruminations 1: The History of Animals." (2006). Accessed February 19, 2017. https://networks.h-net.org/node/16560/pages/32226/history-animals-erica-fudge.

Fudge, Erica. "Renaissance Animal Things." In *Gorgeous Beasts: Animal Bodies in Historical Perspective*, edited by J. Landes, P.Y. Lee and P. Youngquist, 41–56. Pennsylvania: Penn State University Press, 2012.

Gibbs, E.P.J. "The Evolution of One Health: A Decade of Progress and Challenges for the Future." *Veterinary Record* 174 (2014): 85–91.

Gillis, J. "The History of the Patient History since 1850." *Bulletin of the History of Medicine* 80 (2006): 490–512.

Grandin, T. and C. Johnson. *Animals in Translation.* London: Bloomsbury, 2005.

Guerrini, Anita. *Experimenting with Humans and Animals: From Galen to Animal Rights.* London: John Hopkins University Press, 2003.

Haraway, Donna. *When Species Meet.* Minneapolis: University of Minnesota Press, 2008.

Henninger-Voss, M. (ed.). *Animals in Human Histories: The Mirror of Nature and Culture.* Rochester: University of Rochester Press, 2002.

Hochadel, Oliver. "Acculturating Wild Creatures." In *Beastly Natures: Animals, Humans and the Study of History*, edited by D. Brantz, 81–107. London: University of Virginia Press, 2010.

Hribal, J. "Animals, Agency and Class: Writing the History of Animals from Below." *Human Ecology Forum* 14 (2007): 101–12.

Hurren, E. "'Abnormalities and Deformities': The Dissection and Interment of the Insane Poor, 1832–1929." *History of Psychiatry* 23 (2012): 65–77.

Institute for Critical Animal Studies. "About." Accessed 19 February 2017. http://www.criticalanimalstudies.org/about/.

Jones, Susan. "Framing Animal Disease: Housecats with Feline Urological Syndrome, their Owners, and their Doctors." *Journal of the History of Medicine and Allied Sciences* 52 (1997): 202–35.

Kalof, L. and B. Resl (eds.). *A Cultural History of Animals.* Oxford: Berg, 2007.

Kean, Hilda. "Challenges for Historians Writing Animal–Human History: What Is Really Enough?" *Anthrozoos* 25 (2012): 57–72.

Kete, K. *The Beast in the Boudoir: Pet-keeping in Nineteenth Century Paris.* London: University of California Press, 1994.

Kirk, R.G.W. and M. Worboys. "Medicine and Species: One Medicine, One History?" In *The Oxford Handbook of the History of Medicine*, edited by Mark Jackson, 561–77. Oxford: Oxford University Press, 2011.

Kirk, R.G.W. "The Invention of the 'Stressed Animal' and the Development of a Science of Animal Welfare, 1947–86." In *Stress, Shock, and Adaptation in the Twentieth Century*, edited by D. Cantor and E. Ramsden, 241–62. Rochester: University of Rochester Press, 2014.

Kirk, R.G.W. "Animals in Science. Laboratory Life from the Experimental Animal to the Model Organism." In *Routledge Companion to Animal-Human History*, edited by Hilda Kean and Phillip Howell. London: Routledge, 2017.

Kohler, R. *Lords of the Fly*. Chicago: University of Chicago Press, 1994.

Latour, Bruno. *The Pasteurization of France*. Translated by Alan Sheridan and John Law. London: Harvard University Press, 1988.

Latour, Bruno. *We Have Never Been Modern*. Translated by Catherine Porter. London: Harvester Wheatsheaf, 1993.

Latour, Bruno. *Reassembling the Social: An Introduction to Actor-Network-Theory*. Oxford: Oxford University Press, 2005.

Law, John and Annemarie Mol. "The Actor-Enacted: Cumbrian Sheep in 2001." In *Material Agency Towards a Non-Anthropocentric Approach*, edited by Carl Knappett and Lambros Malafouris, 57–77. London: Springer, 2008.

Lorimer, J. "Posthumanism/Posthumanistic Geographies." In *International Encyclopedia of Human Geography*, edited by R. Kitchin and N. Thrift, 344–54. Elsevier Science, 2009.

Löwy, Ilana. "The Experimental Body." In *Companion Encyclopedia of Medicine in the Twentieth Century*, edited by Roger Cooter and John Pickstone, 435–49. London: Routledge, 2003.

Löwy, Ilana. "Historiography of Biomedicine: 'Bio,' 'Medicine,' and In Between." *Isis* 102 (2011): 116–22.

Marvin, G. and S. McHugh (eds.) *Routledge Handbook of Human-Animal Studies*. London: Routledge, 2014.

McFarland, S. and R. Hediger. *Animals and Agency: An Interdisciplinary Exploration*. Leiden: Brill, 2009.

McLean, Chris and John Hassard. "Symmetrical Absence/Symmetrical Absurdity: Critical Notes on the Production of Actor-Network Accounts." *Journal of Management Studies* 41 (2004): 493–519.

McNeill, John. *Something New under the Sun: An Environmental History of the Twentieth-Century World*. London: Allen Lane, 2000.

Michell, A. "Only One Medicine: The Future of Comparative Medicine and Clinical Research." *Research in Veterinary Science* 69 (2000): 101–6.

Mitchell, Timothy. *Rule of Experts: Egypt, Technopolitics, Modernity*. London: University of California Press, 2002.

Nance, Susan (ed.). *The Historical Animal.* New York: Syracuse University Press, 2015.

Nash, Linda. "The Nature of Agency or the Agency of Nature." *Environmental History* 10 (2005): 67–9.

One Health Initiative. "One Health Initiative Will Unite Human and Veterinary Medicine." Accessed February 19, 2017. http://www.onehealthinitiative.com/.

Pearson, Chris. "Dogs, History, and Agency." *History and Theory* 52 (2013): 128–45.

Pearson, S.J. and M. Weismantel. "Does 'The Animal' Exist? Toward a Theory of Social Life with Animals." In *Beastly Natures: Animals, Humans and the Study of History*, edited by D. Brantz, 17–39. London: University of Virginia Press, 2010.

Pettit, Michael, Darya Serykh and Christopher D. Green. "Multispecies Networks: Visualizing the Psychological Research of the Committee for Research in Problems of Sex." *Isis* 106 (2015): 121–49.

Philo, Chris and Chris Wilbert. "Animal Spaces, Beastly Places: An Introduction." In *Animal Spaces, Beastly Places: New Geographies of Human-Animal Relations*, edited by Chris Philo and Chris Wilbert, 1–34. London: Routledge, 2000.

Pooley-Ebert, Andria. "Species Agency: A Comparative Study of Human-Horse Relationships in Chicago and Rural Illinois." In *The Historical Animal*, edited by Susan Nance, 148–65. New York: Syracuse University Press, 2015.

Porter, Roy. "The Patient's View: Doing Medical History from Below." *Theory and Society* 14 (1985): 175–85.

Porter, Roy. "Man, Animals and Medicine at the Time of the Founding of the Royal Veterinary College." In *History of the Healing Professions, volume 3*, edited by A. R. Mitchell, 19–30. Wallingford: CABI, 1993.

Rader, K. "Scientific Animals: The Laboratory and its Human-Animal Relations, from Dba to Dolly." In *A Cultural History of Animals, Vol. 6. The Modern Age (1920–2000)*, edited by L. Kalof and B. Resl, 119–37. London: Bloomsbury, 2007.

Ritvo, Harriet. *The Animal Estate: The English and Other Creatures in the Victorian Age.* London: Harvard University Press, 1987.

Ritvo, Harriet. "Border Trouble: Shifting the Line between People and Other Animals." *Social Research* 62 (1995): 481–500.

Ritvo, Harriet. "History and Animal Studies." *Society and Animals* 10 (2002): 403–6.

Ritvo, Harriet. "On the Animal Turn." *Daedalus* 136 (2007): 118–22.

Rothfels, N. (ed.). *Representing Animals.* Bloomington: Indiana University Press, 2002.

Rupke, Nicolaas (ed.). *Vivisection in Historical Perspective.* London: Croon Helm, 1990.

Schlich, Thomas and Martina Schlünder. "The Emergence of 'Implant-Pets' and 'Bone-Sheep:' Animals as New Biomedical Objects in Orthopedic Surgery (1960s–2010)." *History and Philosophy of the Life Sciences* 31 (2009): 433–66.

Schlich, Thomas, Eric Mykhalovskiy and Melanie Rock. "Animals in Surgery—Surgery in Animals: Nature and Culture in Animal-Human Relations and Modern Surgery." *History and Philosophy of the Life Sciences* 31 (2009): 321–54.

Schrepfer, Susan and Phillip Scranton (eds.) *Industrializing Organisms: Introducing Evolutionary History.* London: Routledge, 2003.

Schwabe, Calvin. *Veterinary Medicine and Human Health.* 3rd rev. edn. London: Williams & Wilkins, 1984.

Shaw, D.G. (ed.). "Does History Need Animals?" *History and Theory* 52 (2013a): 45–67.

Shaw, G. "A Way with Animals." *History and Theory* 52 (2013b): 1–12.

Sivasundaram, Sujit. "Imperial Transgressions: The Animal and Human in the Idea of Race." *Comparative Studies of South Asia, Africa and the Middle East* 35 (2015): 156–172.

Swart, Sandra. "'But Where's the Bloody Horse?' Textuality and Corporeality in the 'Animal Turn.'" *Journal of Literary Studies* 23 (2007): 271–92.

Swart, Sandra. "Zombie Zoology: History and Reanimating Extinct Animals." In *The Historical Animal*, edited by Susan Nance, 54–71. New York: Syracuse University Press, 2015.

Taylor, Nik and Richard Twine (eds.). *The Rise of Critical Animal Studies. From the Margins to the Centre.* Abingdon: Routledge, 2014.

Thomas, Keith. *Man and the Natural World: Changing Attitudes in England, 1500–1800.* London: Penguin Books, 1983.

Todes, Daniel. "Pavlov's Physiology Factory." *Isis* 88 (1997): 205–46.

Tortorici, Zeb. "Animal Archive Stories: Species Anxieties in the Mexican National Archive." In *The Historical Animal*, edited by Susan Nance, 75–98. New York: Syracuse University Press, 2015.

Vandersommers, Dan. "The 'Animal Turn' in History." American Historical Association Blog. Accessed 19 February 2017. http://blog.historians.org/2016/11/animal-turn-history/.

Warner, J.H. "The Uses of Patient Records by Historians – Patterns, Possibilities and Perplexities." *Health & History* 1 (1999): 101–11.

Wolfe, C. (ed.). *Zoontologies: The Questions of the Animal.* Minneapolis: University of Minnesota Press, 2003.

Woods, Abigail. "Animals and Disease." In *Routledge History of Disease*, edited by Mark Jackson, 147–64. London: Routledge, 2016.

Woods, Abigail. "Animals in Surgery." In *Handbook of the History of Surgery*, edited by Thomas Schlich, forthcoming. Basingstoke: Palgrave Macmillan, 2017a.

Woods, Abigail. "Animals in the History of Human and Veterinary Medicine." In *Routledge Companion to Animal-Human History*, edited by Hilda Kean and Phillip Howell. London: Routledge, 2017b.

Woods, Abigail. "From One medicine to Two: The Evolving Relationship between Human and Veterinary Medicine in England, 1791–1835." *Bulletin of the History of Medicine* 91 (2017c), 494–523.

Woods, Abigail and Michael Bresalier, "One Health, Many Histories." *Veterinary Record* 174 (2014), 650–4.

Zinsstag, J., E. Schelling, D. Waltner-Toews and M. Tannera. "From 'One Medicine' to 'One Health' and Systemic Approaches to Health and Well-being." *Preventive Veterinary Medicine* 101 (2011): 148–56.

CHAPTER 2

Doctors in the Zoo: Connecting Human and Animal Health in British Zoological Gardens, *c*.1828–1890

Abigail Woods

In 1865, the Royal Zoological Society of Ireland (RZSI) announced the death of a three-year-old male Indian rhino in its Dublin Zoological Gardens. The event was a considerable blow to the society, which had paid £160 for the unusual creature in the hope of inspiring scientific and public interest in the zoo. However, on arrival from Calcutta just eight months previously, the rhino was already sickly and suffering from fits. It was attended by three medical members of the RZSI, including the secretary, Reverend Professor Samuel Haughton, of Trinity College Dublin (TCD), who recommended the administration of three pints of boiled rice with bran, and a gallon of milk with some tonic mixed in. However, the fits continued. Haughton elected to increase the dose of tonic and remove cabbage from the diet. This brought about a temporary improvement, but in April 1865 the animal was found in pain with a prolapsed rectum. Haughton, two other doctors and two vets were summoned. They administered castor oil, opium, aromatic spirits of ammonia and turpentine, but to no avail.[1]

After its death the rhino continued to attract attention. The Royal Dublin Society offered £15 for the body in the hope of adding to its collection of comparative anatomy specimens. It was outbid by Haughton, who habitually dissected animals that died in the zoo.[2] His post-mortem

[1] de Courcy (2010). See also de Courcy (2009).

[2] de Courcy (2010), *Proceedings of the Royal Zoological Society of Ireland* (1863–1864) p. 13.

A. Woods et al., *Animals and the Shaping of Modern Medicine*, Medicine and Biomedical Sciences in Modern History,
https://doi.org/10.1007/978-3-319-64337-3_2

examination of the rhino's pathology and anatomy was attended by anatomists, medical men and the queen's veterinary surgeon for Ireland, with assistance provided by medical students and the demonstrator in anatomy at the Royal College of Surgeons, Ireland. By then, the rhino had begun to decompose and the stench from its body was almost intolerable, causing several of the attendants to suffer typhoid diarrhoea. Examination revealed that its rectum had prolapsed and ruptured, and its stomach was distended almost to bursting with fermenting Indian corn. This had exerted pressure on the diaphragm, leading to death by suffocation. A furious Haughton instructed the council of the RZSI to institute a searching enquiry as to why the rhino had been fed corn when it was not listed on the society's formally prescribed dietary.[3] Proceeding to dissect the remainder of the body, he wrote a lengthy report on the rhino's muscles, which he published alongside his pathological findings in the *Proceedings of the Irish Academy*. As number 16 in his series of 18 'Notes on Animal Mechanics', the report informed his 1873 volume, *Principles of Animal Mechanics*, which compared and contrasted the bodies of various species including humans, and argued—contrary to Darwin—for a teleological view of nature.[4] What remained of the rhino was sent to a taxidermist and then displayed alongside other animals in the zoological museum of TCD.[5]

This vignette of the life, death and afterlife of the unfortunate Dublin rhino introduces several key themes that will be investigated further in this chapter. First, it offers a glimpse of the illness experiences of animals that were confined to nineteenth-century zoological gardens for their frequently short and sickly lives. Second, it reveals the sorts of human responses that those illnesses inspired. Sick animals were fashioned into patients, pathological specimens, victims of their environments and points of interspecies comparison, and subjected to medication and dietary modifications in life, and dissection after death. Third, it shows that these responses were led not, as one might expect, by veterinary surgeons but by medical men. Finally, it illustrates how, in stimulating such responses, sick animals were able to shape medical knowledge and practice, and how the zoo was run. Through exploring these themes in relation

[3] Haughton (1864–1866).

[4] Haughton (1864–1866, 1873), Adelman (2009).

[5] de Courcy (2010).

to the London and Dublin Zoological Gardens (established in 1828 and 1831, respectively), with occasional references to Bristol (1835) and Manchester Belle Vue Zoological Gardens (1836), this chapter demonstrates the mutual shaping of animals, medicine and zoological gardens in the middle decades of the nineteenth century.

This period saw many zoological gardens established across Western Europe. Symbolizing colonial possession and mastery over nature, they were intended as bourgeois institutions, distinct from existing menageries. Engaging in new modes of animal display, public education and entertainment, zoos sought to advance knowledge of taxonomy, natural history, acclimatization, animal behaviour and comparative anatomy. These aspects of their histories are well documented. However, the health of their animal inhabitants is not.[6]

While animal historians have explored the lives and afterlives of certain zoo animals, and their contributions to human history, they have paid little sustained attention to their health.[7] This is surprising given the extraordinarily high incidence of disease and death reported by mid-nineteenth-century zoos. In London, for example, mortality rates approached 33% per year,[8] which suggests that ill health was fundamental to the lived experiences of its animals. This chapter aims to shed light on those experiences, and how animals were affected by human responses to them. It thereby addresses issues neglected by zoo historians, who are generally more concerned with the humans who founded, ran and visited zoological gardens than the animals that lived within them. On the occasions that these authors refer to animal health, they make retrospective, negative assessments of human responses to it.[9] This chapter challenges such assessments by revealing the considerable attention

---

[6] Green-Armytage (1964), Akerberg (2001), Keeling (2001), Baratay and Hardouin-Fugier (2002), Burkhardt (2002), de Courcy (2009), Nyhart (2009) pp. 79–124, Ito (2014).

[7] Ritvo (1987) pp. 205–42, Rothfels (2002), Benbow (2004), Adelman (2009), Alberti (2011), Flack (2013), Miller (2013), Flack (2014), Nance (2015).

[8] Murie (1866).

[9] For example: Akerberg (2001) pp. 186–94, Hancocks (2001) pp. 50–1, 73–6, Baratay and Hardouin-Fugier (2002) pp. 131–9, Burt (2002), Cowie (2014) pp. 94–8. Many of these authors rely on Chalmers Mitchell (1929), who as secretary of the Zoological Society of London, 1903–1935, claimed to have taken the first real steps to improve zoo animal health.

that diseased animals attracted during this period, and the many ways in which medical men attempted to understand and promote their health.

The health of zoo animals is equally overlooked by medical historians. As noted in Chapter 1, disciplinary traditions hold that medical history is a field concerned primarily with human health, which considers animals only in their relations to humans. It positions sick animals within the sub-field of veterinary history, and the study of animal life within the history of biology. While these two fields have paid some attention to the bodies and diseases of zoo animals,[10] the absence of these animals from medical history scholarship implies that their health had no bearing on human lives. This chapter demonstrates to the contrary. It reveals doctors' efforts to advance zoo animal health for its own sake, how their efforts intersected with veterinary practice and the study of comparative anatomy, and how zoo animals contributed to knowledge of human health. It thereby challenges historians' very notions of medicine as a human-focused endeavour.

The history recorded in this chapter derives from the traces that zoo animals left on the medical historical record.[11] These traces survive in museum collections and catalogues, press reports, records of medical society meetings, medical journals and textbooks, medical biographies and the zoos' institutional archives. They include the material changes that disease inflicted on animal bodies, and their representation in images, verbal reports and statistics. They also encompass human responses to those changes, which left imprints on human and animal bodies and relationships, the zoos' natural and built environments, and on the careers of medical investigators. Through analysing these traces and the circumstances of their production, the chapter sheds new light on animals' health histories, and on the historical co-constitution of animals, zoos and medicine.

The chapter is divided into halves. Each is structured around a different reason why zoo animal health attracted the attention of human

---

[10] Veterinary accounts include: Jones (1976), Furman (1996). For the history of biology, see Desmond (1985), Burkhardt (1999), Hochadel (2005), Hochadel (2011), Nyhart (2009) pp. 110–7. Nyhart argues that a sense of moral obligation to animals provided an important motivation for maintaining their health, but this was not evident in British zoos at the time.

[11] Benson (2011).

doctors, and explores the interventions they made, and the implications for animals and medicine. The first half revolves around the threat that diseased animals posed to zoos as financially viable institutions devoted to the scientific study of comparative anatomy. It recounts how medical members of the zoological societies that ran the zoos attempted to prevent, manage and learn about animal diseases through the use of three modes of medicine that were typically applied to humans: public health, bedside medicine and hospital medicine.[12] Their use in the zoo awarded diseased animals a quasi-human status, and refashioned them—in ways shaped by the animals' physical and behavioural characteristics—into victims of their environments, patients and pathological specimens, with some unanticipated implications for human health.

The second half of the chapter explores the zoo's appeal to medical men who were not involved in its maintenance. This appeal lay in the diversity of species, the presence of monkeys (whose zoological proximity to humans was acknowledged long before Darwin) and the zoo's status as a total institution in which animal bodies, behaviours, lifestyles and environments were centrally controlled by humans. Refashioning animals into points of comparison with humans, these doctors used them to gather insights into human health, the general nature of disease, and relationships between species.[13] This agenda became known as 'comparative pathology'. Emerging at the nexus of medicine, veterinary medicine and comparative anatomy, it was a quite different form of comparative pathology to the experimental, laboratory-based comparative pathology pursued by Pasteur, Koch and others, which dominates existing medical historical literature.[14] Like the health interventions documented in the first half of the chapter, its analysis reveals that zoo animals exerted a far greater influence on medical knowledge and practice than historians have previously realized.

---

[12]There is copious medical historical literature on these regimes. Key works include: Foucault (1973), Jewson (1976), Hamlin (1998). For an overview, see Bynum (1994).

[13]The concept of 'total institution' is usually attributed to Goffman, who described it as 'a place of residence and work where a large number of like-situated individuals, cut off from the wider society for an appreciable period of time, together lead an enclosed, formally administered round of life' (Goffman 1968) p. 11. While this is a human-centred definition, which Goffman applied to mental hospitals, it resonates with animal life in zoos.

[14]Wilkinson (1992).

2.1 Disease and Death in the Zoo

It was not long before the governing councils of the Zoological Society of London (ZSL) and the RZSI discovered the difficulties inherent in maintaining animals exotic to Britain in life and health. Following their creation, in 1828 and 1831 respectively, the societies raised funds by subscription, selected suitable sites for the establishment of zoological gardens, and populated them with animals purchased from overseas suppliers or awarded as gifts. However, these animals were soon beset by disease and death. Despite the day-to-day care provided by zookeepers, the traumatic circumstances of animal capture, long voyages under unsuitable conditions and the conditions of life in the gardens took their toll. Bristol's first elephant cost £270 but died within two years. Chimps and monkeys were purchased but soon died and were not replaced.[15] In Dublin, deaths from distemper, heart disease, fighting and 'decline' were reported,[16] while the inhabitants of London Zoo suffered inflammation, enteritis, lameness, wasting and cold.[17]

The zoological societies did not necessarily regard all of these deaths as problematic. The RZSI attributed some to accidents and others to old age, although the lack of information about natural lifespans made it difficult to define the latter. Council members expected exotic animals to suffer as a result of the British climate and their unnatural surroundings.[18] Consequently they often assessed mortality in relative rather than absolute terms: the fact that in 1840, deaths in Dublin Zoo were fewer than in London was cause for self-congratulation.[19] Societies typically drew distinctions between losses that were 'not of importance'—such as small animals and birds, whose individual disappearance had few implications for visitors or the societies' bank balances—and those of greater significance. The latter comprised cases of 'unusual' mortality in which a number of animals died unexpectedly, and so-called 'major' deaths of valuable, popular animals, such as elephants, primates and large carnivores.[20]

---

[15] Green-Armytage (1964) pp. 15, 33.

[16] de Courcy (2009) p. 24.

[17] Medical Superintendent (1838–1841).

[18] *Proceedings of the Royal Zoological Society of Ireland*, passim. Early attempts by the ZSL to acclimatize certain animals to British soils failed. See Ito (2014) pp. 138–62.

[19] For example: *Proceedings of the Royal Zoological Society of Ireland* (1840) p. 1.

[20] *Proceedings of the Royal Zoological Society of Ireland* (1840) p. 1, (1846) p. 38, (1848) p. 52.

In some ways, these deaths benefited zoological societies by providing their members with exciting opportunities to dissect animal bodies and compare anatomies. Comparative anatomy was a cutting-edge mode of enquiry in the late eighteenth and early nineteenth centuries, which drew on and contributed to ideas about divine providence, man's unique place in nature and how society should be organized. It was grounded in the assumption that unity existed in the midst of diversity; and that there were laws of bodily structure and function that applied equally to humans and animals and could be identified by comparing anatomical similarities and differences across species. There was no uniform approach to comparative anatomy. Perceptions of the relationships between species resonated with ideas about the ideal relationships between different classes of society, the state and its citizens, and God and his subjects. Consequently, the field was often beset with controversy. Prior to the late nineteenth-century transformation of biology and zoology into academic disciplines, formal training in comparative anatomy was delivered primarily through the medical curriculum, and its key sites of investigation were museums and zoological gardens. Indeed, the advancement of comparative anatomy was a prime motivation for the zoos' establishment.[21] These circumstances help to explain why many medical men became involved in running zoological societies. The opportunities these societies offered for mingling with learned gentlemen and aristocrats who were similarly interested in comparative anatomy provided an additional draw to members of this socially aspiring profession.[22]

Some historians have argued that the zoological societies' enthusiasm for comparative anatomy meant that they welcomed animal death and did little to prevent it.[23] This claim is not supported by historical evidence. Although dead animals were often of great scientific interest, they had definite drawbacks for the societies' finances. Within a few years of their foundation, the zoological societies of London, Ireland and

---

[21] Cave (1976), Desmond (1985), Desmond (2001), Cunningham (2010) pp. 295–355. Akerberg notes that c.40% of scientific reports emanating from London Zoo in the period 1830–1900 were anatomical in character (Akerberg 2001) pp. 174, 186–90.

[22] Desmond (1989), Brown (2011).

[23] Akerberg (2001) pp. 186–94, Hancocks (2001) pp. 50–1, 73–6, Baratay and Hardouin-Fugier (2002) pp. 131–9, Cowie (2014) pp. 94–8.

Bristol all faced financial difficulties, to the extent that replacing dead animals threatened their very survival.[24] According to William Rees, assistant secretary to the ZSL, the deaths of at least one large carnivore each month in 1841–1843 had cost the society £200 per annum, the equivalent to an investment of £5000 at 4% per annum.[25] While societies could decide not to replace dead animals, this would ultimately rebound on their comparative anatomical projects. It would also reduce income from visitors, who paid to enter London and Bristol Zoos in the hope of encountering rare, exotic animals, some of which had become national celebrities.[26] Animal disease was similarly problematic because it rendered animals unappealing to visitors but no less costly to maintain.[27] In order to address this situation and improve the abilities of zoo animals to perform their human-designated roles as public attractions, sources of revenue and scientific specimens, medical members of the zoological societies took steps to improve their health.

The fashioning of zoo animals into medical subjects built on a long tradition of medical engagement with animals in health and disease. It was not unusual for nineteenth-century doctors to dissect and experiment on animals, both to learn about humans and human–animal relationships, and to promote the health of animals as an end in itself. In a horse-drawn society, half of whose members still lived in rural areas in the mid-nineteenth century, there were definite personal benefits to being able to manage animal health. During the eighteenth century, elite equine farriery had attracted converts from human surgery, while physicians and surgeons were drawn to study outbreaks of contagious animal diseases and to promote the improvement of livestock. They also championed the 1791 foundation of Britain's first veterinary school in London, and participated in its activities for decades afterwards.[28] The zoos provided a new institutional setting and an additional rationale for the expression of these existing interests. Perceiving no obvious distinction between the medicine of humans and animals, medical members

---

[24] Green-Armytage (1964), de Courcey (2009), Ito (2014).

[25] Zoological Society of London (1844) pp. 10–11.

[26] Dublin Zoo was free to enter but relied on visitors for special fundraising events. Probably the most famous celebrity was Jumbo the elephant at London Zoo (Nance 2015).

[27] Zoological Society of London (1848) p. 14.

[28] Woods (2017).

of the zoological societies responded to sick zoo animals through the application of three regimes that they also applied to the management of human health. These will be addressed in turn.

2.1.1 *Public Health*

Growing interest in the health of zoo animals coincided with the emergence of public health as a human medical regime that addressed the health of human populations, especially the urban poor. During the 1830s and 1840s, the causes of an apparent deterioration in public health were investigated by various medical men and by lawyer Edwin Chadwick, secretary to the Poor Law Commission, whose *Report on the Sanitary Condition of the Labouring Population of Great Britain* (1842) documented the poor housing and insanitary lives of urban slum dwellers. In attributing disease to dirt, which gave rise to unhealthy miasmas, Chadwick's report constructed the urban poor as victims of their environments, and precipitated the passage of the British government's first Public Health Act in 1848, which awarded powers to clean up nuisances and provide clean water to towns.[29]

Similarly, from the 1830s, the zoological societies' annual reports reveal ongoing concerns about the sanitary condition of zoo animal populations, and perceptions that these creatures were victims of their unhealthy environments. In 1832, physician J.C. Cox probed the relationship between climate and animal constitutions,[30] making recommendations for the humidity, temperature and vegetation of their enclosures that he later drew on when advising on human health in his volume *Hints for Invalids about to Visit Naples.*[31] John Houston, curator of the museum of the Royal College of Surgeons in Ireland, passed on similar observations to the RZSI following his investigations into the causes of zoo animal deaths.[32] Meanwhile, a correspondent to *The Times* drew attention to the substandard buildings and damp, muddy enclosures in the ZSL's gardens, and their likely effect on the health of animal inhabitants.[33]

[29] Hamlin (1998).

[30] Cox (1832) pp. 33–8.

[31] Cox (1841).

[32] Houston (1834).

[33] Spectator (1836).

In response to these observations, the ZSL council began, in the 1840s, to plan new buildings 'with reference to the primary object of preserving the animal in health'.[34] This meant that without intending to do so, diseased animals shaped the structures that were erected to accommodate them, thereby leaving their traces in the zoo's architecture. Previously, council members had believed that exotic animals had to be protected from the environment, and therefore confined them in heated rooms with a close atmosphere. Now, however, they emphasized the merits of fresh air and ventilation. Their views may have been informed by concurrent proposals to improve the ventilation and cleanliness of hospitals, which also housed large number of bodies in close proximity and were experiencing high death rates.[35] Certainly, the mid-century drive for fresh air long preceded the work of late nineteenth-century zoo reformers such as Peter Chalmers Mitchell in London and Carl Hagenbeck in Hamburg, who later claimed to have introduced the concept.[36]

In the early 1840s, the ZSL followed the same principle when constructing a new 'carnivore house', with dens open to the fresh air and no artificial heat. It reported that as a result of this 'bold experiment',[37] the death rate fell, leopards grew fatter, females began to exhibit symptoms of breeding, and appetites increased to such an extent that a tigress and puma unfortunately devoured their companions. Inspired by this result, members turned their attention to the monkey house, where ventilation was restricted and mortality extremely high. They suspended the use of hot-water apparatus and limited the application of artificial heat. Reportedly, this led to a great improvement in health.[38] Similar interventions were performed in Dublin Zoo, with the same result.[39]

Some thirty years later, in his 1875 lectures on state medicine, Surgeon-Major De Chaumont, the Assistant Professor of Military Hygiene at the Army Medical School, Netley, noted that ventilation in many human dwellings was still just as defective as it had been in the ZSL's unimproved monkey house.[40] Such statements, like Cox's earlier *Hints*

---

[34] Zoological Society of London (1851) p. 11.

[35] Granshaw (1992).

[36] Chalmers Mitchell (1929) pp. 189–203, Rothfels (2002).

[37] Zoological Society of London (1844) p. 10.

[38] Zoological Society of London (1845) pp. 12–3.

[39] *Proceedings of the Royal Zoological Society of Ireland* (1847) p. 47.

[40] 'State Medicine' (1875).

for Invalids about to Visit Naples, show that the movement of ideas and practices between human and animal health was not entirely one way. In the meantime, however, the ZSL had backtracked on its enthusiasm for open air following numerous deaths from exposure. In 1854–1855, it erected a glazed screen and blinds in an attempt to protect lions from the wind, damp and sudden changes in temperature.[41] In 1861, ZSL Secretary Philip Sclater was forced to write to the *Morning Post* to deny public accusations that animals were dying of cold. He claimed that the only 'really valuable' animals lost were three antelopes, and a new house was being constructed for the protection of those remaining.[42]

The notion of miasma as a cause of disease also directed zoological societies' attention to the wider zoo environment, whose subsequent refashioning enabled diseased animals to leave their traces on zoo landscapes and water supplies. From 1848, the ZSL lobbied the Commissioners of Sewers to order the drainage of its site in Regent's Park on the grounds that dampness was giving rise to fogs that injured human and animal inhabitants alike.[43] On completion of this work in 1853, members eagerly anticipated an improvement in animal health.[44] The reservoir that supplied the gardens was also reconstructed to manage the 'accumulation of decayed vegetable matter and other impurities … which … may possibly have generated some of the attacks of disease which have occurred at various periods and have baffled all other conjecture as to their origin'.[45] In the later nineteenth century, this sanitary mode of thinking was supplemented and then marginalized by emerging germ theories, which located the source of disease within contaminated bodies rather than environments.[46] Nevertheless, close confinement and bad air continued to be cited as causes of ill health and death in the London, Dublin and Manchester zoological gardens, and a succession of new houses were erected in efforts to combat the problem.[47] Writing in 1887, ZSL

[41] Zoological Society of London (1855) p. 12.

[42] Sclater (1861) p. 5.

[43] Zoological Society of London (1849) pp. 13–4, (1851) p. 16.

[44] Zoological Society of London (1853) p. 13.

[45] Zoological Society of London (1857) p. 6.

[46] Worboys (2000).

[47] Flower (1887), Jennison (1929), de Courcy (2009) pp. 31–42.

Secretary, Professor W.F. Flower, claimed that such improvements contributed not only to the health and strength of animals, but also to their happiness, and therefore to the enjoyment that visitors gained from watching them.[48]

As another aspect of public health, diet attracted considerable attention in mid-nineteenth-century Britain. Newspaper reporting on the Great Famine in Ireland (1845–1852), the Lancashire Cotton Famine (1861–1865) and workhouse dietaries framed hunger as a public rather than a private problem, while German chemist, Justus Liebig, crafted a new science of nutrition which informed medical understandings of dietary intake.[49] These insights and concerns spilled over to the zoo, where the nutritional needs of zoo animals moulded the activities of keepers and zoological society doctors.[50] When selecting animal diets, these men took their lead from the classification of animals into carnivores and herbivores. This laid open the possibility of misclassification, as suggested in the case of a ZSL walrus whose failure to thrive was reported in 1868.[51] Feeding practices also took food type, quality, variety and texture into consideration. However, efforts to provide suitable diets were complicated by a lack of knowledge about, or inability to obtain the foods consumed in the wild, and by the difficulty of preventing feeding by visitors.[52]

In both humans and animals, diet was understood to impact on health in various ways—indirectly, through undermining bodily constitutions,[53] and also directly, as illustrated in the opening vignette. The post-mortem examination of dead animals revealed its effects. While the rhino's demise was attributed to the misfeeding of Indian corn,[54] other animals died of scurvy[55] and emaciation.[56] Foreign bodies in the digestive tract were not uncommon. A ZSL sea bear was killed by fish hooks, and an ostrich by

[48] Flower (1887) p. 67.

[49] Vernon (2007) pp. 17–22.

[50] Bartlett (1899).

[51] Murie (1868) pp. 67–71.

[52] Bartlett (1899).

[53] Vernon (2007), Hamlin (1996).

[54] Haughton (1864–1866) p. 516.

[55] 'Proceedings of the Pathological Society' (1865) p. 201.

[56] Clark (1872).

half a gallon of stones and copper coins in its stomach.[57] Other animals suffered because they were unable to eat the diet provided. The mother of lion cubs born with cleft palates in Dublin in 1873 had received horse bones that were too hard for her to chew. On the recommendation of Dr Samuel Haughton, rabbits were fed instead and the problem did not recur. In an 1873 introductory address to University College Hospital, the surgeon, Mr Erichsen, referred to this episode as an important lesson in how to prevent such defects in human children.[58] As discussed below, this issue attracted further attention in London during the 1880s.

2.1.2 *Bedside Medicine*

Another medical regime that found expression in Britain's nineteenth-century zoos was that which historians have termed 'bedside medicine'. This was an individualized system of clinical care applied particularly to elite patients who could afford private medical attention in their homes. It was not the only mode of treating disease. Just as sick people turned usually to family, friends or trusted members of local communities for remedies and advice, so the day-to-day care of sick animals was provided by zookeepers and superintendents. In mid-century Dublin, keepers had their wages docked if animals died or escaped,[59] while in London they were expected to 'as far as possible obtain a knowledge of the structure and acquaint themselves with the disorders of the animals'.[60] Many keepers were former farm labourers. From informal exchanges of knowledge and close acquaintance with the animals in their care, they learned to identify symptoms of illness and to handle sick animals in ways that sometimes permitted inspections, drug administration and the management of physical injuries.[61] The expertise of Abraham Dee Bartlett, superintendent of London Zoo from 1859 to 1897, was legendary and extended to surgical interventions, such as the tricky dental operation performed on Obaysch the celebrity hippo, and the removal of broken fangs causing abscesses from the mouths of poisonous serpents—an

[57] Murie (1867) pp. 243–44, Darwin and Garrod (1872) pp. 356–63.

[58] Erichsen (1873) p. 413.

[59] de Courcy (2009) p. 20.

[60] 'Zoological Society of London, Meeting of Council' 22 May 1833.

[61] Burt (2002), Hochadel (2011).

operation that once left fatal marks on the body of a drunken keeper who was attempting to restrain them.[62]

In awarding animals the roles of patients, 'bedside medicine' was superimposed on this regime. Between 1829 and 1842, the ZSL employed a 'surgeon' or 'medical superintendent' to treat their diseases. The post-holder was actually a veterinary surgeon. The first appointee, Charles Spooner, had recently qualified from the London (later Royal) Veterinary College and was known for his anatomical prowess. He agreed to attend the gardens three times a week, and more often when necessary, for a fee of £60 per annum.[63] Reportedly, his relationship with the keepers was not entirely amicable and he was replaced in 1833 by William Youatt, a fellow of the ZSL who received £100 per annum. Youatt was a highly respected though unqualified vet. He ran a large clinic in London's Oxford Street and lectured at London University on the diseases of domestic animals. He and the head keeper inspected the menagerie together twice a week and issued regular, joint reports to council.[64] Medical members of the ZSL council sometimes attended these inspections and offered their own opinions, diagnoses and suggested remedies—to the irritation of Youatt, who was working with other veterinary reformers to separate the domain of veterinary from human medicine and to limit medical participation in it.[65]

Traces of Spooner's and Youatt's animal patients—who were mostly mammals or valuable birds—are left in their journals, which itemize each patient, their disease, their clinical condition (as deduced largely from symptoms, outward appearances and keepers' reports of recent behaviour) and recommendations for treatment. Usually applied by keepers, therapies ranged from nursing to ointments and medicines aimed at symptomatic relief.[66] Youatt also published a series of individual case reports in his periodical, *The Veterinarian,* under the heading 'comparative pathology' (although they featured little in the way

---

62 Bartlett (1899).

63 'Zoological Society of London, Meeting of Council' 1 July 1829.

64 'Zoological Society of London, Meeting of Council' 22 May 1833.

65 Youatt (1836d, 1836e), Woods (2017).

66 'Surgeon's Journal' (1829–1831), Medical Superintendent (1838–1841).

of comparison).[67] These records offer rare insights into the health experiences of animal patients, as perceived by their human healers. Youatt diagnosed conditions such as mange, moulting, lameness, paralysis, phthisis, wasting, enteritis, diarrhoea, wounds and abscesses. He documented the demeanour, appetites and appearances of his patients, and expressed humanitarian concern for them, as befitted a supporter of the Royal Society for the Prevention of Cruelty to Animals. He routinely referred to a sick animal as a 'poor fellow'. When ordering the application of yet another caustic blister to a pheasant's skin, he was 'loath to punish the poor bird any more'.[68] His lengthy account of the decline and death of a chimpanzee—which appeared also in the medical press—was shot through with emotion at the animal's plight.[69]

Youatt's reports show that animals did not always cooperate with 'bedside medicine'. For example, a moose deer that he examined on 19 April 1835 was reportedly 'a sadly ferocious fellow, and cannot be handled'. By the 28th of the month the deer would 'no longer take his powders' and two days later was reportedly 'very suspicious of his food and will not eat anything in which medicine is concealed'. His condition fluctuated over the next two months until 'unexpected by any of us' he died.[70] Another of Youatt's patients, a rhinoceros with colic, did not respond to having his belly rubbed, although he gained some relief from calomel, which Youatt tricked him into consuming by concealing it in a carrot. When the pains resumed, keepers tried to roll the rhino with the aid of ropes and a collar placed around his neck. They also forced three pints of castor oil and half a pint of laudanum down his throat. He struggled to exhaustion and did not respond to the medicine. Youatt thought of administering an enema but it proved 'utterly impossible', and when men tried to drench the rhino with Epsom salts he broke his collar. Nevertheless, he gradually recovered—presumably in spite of rather than as a result of Youatt's interventions.[71]

---

[67] For example: Youatt (1836a).

[68] Medical Superintendent, 14 March 1838, Case 1130.

[69] Youatt (1836d, 1836e).

[70] Youatt (1836a).

[71] Youatt (1836).

Youatt remained in post until 1842, when deteriorating finances led the council to award his responsibilities to the head keeper, reportedly 'without in any degree impairing the general efficiency of that department'.[72] From then until the twentieth century, veterinarians made only occasional contributions to the health of animals in the gardens, primarily in the surgical treatment of valuable animals, as in 1850, when Royal Veterinary College Principal, J.B. Simonds, worked with a human surgeon to amputate a leopard's leg using chloroform.[73] 'Bedside medicine' was still provided to valuable, high-profile animals but by medical members of the zoological societies, who occasionally summoned aid from leading members of their profession. In 1850s Dublin, sick animals were identified, diagnosed and treated by whichever RZSI council member was responsible for conducting the weekly inspection of the gardens. Subsequently, this responsibility was assumed by surgeon, RZSI council member and its future secretary the Reverend Professor Samuel Haughton.[74] In 1860s London, the naturalist and surgeon Frank Buckland doctored the ZSL's animals in conjunction with Superintendent Bartlett, and turned his house into an honorary animal hospital.[75] Care was also provided by surgeon James Murie who as shown below, was appointed in 1865 as the ZSL's first prosector.[76] This was a post that existed in many human hospitals, and involved the performance of post-mortem examinations on human (or, in this case, animal) bodies.

These medical men were clearly convinced that their experiences at the human bedside formed a useful guide to 'cage-side' treatments, and that as a consequence, dedicated veterinary care was rarely required. Their applications of bleeding, medicines and nursing care closely resembled those applied to human patients.[77] For surgical problems such as tooth abscesses, swollen joints, cataracts and wounds, they applied the principles and techniques of human surgery, and possibly also their knowledge of comparative anatomy. For example, in 1835, Phillip Crampton, surgeon-general of Ireland and fellow of the RZSI,

[72] Zoological Society of London (1855) p. 4.

[73] 'A Leopard' (1850) p. 4.

[74] de Courcy (2009) pp. 33, 41–3.

[75] Bompas (1885).

[76] For example: Murie (1870) pp. 611–5.

[77] Jewson (1976).

performed a tracheotomy on a wapiti after noticing during a visit that it had difficulty breathing.[78] His colleague, Dr Houston, performed an eye operation to relieve an ostrich suffering from an injury-induced abscess.[79] Surgeons quickly discovered that animals were more resistant to such interventions than human patients. In 1840, a sick leopard had to be restrained in a net so that a Dr Corrigan could auscultate its chest with a stethoscope.[80] A decade later, when Dr John Snow attempted to apply newly discovered chloroform anaesthesia to a bear so that William White Cooper (later surgeon-oculist to Queen Victoria) could operate on its cataracts, it took several men more than ten minutes to manoeuvre the bear into a position where anaesthesia could be applied.[81] Likewise, in attempting to perform minor operations on monkeys in London during the 1880s, surgeon John Bland Sutton was impeded by their propensity to struggle and bite.[82] In these ways, animals moulded their relationships with medical men, and the clinical interventions that were performed on them.

2.1.3 *Hospital Medicine*

Doctors' interest in the health of zoo animals did not end with the failure of preventive or curative interventions. After animals died, they awarded them additional roles as pathological specimens. In London, post-mortem inspection of animals' morbid anatomy was conducted initially on a limited scale by the veterinarians Spooner and Youatt, with the aim of determining why valuable animals had died.[83] Subsequently, the practice expanded to resemble what historians of human medicine have described as 'hospital medicine'. Emerging in revolutionary Paris and spreading later to England, hospital medicine proceeded through extensive post-mortem examinations on hospital patients. From examining pathological anatomical changes after death and correlating them with the signs and symptoms of disease displayed in life, doctors developed

[78] 'Novel Operation' (1835) p. 2.

[79] Houston (1834) pp. 287–8.

[80] 'Royal Zoological Gardens' (1840).

[81] 'An Account of Operations' (1850).

[82] Bland Sutton (1931) p. 142.

[83] Spooner (1832, 1833), Medical Superintendent (1838–1841).

new insights into the identities and relative frequencies of diseases, and how to diagnose them.[84]

Zoos offered unique opportunities for the practice of hospital medicine. The control that they exerted over animals' living conditions and the regular surveillance performed by keepers and the zoological societies generated intimate knowledge of the circumstances and manifestations of disease in life. The examination of animal bodies after death was facilitated by high death rates, the absence of the social taboos that impeded dissection of human bodies, and the zoological societies' existing interest in animal dissection for comparative anatomical purposes. However, 'hospital medicine' in the zoo did not map exactly onto that performed on humans, partly because, as shown above, animals sometimes resisted efforts to examine them clinically in life, which made it difficult to perform anatomo-clinical correlations after death. In addition, animal bodies were sometimes so appealing to the societies' comparative anatomy enthusiasts that attempts to investigate their pathologies were sidelined. In theory, both activities could be performed on the same body, but in practice, they had quite different objectives: pathological anatomical changes showed why an individual animal had died, but its comparative anatomy represented its general zoological type. For the zoological societies, the generation of universal knowledge took precedence over the particular, and so where tensions arose, they privileged comparative over pathological anatomy.

This situation impacted on Youatt's efforts to fashion animals into pathological specimens. Reportedly, the ZSL sometimes asked him to desist his post-mortems in order to preserve certain bodies 'for more detailed dissection, or as a specimen for the museum'.[85] The post-mortem inspection of a tiger had to be delayed until ZSL members interested in its comparative anatomy had assembled. By the time Youatt opened the body, it gave off a 'stench … of a particularly oppressive character' that 'exceeded anything I had ever experienced'.[86] On another occasion, members could not wait, and had opened the thorax of a lioness and buried the contents before

[84] Bynum (1994).

[85] 'Zoological Society of London, Meeting of Council' 22 May 1833, Youatt (1836a).

[86] Youatt (1834).

Youatt arrived on the scene, thereby preventing him from confirming or refuting the diagnosis of phthisis that he had made in life.[87]

Surgeon James Murie, who was appointed in 1865 as the ZSL's first prosector, also fell foul of its prioritization of comparative over pathological anatomy. Like Spooner and Youatt, he owed his role at the zoo to its animals' propensity to disease and death. He was required to attend daily and dissect all of the zoo's dead animals in a new room constructed specially for the purpose. As well as determining why animals had died, he had to study their comparative anatomies, and organize the sale of their body parts to dealers, museums, and members of the scientific and medical communities. As revealed by the aforementioned case of the Dublin rhino, the RZSI also engaged in this commercial practice in order to recoup some of the financial losses caused by animal disease and death. In this way, dead zoo animals acquired afterlives beyond the zoo, as subjects of taxidermy, scientific research and museum display.[88]

Murie poured his energies into the development of 'hospital medicine' at the zoo. He kept detailed records of each animal he examined, their symptoms in life where ascertainable, and their pathology after death. He transformed individual cases into collective statistics, which laid bare the immense mortality in the zoo: in 1866, 684 (33%) out of a total 2073 animals perished. Murie also started to develop epidemiological perspectives on zoo animal diseases by identifying the commonest causes of death among different classes of animal, and their seasonality and distribution by age and length of time spent in the gardens. Perceiving no distinction between the causes of death in humans and animals, he analysed the latter using the disease categories drawn up by William Farr at the Registrar General's Office.[89] He went on to draw lessons for how to improve animal health through public health interventions, such as housing and feeding.[90] However, the ZSL's Prosectorial Committee was not satisfied with his construction of intricate pathological and statistical analyses of animals and demanded that he turn his attention to comparative anatomical descriptions 'for the interest of

[87] Youatt (1836c).

[88] See also Alberti (2011).

[89] Eyler (1979).

[90] 'Prosector's Report' (1865–1868).

science and the credit of the society'.[91] Murie proved unable to complete these to the required timetable. After much correspondence, he resigned in 1870 citing ill health.[92] His successors—A.H. Garrod, W.A. Forbes and F.E. Beddard—neatly sidestepped the tensions between comparative and pathological anatomy by largely ignoring the latter. Appointed on account of their anatomical prowess, they were given a free rein to pursue their interests. The Prosectorial Committee lost interest and hardly met following Beddard's appointment in 1884.[93]

The tensions between pathological and comparative anatomy were not inevitable. As shown in the opening vignette, the Reverend Professor Samuel Haughton succeeded in pursuing these activities simultaneously. He already held the chair of geology at TCD when in 1859 he decided to read medicine. He joined the council of the RZSI in 1860, became honorary secretary in 1864 and then was president from 1885 to 1889.[94] From 1859 he decided to examine all the animals that died in the Dublin gardens. This enabled him to identify causes of death and their frequency, and to make preventive recommendations, for example by changing diets or improving ventilation.[95] At the same time he used the bodies to pursue a less utilitarian programme of comparative anatomical research that created traces of animal musculature, as documented in his 1873 volume *Principles of Animal Mechanics*.[96] Haughton's ability to avoid the tensions that destroyed Murie may have resulted from his position at the zoo. As secretary and president, he possessed considerably more power than Murie, who was a mere employee.

2.2 Comparative Perspectives

The activities described above were primarily performed or directed by medically qualified fellows of the zoological societies. Applying the ideas and practices of human medicine, they awarded animals roles as victims of their environments, patients and pathological specimens.

[91] 'Prosectorial Committee: Meetings' 11 November 1869.

[92] 'Prosectorial Committee: Meetings' 17 November 1869, 22 February 1870.

[93] 'Prosectorial Committee: Meetings' passim.

[94] Jessop (1973).

[95] 'Proceedings of the Pathological Society of Dublin' (1865), Haughton (1864–1866), *Proceedings of the Royal Zoological Society of Ireland* (1864) p. 12, (1865) p. 18.

[96] Haughton (1873).

They performed interventions in order to protect the societies' finances, and to ensure that the zoos continued to function as sites for the comparative anatomical investigation of exotic animal bodies. Running alongside these 'in-house' activities were other investigations pursued for quite different purposes, by medical men who were not formally associated with the zoological societies and were often marginal to their profession. These men deliberately sought out dead and diseasedzoo animals and worked to refashion them into points of comparison with humans in the hope of advancing medicine and potentially their careers. In comparison with 'in-house' activities, their work was less concerned with using medicine to shape animals, than using animals to shape medicine.

Their efforts to develop comparative perspectives on disease drew on prevailing approaches to comparative anatomy. As outlined above, this activity was rooted in the premise that unity existed in the midst of species diversity, and sought, through comparative studies of diverse species, to identify underlying laws of bodily structure and function. As the nineteenth century progressed, it drew strength from successive, overlapping scientific and intellectual traditions, notably natural theology at the turn of the nineteenth century, Romantic naturphilosophie, cell theory (as developed by Schwann and elaborated by Virchow), Charles Darwin's theory of evolution and, in the 1870s, Ernest Haeckel's evolutionary morphology (which sought to determine relations between organisms by tracing them back to common ancestors).[97] Meanwhile, a general physiology that evolved separately from medically oriented physiology likewise attempted to extract general laws from the diversity of animal life.[98] The notion of disease as 'life gone wrong', which gained strength mid-century through Virchow's work, facilitated the incorporation of pathology into this comparative, biological project, while

[97] Darwin (1868) pp. 1–27, Jacyna (1984a, 1984b), Desmond (1989), Nyhart (1995).

[98] Nyhart (1995), Logan (2002). London Zoo merits further study as a site of medical physiological enquiry. Richard Quain and John Sibbald used its reptiles to work out the source of heart sounds, while Alfred Wiltshire, lecturer in obstetrics at St Marys Hospital London, used a range of species to study menstruation. Wiltshire (1883) pp. 446–8, 500–2, Wiltshire (1884) pp. 301–5, 'Obituary' (1905).

Darwin's musings on the inheritance of disease brought an additional, evolutionary dimension to it.[99]

Proceeding through the dissection, observation and comparison of animal bodies, the activity known as 'comparative pathology' bridged medicine and the increasingly professionalized and institutionalized discipline of biology. It encompassed attempts to work out the general nature of disease, to identify species differences in the expression of disease, and to learn something about disease in humans from its expression in the lower animals. Its practice meant that as the century progressed, spontaneously diseased animals continued to attract medical attention, and medical men continued to speak authoritatively about them. Its genealogy challenges historians' claims that it was the rise of germ theory in the 1860s and 1870s that brought human and animal diseases within the same frame of reference by demonstrating that infectious agents could spread between them.[100] While bacteriology did stimulate a new form of 'comparative pathology', which attempted to work out, through laboratory-based experiment, the relationships between infectious diseases in humans and animals, there was already a rich observational tradition that went by the same name. Largely overlooked by historians, it continued to be practised alongside the experimental version.[101]

The zoo was a key site for the pursuit of this comparative pathology. Its scientific mission and eminent medical figures meant that medical investigators found it easier to access than other centres of animal populations such as farms, stables and dairies. Comparative work was facilitated by the unparalleled diversity of animal inhabitants, by the presence of primates which were zoologically proximate to humans, and by the fact that zoo animals—like many humans—lived 'unnatural' lives in overcrowded, unhealthy environments, and died frequently from disease. Interest in comparative pathology was not confined to the medical men who conducted investigations in the zoo. These investigators often presented specimens of diseased zoo animal bodies to meetings of medical societies, particularly the pathological societies that sprang up across Britain from the 1830s in

[99] Virchow (1860), Aitken (1888), Pagel (1945), Churchill (1976).

[100] Wilkinson (1992), Hardy (2003a).

[101] A rare account is offered by Li (2002).

response to the development of hospital medicine.[102] From here, some specimens found their way into medical museums, where they were used to illustrate general pathologies that occurred in all mammals, such as arthritis or fracture repair.[103] Verbal descriptions entered medical lectures, textbooks and articles published in the medical press. This shows how even after their deaths, diseased animals retained the capacity to make a difference to human medicine.

2.2.1 *The Pursuit of Comparative Pathology*

One of the earliest practitioners of zoo-based comparative pathology was John Houston, surgeon to the city of Dublin hospital and curator of the museum of the Royal College of Surgeons in Ireland. Before his untimely death in 1845, he made numerous dissections of animals that had died in Dublin Zoo. Drawing analogies between the pathologies they displayed and those found in humans,[104] he incorporated specimens of their bodies into his museum, including a 'series of the comparative pathology of the lungs ... so far complete as to afford examples, in the lower animals, of most of the diseases to which the lung of the human being is liable'. This featured a lynx, two deer, two seals, a wild boar, a goose, a bear and a spider monkey.[105]

In London, enquiries of a similar nature were pursued during the 1850s by Edwards Crisp, a general practitioner, whose failed attempt to elevate his status to consulting physician led him to wage war on the medical establishment. Unable to secure the hospital position he needed to advance his career, he looked instead to diseased animals. He kept a small menagerie in his Chelsea garden, used his farming background to gain access to livestock, and sought out the rich resources of London zoo.[106] Later dubbed a 'pioneer of the study of comparative pathology',[107] he was convinced that 'the nature of the diseases of man will not

[102] For example, see *Transactions of the Pathological Society of London*, which from 1854 contained a section entitled 'Diseases of the Lower Animals'.

[103] For example: Clarke (1891), Keith (1910).

[104] Houston (1834) pp. 287–8.

[105] 'Scientific Intelligence' (1843) pp. 209.

[106] Dobson (1952).

[107] 'Annual Report of Council' (1883) p. xix.

be thoroughly understood, nor appropriately treated, until the deviations from normal structure are fully investigated in plants and in the lowest grade of animals'.[108] Although he did not actually conduct experiments on animals, Crisp used their rising prominence within continental physiology to generate rhetorical support for his activities,[109] claiming in 1852 that 'All the great discoveries in physiology have been made by experiments upon living animals in a state of health; but why should not their diseased conditions be turned to account? Why may not brute pathology hereafter clear up some of the doubts and difficulties of our art?'[110]

In 1851, the ZSL granted Crisp permission to examine all of its dead animals. He acted in the capacity of honorary pathologist for at least a decade before Murie's appointment as prosector. Simultaneously, he pursued many anatomical and physiological enquiries. He presented his findings frequently to the ZSL, various medical societies and in numerous publications, including his lengthy 1855 account of the spleen, which recounted the size and appearance of 334 spleens obtained from mammals, birds, fish and reptiles.[111] His systematic recording of the causes of death and their relative frequency resembled hospital medicine, but his stated ambition (which was only partially realized) was to work out how animal pathology differed from that of humans.[112]

Crisp's stay at London Zoo overlapped with that of parasitologist Thomas Cobbold, another marginal medical man who was struggling to make his mark through the study of parasitic animals, which he regarded as contributors to, but rarely the sole causes of, death.[113] He spent 1857–1860 attempting to harvest and classify parasites found in the bodies of their zoo animal hosts.[114] Meanwhile, in Manchester, Samuel Bradley, a young lecturer in comparative anatomy and author of a manual on the subject, was drawn to examine the bodies of animals that had died in Manchester's Belle Vue Zoological Gardens. He echoed Crisp in his stated rationale: 'So much light has been thrown upon

108 Crisp (1860).

109 Coleman and Lawrence (1988).

110 Crisp (1860) p. 176.

111 Crisp (1855).

112 Crisp (1860).

113 Foster (1961).

114 Cobbold (1861).

human physiology by the study of comparative physiology and experiments ... that we may reasonably expect that a proportionate increase of light will be thrown upon the knowledge of human pathology by the observation of the diseases which affect the lower animals.' His investigations were particularly concerned with disease aetiology. Referring to the 'unnatural lives' of many zoo animals, he identified bad air and improper food as key factors in the deaths of many mammals, birds, reptiles and fish.[115] This finding drew on, and perhaps informed his work among the Manchester poor, which led to clashes with the Poor Law Guardians over their treatment.[116]

A decade later, new investigations were launched within the zoo by the Pathological Society of London (PSL). Established in 1846 for the 'cultivation and promotion of pathology by the exhibition and description of specimens, drawings, microscopic preparations, casts or models of morbid parts', the PSL was one of London's most popular medical societies, with members drawn from all ranks of the profession.[117] Its meeting reports and annual *Transactions* reveal a long tradition of fashioning animals into pathological material. In 1879, its president, Jonathan Hutchinson (a senior London surgeon who was convinced that comparative pathology could shed light on the diseases of humans[118]) proposed to take forward suggestions made by his recently deceased predecessor, Charles Murchison, to pay more dedicated attention to them.[119] The men were partly inspired by recent epidemiological and bacteriological investigations that had implicated animals in a series of human diphtheria outbreaks.[120] However, since the PSL was a generalist society populated by clinicians, its members preferred to conduct enquiries not in the laboratory, where an experimental form of comparative pathology was emerging, but in the zoo, an institution they saw as

---

[115] Bradley (1869).

[116] 'Bradley, Samuel Messenger'.

[117] Butlin (1896).

[118] Hutchinson was best known for his work on dermatology, neurology and syphilis. As editor of the *British Medical Journal*, 1869–1871, he established a regular column on comparative pathology. Hutchinson (1865) p. 296, Hutchinson (1946).

[119] 'Pathological Society of London: Annual General Meeting' (1879).

[120] Power (1879) pp. 546–51.

analogous to the human hospital. A PSL committee was appointed and charged with 'exhibiting and reporting on specimens of diseases and injuries in the lower animals'.[121] Crisp was instated as a member but died shortly afterwards.[122] W.H. Flower, president of the ZSL, expressed support for the initiative,[123] as did the *British Medical Journal*,[124] which echoed the PSL's hopes that 'soon much further light will be thrown on some diseases of man'.[125]

The PSL appointed recently qualified surgeon, John Bland Sutton, to conduct investigations on its behalf. The son of a taxidermist, who had paid his way through medical school by working as a demonstrator and private teacher in anatomy, he was attracted to dead animals by his interest in pathological anatomy and his desire to advance his career.[126] He incorporated the zoo's animal inhabitants into a wider research programme that involved the dissection of some 12,000 human and animal subjects between 1878 and 1886. The investigation enabled him to mingle with socially elevated members of the ZSL and to win invitations to present at their meetings and to London's many medical societies, whose published reports brought his name before the wider profession.[127] Diseased animals thereby contributed to his career progression. In 1886 he was appointed assistant surgeon to the Middlesex Hospital, and laid aside his work at the zoo. Subsequently, he became consulting surgeon, president of the Royal College of Surgeons from 1923 to 1925, and a baronet.[128]

Initially, Bland Sutton echoed the PSL in emphasizing that the goal of his research programme was to advance human, not animal health: 'In merely recording the diseases of wild animals in confinement little is to be gained, but in elucidating the diseases of man Comparative Pathology will act as a side light of no mean power'.[129] He approached

[121] 'Pathological Society of London: Sub-committee meeting' (1881).

[122] 'Pathological Society of London: Council meeting' (1881).

[123] Flower (1881).

[124] 'Medical Societies' (1882).

[125] 'Pathological Society of London' (1882).

[126] Bland Sutton (1931).

[127] For example: Bland Sutton (1884b) pp. 177–87, (1884c) pp. 88–145.

[128] Bland Sutton (1931).

[129] Bland Sutton (1883b).

disease anatomically, by organ system: dental, circulatory, reproductive, and so on. For each system he described the types of pathology displayed by mammals, particularly monkeys, with occasional references to fish, reptiles, amphibians and birds. His findings reinforced the human–animal analogy by illustrating how, when subjected in the zoo to living conditions that approximated those of humans, animals suffered from varieties of the same diseases.[130]

Subsequently, Bland Sutton adopted a less human-centred outlook. Influenced by Haeckel's evolutionary morphology, by debates between Virchow and Weismann on the inheritance of acquired (pathological) characteristics,[131] and by observations on animals which suggested that conditions regarded as pathological in one species might be natural in another,[132] he began to conceive of disease as a product of evolutionary forces: 'The same laws which regulate physiology rule pathology … therefore the laws of evolution apply to pathology as well as to the ordinary events of animal life'.[133] Disease could also potentially drive evolution. For example, pathological processes such as hypertrophy (overgrowth of tissues), which were—according to the widely held belief in the inheritance of acquired characteristics—passed on to the next generation, could play a role in the differentiation of species.[134] Bland Sutton described the study of such matters as 'zoological pathology', and 'general pathology in its fullest sense'. It was a branch of biology that could only be advanced through looking at species other than humans.[135] Like the comparative pathology which informed it, this 'evolutionary pathology' was not exclusive to Bland Sutton, but his findings were uniquely informed by his relationships with zoo animals.[136]

[130] 'Pathological Society of London' (1887).

[131] Churchill (1976).

[132] Bland Sutton (1890) p. 4.

[133] Bland Sutton (1886) p. 376.

[134] Bland Sutton (1885).

[135] Bland Sutton (1890) p. 12.

[136] Other iterations include Williams (1888) and Hutchinson (1892). There was another form of evolutionary pathology that was primarily concerned with the evolution of germs. It can be viewed as the corollary of the other, experimental form of comparative pathology. See Bynum (2002), Zampieri (2006), Buklijas and Gluckman (2013).

2.2.2 *Tuberculosis and Rickets*

Medical men were most interested in the diseases of zoo animals that were analogous to important human diseases. Cancer, reproductive, dental, respiratory and bone diseases were all noted, but tuberculosis and rickets attracted particular attention. Tuberculosis or phthisis was the commonest cause of death in humans during the mid-nineteenth century. Prior to its definition as a bacterial disease in the 1880s, it was typically identified through the post-mortem appearance of characteristic 'tubercules' in the lungs and elsewhere in the body.[137] Described in 1846 as the 'bane of the zoological gardens',[138] it was discovered through post-mortem examination to be the cause of death of virtually every monkey in captivity.[139] This finding reinforced perceptions of monkeys' proximity to humans on the zoological scale, and led John Simon, the Medical Officer of Health for London, to comment in 1850 that with 'the dignity of standing next to man' came the 'inconvenience of this very human liability'.[140]

Investigators detected certain differences in the appearance of monkey lungs compared with those of humans who died from tuberculosis, which led the editor of *The Lancet* to apply ideas about comparative anatomy to pathology: 'was there a certain order in the series of diseases through which the human form passes, bearing some analogy with the gradual evolution of its organization?'[141] Others were less concerned with the differences than the similarities. Houston's colleague Dr Harrison suggested that tuberculosis in captive monkeys was 'a sort of analogous experiment' that permitted the extrapolation of observations to humans, and vice versa'.[142] He also showed that monkeys were not the only victims of 'tubercle'. Listing the various mammals and occasional birds that he had identified as having died from the disease in Dublin Zoo, he blamed the 'unnatural' conditions of confinement such as poor food and lack of exercise, and claimed that the solution lay in

137 Worboys (2000) pp. 193–234.

138 Bulley (1846).

139 Harrison (1837).

140 Simon (1850).

141 Editorial (1834) p. 147, Houston (1834) pp. 285–6.

142 Harrison (1837) p. 227.

improved diet and housing. He went on to argue for the further cultivation of comparative pathology, which promised, like comparative anatomy, to extend and confirm knowledge of the human species.[143]

During the 1860s, as post-mortem examinations on zoo animals became more systematic, and pathological understandings of 'the tubercle' more restricted, the belief that tuberculosis was the commonest cause of monkey death in captivity began to be challenged.[144] Nevertheless, it remained an important reference point for the disease in humans, and was used to draw attention to the poor conditions in which both human and animal victims lived. For the asylum doctor, William Lauder Lindsay, there was a clear parallel between its occurrence in humans living in overcrowded dwellings, workhouses, barracks and asylums, and in monkeys in the zoo. Elsewhere, the zoo was compared to a factory whose lack of light and air rebounded on the health of its inhabitants.[145] When a Royal Commission sat in 1875 to consider the regulation of animal experiments, its members suggested to Alfred Garrod, ZSL prosector, that the zoo was a gigantic pathological experiment, of which death by tuberculosis was the result. Garrod admitted that the disease was extremely common and was generated by the conditions in which animals lived.[146] Their habitation in the zoo had transformed them from wild, foreign creatures into domesticated slum dwellers, analogous to the urban poor. While such ideas about the causation of tuberculosis did not disappear, the zoological breadth of its expression was subsequently eclipsed by Koch's 1882 discovery of a bacterial cause, which focused attention more narrowly on its transmission between humans, cows and birds.[147]

Rickets, which caused softening and deformities of the bones, was another major human health problem, especially among poor children residing in industrial towns. Heredity, early weaning, improper diets, poor hygiene, and a lack of fresh air and sunlight were all implicated, as was syphilis in the 1880s, but much uncertainty surrounded their

---

[143] Harrison (1837).

[144] Crisp (1860) p. 178, 'Proceedings of the Pathological Society of Dublin' (1865).

[145] Lauder Lindsay (1878), Alexander (1879).

[146] Garrod (1876).

[147] Worboys (2000).

relative contributions.[148] By mid-century, rickets had been identified in animals and similar causes invoked.[149] Drawing no distinction between the disease in humans and monkeys, George Humphrey used a monkey skeleton to illustrate its human pathology in his 1850 surgical lectures to Cambridge University.[150] Subsequently, the PSL received reports of rickets in dogs,[151] pheasants, and an ostrich from London Zoo.[152] In 1880, it held a lengthy discussion about the disease, and invited Edwards Crisp to comment on how it affected the lower animals. Crisp reported that domestic animals were rarely affected because they were generally better fed and cared for than the human poor. However, he noted that nearly all of the lions born at the zoo had soft bones, and most died before reaching maturity.[153]

On commencing his investigations at London Zoo, Bland Sutton was astonished by the frequency of rickets.[154] It proved to be the second most common cause of death in the 100 monkeys he examined in the 14 months from December 1881.[155] Subsequently he reported its presence in half of the zoo's dead carnivores, as well as in many rodents, birds and lizards.[156] He concluded that its incidence among wild animals in captivity was similar to, if not greater than that in human children.[157] By this time, medical scientists working in laboratories had made various attempts to transform animals into experimental 'models' of rickets in the hope of using them to learn more about the disease in humans. However, the results were either negative or confusing.[158] Zoo animals—particularly monkeys—that suffered spontaneously from the disease seemed to offer more promising opportunities to advance

[148] Hardy (2003b) pp. 337–40.

[149] 'Birmingham Pathological Society' (1843).

[150] Humphry (1850).

[151] Dick (1863).

[152] 'The Pathology of Rickets' (1881) p. 332.

[153] 'The Pathology of Rickets' (1881) pp. 313–91.

[154] Bland Sutton (1883a) pp. 312–22.

[155] Bland Sutton (1883b).

[156] Bland Sutton (1884a).

[157] Bland Sutton (1884a) p. 364.

[158] 'The Pathology of Rickets' (1881).

knowledge. In reporting about them, Bland Sutton also awarded them roles as disease victims and described their disease experiences. He noted that the first sign of the disease in monkeys was reduced activity. Then the lower limbs became paralysed. Monkeys responded by using their arms as crutches until these began to bow under the weight. Eventually they became paraplegic, and suffered incontinence and priapism. Death intervened after three to four months, usually from bronchitis.[159]

As pathological specimens, monkeys revealed to Bland Sutton the different forms of rickets occurring at different ages. From the microscopic appearances of their bones, he drew parallels with the disease as it developed in humans.[160] He also developed epidemiological analogies between the conditions of animal life in the zoo and those experienced by human sufferers, and attempted clinical interventions on lions, which he awarded dual roles as patients and human analogues. Whereas Dublin Zoo's lion-breeding 'industry' was celebrated for the prolificacy of its dams and ability to rear cubs to maturity, in London, many cubs were born with cleft palates and did not survive for long. Others developed signs of rickets after keepers removed them from their mothers for fear of harm. Bland Sutton noted that both adults and cubs were typically fed on old horse carcasses, the bones of which were generally too tough for their teeth. When he fed pregnant lions with goat flesh and soft bones, cleft palates in the offspring did not occur. Moreover, rickety cubs quickly recovered when pounded bones and cod liver oil were added to their diet. Their environment was kept constant in all other ways, with the same amount of air, light and warmth as before.[161]

Bland Sutton did not publish a formal account of these findings, perhaps because from the zoo's perspective, cod-liver oil supplements cost as much as a replacement lion.[162] There were no long-term changes in feeding practices, and the disease continued to occur, as shown by the continuing deposition of rickety lion skeletons in the Royal College of Surgeons museum.[163] However, some medical men became very excited

[159] 'Pathological Society of London' (1883).

[160] Bland Sutton (1883a) pp. 312–22.

[161] Cheadle (1882).

[162] Bland Sutton (1931).

[163] For example: 'Skull, Rickets, Osteomalacia' (1947).

by his findings. Speaking at the Diseases of Children section of the British Medical Association's 1888 Annual Meeting, Dr Cheadle, senior physician to the Great Ormond Street Hospital for Sick Children, declared Bland Sutton's dietary experiment 'a crucial one, and … conclusive as to the chief points in the aetiology of rickets'.[164] It showed that rickets occurred when diets were deficient in fat and bone salts. This became the accepted view of the disease. Rickety lions began to feature in discussions of human rickets and infant feeding practices. They also provided the jumping-off point for Edward Mellanby's subsequent discovery that the key antirachitic component was a substance found particularly in animal fat, later named fat-soluble vitamin D.[165] In this way, spontaneously diseased zoo animals became unwitting contributors to human health.

2.3 Conclusion

This chapter has provided an overview of the health and medicine of the animals that inhabited Britain's zoos during the mid- to late nineteenth century. Contrary to existing historical accounts, which claim that animal health was neglected in this period and that few medical interventions took place, it reveals wide-ranging, ongoing attempts by medical men to understand, prevent and treat animal disease. By turning the spotlight onto these interventions, the circumstances that gave rise to them, and their implications for participating humans and animals, it offers new perspectives on the interlinked histories of zoos, animals and medicine.

We have seen how zoos impacted on, and were moulded by, the health experiences of their animal inhabitants. Methods of animal housing, feeding and management precipitated ailments such as rickets, tuberculosis and digestive upsets, which caused much animal suffering and frequently death. To the zoological societies, these events threatened the zoos' finances and its scientific activities, while to certain external medical men, they offered prospects of scientific and career advancement. The unanticipated occurrence of these diseases prompted the medicalization of zoos—their transformation into sites for medical

[164] Cheadle (1882) p. 1146.

[165] Chesney and Hedberg (2010).

research and practice. This, in turn, prompted wider transformations—in the zoos' physical structures as post-mortem rooms and more sanitary animal enclosures were built; in their 'natural' landscapes as unhealthy swamps were drained; and in their social organization, as new staff were employed to manage health and investigate disease. The health of zoo animals therefore provides a unique perspective on the history of the zoo and its animal inhabitants.

In health, disease and death, zoo animals inspired medical men to engage with them, both directly within the zoo, and remotely via the traces they left on the medical record. This chapter has revealed how both humans and animals were produced through these relationships. Animals were transformed into patients, victims of their environments, pathological material, and points of comparison across species, while human doctors became healers and investigators of animals. In the process, perceptions of what it meant to be human or animal changed. 'In-house' efforts to improve animal health proceeded on the basis that animals were sufficiently close to humans to permit the application, by doctors, of ideas and practices drawn from human medical contexts. In practice, however, animals' resistance to handling and their unusual anatomies—which attracted medical attention independently of the pathologies they displayed—placed limits on the wholesale importation of human medicine into the zoo. Likewise, while investigations into comparative pathology reinforced notions that humans and animals (particularly monkeys) were sufficiently similar to allow deductions about the former to be drawn from the latter, they also highlighted key differences that were attributed to, and served to consolidate ideas about, their evolutionary relationships. In these ways, the practice of medicine within the zoo simultaneously brought humans and animals closer together, and demarcated the distances between them.

Medical interventions in the zoo also had implications for animal, and to a lesser extent, human health. Some of the zoos' more valuable mammalian inhabitants probably did benefit from zoological society efforts, especially those directed towards environmental improvements. Mortality statistics are not particularly useful in revealing such benefits because they refer to all species. Also, it should be noted that without medical interventions, mortality rates may have been even higher. Rickets provides the best example of a disease whose management in humans was advanced through investigations performed on zoo animals. However, this chapter has provided many other examples of doctors drawing unanticipated lessons for human health from their experiences in the zoo.

As the zoo became medical, so medicine became zoological, extending beyond its typical human targets to encompass an array of vertebrate species, which shaped medicine in ways that are not captured by its existing histories. In attempting to promote the health of animals as an end in itself, medical members of zoological societies engaged in activities that historians have tended to regard as 'veterinary' in character. However, they were not viewed in this way at the time: while zoological societies sometimes relied on vets such as Spooner and Youatt, leadership in the management of animal health was provided by their medical members, whose actions suggest that they did not perceive medicine to be bounded by species. Nor did medical visitors to the zoo, who studied diverse spontaneously diseased animals in their efforts to identify the fundamental processes of disease and its similarities and differences across species. Emerging from comparative anatomy and physiology, and straddling the border between medicine and biology, their 'comparative pathology' was much more zoological than the experimental version that features in the existing historical literature. The latter focused largely on rodents, dogs and monkeys, whose similarities with humans were assumed rather than subjected to empirical investigation.

This analysis of health and medicine in the zoo therefore reveals the multispecies dimensions of British medicine in the mid- to late nineteenth century, the fluidity of its boundaries with veterinary medicine and biology, and its historically significant—yet almost completely overlooked—spaces, practices and participants. It shows that in this period, medicine was not a purely human-centred endeavour; nor was its interest in animals restricted to what their experimentally manipulated bodies could reveal about human health and disease. Within the zoo, animals were medical subjects in their own right, whose management brought changes to the institution. Their similarities to and differences from humans both informed, and emerged through their investigation and treatment, while their participation in human medicine had important implications for its ideas, practices and personnel. Animals, medicine and zoos thereby shaped and reshaped each other, to the extent that studying any one in isolation from the others can provide only a partial understanding of history.

Bibliography

"A Leopard Under The Influence Of Chloroform." *Times*, June 15, 1850: 4.

Adelman, Juliana. "Animal Knowledge. Zoology and Classification in Nineteenth-century Dublin." *Field Day Review* 5 (2009): 109–21.

Aitken, William. "On the Progress of Scientific Pathology." *British Medical Journal* 2 (1888): 348–58.

Akerberg, S. *Knowledge and Pleasure at Regent's Park: The Gardens of the Zoological Society of London During the Nineteenth Century*. Sweden: Umea University, 2001.

Alberti, Samuel (ed.). *The Afterlives of Animals: A Museum Menagerie.* University of Virginia Press: Charlottesville, 2011.

Alexander, R. "Practical Notes on the Treatment of Phthisis." *Lancet* 114 (1879): 760–1.

"An Account of Operations for Cataract on Bears." *Morning Post*, December 13, 1850: 2.

"Annual Report of Council." *Transactions of the Pathological Society of London* 34 (1883): xix.

Baratay, Eric and Elizabeth Hardouin-Fugier. *Zoo: A History of Zoological Gardens in the West.* London: Reaktion, 2002.

Bartlett, A.B.E. *Wild Animals in Captivity: Being an Account of the Habits, Food, Management and Treatment of the Beasts and Birds at the Zoo.* London: Chapman and Hall, 1899.

Benbow, S.M.P. "Death and Dying at the Zoo." *Journal of Popular Culture* 37 (2004): 379–98.

Benson, Etienne. "Animal Writes: Historiography, Disciplinarity, and the Animal Trace." In *Making Animal Meaning*, edited by L. Kalof and G. M. Montgomery, 3–16. East Lansing, MI: Michigan State University Press, 2011.

"Birmingham Pathological Society." *Provincial Medical and Surgical Journal* 7 (1843): 76–9.

Bland Sutton, John. "Rickets in a Baboon" and "Bone Disease in Animals." *Transactions of the Pathological Society of London* 34 (1883a): 312–5, 315–22.

Bland Sutton, John. "On the Diseases of Monkeys in the Society's Gardens." *Proceedings of the Zoological Society London* (1883b): 581–6.

Bland Sutton, John. "Observations on Rickets, &c., in Wild Animals." *Journal of Anatomy and Physiology* 18 (1884a): 362–87.

Bland Sutton, John. "On the Diseases of the Carnivorous Mammals in the Society's Gardens." *Proceedings of the Zoological Society London* (1884b): 177–87.

Bland Sutton, John. "Comparative Dental Pathology." *Odontological Society Transactions* 16 (1884c): 88–145.

Bland Sutton, John. "On Hypertrophy and its Value in Evolution." *Proceedings of the Zoological Society of London* (1885): 432–45.

Bland Sutton, John. *An Introduction to General Pathology*. Philadelphia: Blakiston & Son, 1886.

Bland Sutton, John. *Evolution and Disease*. London: Walter Scott, 1890.

Bland Sutton, John. *The Story of a Surgeon*. London: Methuen, 1931.

Bompas, George. *Life of Frank Buckland*. 2nd ed. London: Smith, Elder & Co, 1885.

Bradley, Samuel. "Notes on the Diseases of Animals in a State of Confinement." *Lancet* 93 (1869): 708–9.

"Bradley, Samuel Messenger." Platt's Lives of the Fellows online, http://livesonline.rcseng.ac.uk/biogs/E000950b.htm.

Brown, Michael. *Performing Medicine: Medical Culture and Identity in Provincial England, c.1760–1850*. Manchester: Manchester University Press, 2011.

Buklijas, T. and P. Gluckman. "From Evolution to Evolutionary Medicine." In *The Cambridge Encyclopaedia of Darwin and Evolutionary Thought*, edited by Michael Ruse, 505–14. Cambridge: Cambridge University Press, 2013.

Bulley, F.A. "Retrospective Address Read at the Fifth Anniversary of the Reading Pathological Society." *Provincial Medical and Surgical Journal* 10 (1846): 425–8.

Burkhardt, Richard. "Ethology, Natural History, the Life Sciences, and the Problem of Place." *Journal of the History of Biology* 32 (1999): 489–508.

Burkhardt, Richard. "Constructing the Zoo: Science, Society and Nature at the Paris menagerie, 1794–1838." In *Animals in Human Histories: The Mirror of Nature and Culture*, edited by M. Henninger-Voss, 231–57. Rochester, NY: University of Rochester Press, 2002.

Burt, Jonathan. "Violent Health and the Moving Image: The London Zoo and Monkey Hill." In *Animals in Human Histories: The Mirror of Nature and Culture*, edited by M. Henninger-Voss, 258–94. Rochester, NY: University of Rochester Press, 2002.

Butlin, Henry. "An Address on the Jubilee of the Pathological Society of London." *British Medical Journal* 2 (1896): 1221–4.

Bynum, W. *The Science and Practice of Medicine in the Nineteenth Century*. Cambridge: Cambridge University Press, 1994.

Bynum, W. "The Evolution of Germs and the Evolution of Disease: Some British Debates, 1870–1900." *History and Philosophy of the Life Sciences* 24 (2002): 53–68.

Cave, A.J.E. "The Zoological Society and Nineteenth Century Comparative Anatomy." In *The Zoological Society of London 1826–1976 and Beyond*, edited by Professor Lord Zuckerman, 49–66. London: Academic Press, 1976.

Chalmers Mitchell, Peter. *Centenary History of the London Zoological Society.* London: Zoological Society of London, 1929.

Cheadle, Dr. "Introductory Address: A Discussion on Rickets." *British Medical Journal* 2 (1882): 1145–8.

Chesney, Russell and Gail Hedberg. "Metabolic Bone Disease in Lion Cubs at the London Zoo in 1889: The Original Animal Model of Rickets." *Journal of Biomedical Science* 17 (2010): suppl. 1. S36–9.

Churchill, Frederick. "Rudolf Virchow and the Pathologist's Criteria for the Inheritance of Acquired Characteristics." *Journal of the History of Medicine and Allied Sciences*, 31 (1976): 117–48.

Clark, John. "Notes on the Visceral Anatomy of the Hippo." *Proceedings of the Zoological Society of London* (1872): 185–95.

Cobbold, Thomas. "List of Entozoa from Animals Dying at the Society's Menagerie between the Years 1857–60." *Proceedings of the Zoological Society of London* (1861): 117–27.

Coleman, William and Frederick Lawrence (eds). *The Investigative Enterprise: Experimental Physiology in Nineteenth-century Medicine.* Berkeley: University of California Press, 1988.

Cowie, Helen. *Exhibiting Animals in Nineteenth-Century Britain: Empathy, Education, Entertainment.* Basingstoke: Palgrave Macmillan, 2014.

Cox, J.C. "On Atmospheric Causes as Influencing the Health of Exotic Animals Kept in Confinement in England." *Proceedings of the Zoological Society of London* II (1832): 33–8.

Cox, J.C. *Hints for Invalids about to Visit Naples Being a Sketch of the Medical Topography of that City.* London: Longman & Company, 1841.

Crisp, Edwards. *A Treatise on the Structure and Use of the Spleen.* London: The author, 1855.

Crisp, Edwards. "On the Causes of Death of the Animals in the Society's Gardens from 1851 to 1860." *Proceedings of the Zoological Society of London* (1860): 175–83.

Cunningham, Andrew. *The Anatomist Anatomis'd: An Experimental Discipline in Enlightenment Europe.* Ashgate: Farnham, 2010.

Darwin, Charles. *The Variation of Animals and Plants under Domestication, Vol. II.* London: John Murray, 1868.

Darwin, Frank and A.H. Garrod. "Notes on an Ostrich Lately Living in the Society's Collection." *Proceedings of the Zoological Society of London* (1872): 356–63.

de Courcy, Catherine. "Zoology: Trevelyan's Rhinoceros and other Gifts from India to Dublin Zoo." *History Ireland* 18 (2010). Accessed February 16, 2017. http://www.historyireland.com/eighteenth-nineteenth-century-history/zoologytrevelyans-rhinoceros-and-other-gifts-from-india-to-dublin-zoo/.

de Courcy, Catherine. *Dublin Zoo: An Illustrated History.* Cork: Collins Press, 2009.

Desmond, Adrian. "The Making of Institutional Zoology in London, 1822–36." *History of Science* 23 (1985): 153–85, 223–50.

Desmond, Adrian. *The Politics of Evolution.* London: University of Chicago Press, 1989.

Desmond, Adrian. "Redefining the X Axis: 'Professionals,' 'Amateurs' and the Making of Mid-Victorian Biology—A Progress Report." *Journal of the History of Biology* 34 (2001): 3–50.

Dick, H. "Two Italian Greyhounds Suffering from Rickets." *Transactions of the Pathological Society of London* 14 (1863): 289–90.

Dobson, Jessie. "Dr. Edwards Crisp: A Forgotten Medical Scientist." *Journal of the History of Medicine and Allied Sciences* 7 (1952): 384–400.

Editorial. "On Phthisis in Monkeys and Other Animals." *Lancet* 22 (1834): 145–7.

Erichsen, Mr. "Introductory Address." *British Medical Journal* 2 (1873): 413.

Eyler, John. *Victorian Social Medicine: The Ideas and Methods of William Farr.* London: John Hopkins University Press, 1979.

Flack, A.J.P. "Science, 'Stars' and Sustenance: The Acquisition and Display of Animals at the Bristol Zoological Gardens, 1836–c.1970." In *Wild Things: Nature and the Social Imagination*, edited by W.I. Beinart, S. Pooley and K. Middleton, 163–84. Cambridge: White Horse Press, 2013.

Flack, A.J.P. "The Natures of the Beasts: An Animal History of Bristol Zoo since 1835," (PhD diss., University of Bristol, 2014).

Flower, W.H. "Correspondence." May 27, 1881. Council and General Minute Books, Royal Society of Medicine Archive: PSL/A/4.

Flower, Professor. "Address to the General Meeting." *Zoological Society of London. Annual Report* (1887): 55–67.

Foster, W.D. "Thomas Spencer Cobbold and British Parasitology." *Medical History* 5 (1961): 341–8.

Foucault, M. *The Birth of the Clinic.* London: Tavistock, 1973.

Furman, I.B. "The History of Zoos and the Emergence of Zoo Veterinarians." *Veterinary Heritage* 19 (1996): 20–3.

Garrod, A. Evidence to United Kingdom Parliament. Royal Commission on the Practice of Subjecting Live Animals to Experiments for Scientific Purposes. Minutes of Evidence, Vol. XLI, C.1391–1. London: The Stationary Office, 1876: 107.

Goffman, Ernest. *Asylums. Essays on the Social Situation of Mental Patients and Other Inmates.* Harmondsworth: Penguin, 1968.

Granshaw, L. "'Upon this Principle I have Based a Practice:' The Development and Reception of Antisepsis in Britain, 1867–90." In *Medical Innovations in Historical Perspective*, edited by John Pickstone, 17–46. Basingstoke: Palgrave Macmillan, 1992.

Green-Armytage, A.H.N. *The Story of Bristol Zoo.* Bristol: Bristol, Clifton & West of England Zoological Society, 1964.

Hamlin, C. "Edwin Chadwick, 'Mutton Medicine,' and the Fever Question." *Bulletin of the History of Medicine* 70 (1996): 233–65.

Hamlin, C. *Public Health and Social Justice in the Age of Chadwick: Britain, 1800–1854.* Cambridge: Cambridge University Press, 1998.

Hancocks, David. *A Different Nature: The Paradoxical World of Zoos and their Uncertain Future.* Berkeley: University of California Press, 2001.

Hardy, Anne. "Animals, Disease and Man: Making Connections." *Perspectives in Biology and Medicine* 46 (2003a): 200–15.

Hardy, Anne. "Commentary: Bread and Alum, Syphilis and Sunlight: Rickets in the Nineteenth Century." *International Journal of Epidemiology* 32 (2003b): 337–40.

Harrison, Robert. "An Account of Tubercles in the Air-Cells of a Bird, and Some Observations on Tubercles in General." *The Dublin Journal of Medical Science* 11 (1837): 226–36.

Haughton, Samuel. "Notes on Animal Mechanics: No. 16. On the Muscular Anatomy of the Rhinoceros." *Proceedings of the Royal Irish Academy* 9 (1864–66): 515–24.

Haughton, Samuel. *Principles of Animal Mechanics.* Dublin: 1873.

Hochadel, Oliver. "Science in the Nineteenth Century Zoo." *Endeavour* 29 (2005): 38–42.

Hochadel, Oliver. "Watching Exotic Animals Next Door: 'Scientific' Observations at the Zoo (ca. 1870–1910)." *Science in Context* 24 (2011): 183–214.

Houston, Dr. "On the Diseases of the Animals which Died in the Collection." *Dublin Journal of Medical and Chemical Science* 5 (1834): 285–88.

Humphry, George Murray. "A Course of Lectures on Surgery." *Provincial Medical and Surgical Journal* 14 (1850): 141–8.

Hutchinson, Herbert. *The Life and Letters of Jonathan Hutchinson.* London: Wm. Heinemann-Medical Books, 1946.

Hutchinson, Jonathan. "Notes on the Advance of Physic: Being the Annual Oration Before the Hunterian Society, 1864–5." *British Medical Journal* 1 (1865): 296.

Hutchinson, Woods. "Darwinism and Disease." *Journal of the American Medical Association* xix (1892): 147–51.

Ito, Takashi. *London Zoo and the Victorians, 1828–1859.* London: Royal Historical Society, 2014.

Jackson Clarke, J. *Descriptive Catalogue of the Pathological Museum of St. Mary's Hospital.* London: Morton and Burt, 1891.

Jacyna, L.S. "Principles of General Physiology: The Comparative Dimension to British Neuro-science in the 1830s and 1840s." *Studies in the History of Biology* 7 (1984a): 47–92.

Jacyna, L.S. "The Romantic Programme and the Reception of Cell Theory in Britain." *Journal of the History of Biology* 17 (1984b): 13–48.

Jennison, George. *The Making and Growth of the Famous Zoological Gardens, Belle Vue, Manchester.* Disley: Berwick Lodge, 1929.

Jessop, W.J.E. "Samuel Haughton: A Victorian Polymath." *Hermathena* 116 (1973): 3–26.

Jewson, N. "The Disappearance of the Sick-Man from Medical Cosmology, 1770–1870." *Sociology* 10 (1976): 225–44.

Jones, D.M. "The Maintenance of Animal Health in the Collections." In *The Zoological Society of London 1826–1976 and Beyond*, edited by Professor Lord Zuckerman, 204–14. London: Academic Press, 1976.

Keeling, C. "Zoological Gardens of Great Britain." In *Zoo & Aquarium History*, edited by V.N. Kisling, 49–74. Boca Raton: CRC Press, 2001.

Keith, A. *Illustrated Guide to the Museum of the Royal College of Surgeons, England.* London: Royal College of Surgeons, 1910.

Lauder Lindsay, W. "The Artificial Production of Human Diseases in the Lower Animals." *Lancet* 111 (1878): 380–81, 417, 490, 564.

Li, Shang-Jen. "Natural History of Parasitic Disease: Patrick Manson's Philosophical Method." *Isis* 93 (2002): 206–28.

Logan, Cheryl. "Before There Were Standards: The Role of Test Animals in the Production of Empirical Generality in Physiology." *Journal of the History of Biology* 35 (2002): 329–63.

"Medical Societies: The Pathological Society of London." *British Medical Journal* 2 (1882): 1308.

Medical Superintendent. "Journal." 1838–41. Archives of the Zoological Society of London: GB 0814 RAAB.

Miller, Ian. *Nature of the Beasts: Empire and Exhibition at Tokyo Imperial Zoo.* Berkeley: University of California Press, 2013.

Murie, James. "Yearly Report for 1866." In *Prosector's Report* (1865–8). Archives of the Zoological Society of London: GB 0814 RAAC.

Murie, James. "The Cause of Death of the Sea Bear Lately Living in the Society's Gardens." *Proceedings of the Zoological Society of London* (1867): 243–4.

Murie, James. "On the Morbid Appearances Observed in the Walrus Lately Living in the Society's Gardens." *Proceedings of the Zoological Society of London* (1868): 67–71.

Murie, James. "On a Case of Variation in the Horns of a Panolian Deer." *Proceedings of the Zoological Society of London* (1870): 611–5.

Nance, Susan. *Animal Modernity: Jumbo the Elephant and the Human Dilemma.* Basingstoke: Palgrave Macmillan, 2015.

"Novel Operation." *Blackburn Standard*, June 24, 1835: 2.

Nyhart, Lynn. *Biology Takes Form: Animal Morphology and the German Universities, 1800–1900.* Chicago: University of Chicago Press, 1995.

Nyhart, Lynn. *Modern Nature: The Rise of the Biological Perspective in Germany.* London: University of Chicago Press, 2009.

"Obituary: Sir John Sibbald." *British Medical Journal* 1 (1905): 1019–20.

Pagel, Walter. "The Speculative Basis of Modern Pathology: Jahn, Virchow, and the Philosophy of Pathology." *Bulletin of the History of Medicine* 18 (1945): 1–41.

"Pathological Society of London." *British Medical Journal* 1 (1879): 123–5.

"Pathological Society of London." *Lancet* 119 (1882): 27.

"Pathological Society of London." *The Lancet* 122 (1883): 685–6.

"Pathological Society of London." *The Lancet* 129 (1887): 268.

"Pathological Society of London: Annual General Meeting." January 1, 1879. Minute book 3, Royal Society of Medicine Archive, London: PSL/A/3.

"Pathological Society of London: Sub-committee Meeting." March 28, 1881. Council and General Minute Books, Royal Society of Medicine Archive, London: PSL/A/4.

"Pathological Society of London: Council Meeting." October 18, 1881. Council and General Minute Books, Royal Society of Medicine Archive, London: PSL/A/4.

Power, W.H. "Thoughts on the Nature of Certain Observed Relations between Diphtheria and Milk." *Transactions of the Pathological Society London* 30 (1879): 546–51.

"Proceedings of the Pathological Society of Dublin." *The Dublin Quarterly Journal of Medical Science* 40 (1865): 201.

Proceedings of the Royal Zoological Society of Ireland.

"Prosector's Report." 1865–68. Archives of the Zoological Society of London: GB 0814 RAAC.

"Prosectorial Committee: Meetings." 1869–70. Archives of the Zoological Society of London: GB 0814 RBA.

Ritvo, Harriet. *The Animal Estate.* Cambridge: Harvard University Press, 1987.

Rothfels, Nigel. *Savages and Beasts: The Birth of the Modern Zoo.* London: John Hopkins University Press, 2002.

"Royal Zoological Gardens—Management of a Sick Leopard." *Freeman's Journal and Daily Commercial Advertiser*, June 12, 1840: n.p.

"Scientific Intelligence." *The Dublin Journal of Medical Science* 23 (1843): 207–10.

Sclater, P. "The Zoological Gardens." *Morning Post*, February 7, 1861: 5.

Simon, John. "A Course of Lectures in General Pathology." *Lancet* 56 (1850): 138.

"Skull, Rickets, Osteomalacia." 1947. Museum Collections, Royal College of Surgeons, London: RCSOM/G 46.12.

Spectator. "To the Editor of The Times." *The Times*, February 26, 1836: 6.

Spooner, Charles. "Notes of the Post Mortem Examination of a Dromedary." *Proceedings of the Zoological Society of London* II (1832): 126–7.

Spooner, Charles. "Notes on the Post Mortem Examination of a M'horr Antelope." *Proceedings of the Zoological Society of London* I (1833): 2–3.

"State Medicine." *The Lancet* 105 (1875): 774–5.

"Surgeon's Journal." 1829–31. Archives of the Zoological Society of London: GB 0814 RAAA.

"The Pathology of Rickets." *Transactions of the Pathological Society of London* 32 (1881): 313–91.

Vernon, James. *Hunger: A Modern History*. London: Belknap, 2007.

Virchow, Rudolph. *Cellular Pathology*. Translated by Frank Chance. London: 1860.

Wilkinson, Lise. *Animals and Disease: An Introduction to the History of Comparative Medicine*. Cambridge: Cambridge University Press, 1992.

Williams, W. Roger. *The Principles of Cancer and Tumour Formation*. London: John Bale & Sons, 1888.

Wiltshire, Alfred. "Lectures on the Comparative Physiology of Menstruation." *British Medical Journal* I (1883): 446–8, 500–2.

Wiltshire, Alfred. "Lectures on the Comparative Physiology of Menstruation." *British Medical Journal* I (1884): 301–5.

Woods, Abigail and Stephen Matthews. "'Little, If At All, Removed from the Illiterate Farrier or Cow-Leech': The English Veterinary Surgeon, c.1860–85, and the Campaign for Veterinary Reform." *Medical History* 54 (2010): 29–54.

Woods, Abigail. "From One medicine to Two: The Evolving Relationship between Human and Veterinary Medicine in England, 1791–1835." *Bulletin of the History of Medicine* 91 (2017): 494–523.

Worboys, Michael. *Spreading Germs: Disease Theories and Medical Practice in Britain, 1865–1900*. Cambridge: Cambridge University Press, 2000.

Youatt, William. "Illustrations of Disease." *Veterinarian* vii (1834): 428.

Youatt, William. "Contributions to Comparative Pathology no. 1: Inflammation of the Joints—Moose Deer." *Veterinarian* ix (1836a): 23–7.

Youatt, William. "Contributions to Comparative Pathology no. 2: Enteritis—Rhinocerous." *Veterinarian* ix (1836b): 85–8.

Youatt, William. "Phthisis: Lioness." *Veterinarian* ix (1836c): 89–93.

Youatt, William. "Account of the Habits and Illness of the Late Chimpanzee." *The Lancet* 26 (1836d): 202–6.

Youatt, William. "Contributions to Comparative Pathology no. 5: Intestinal Fever and Ulceration in a Chimp." *Veterinarian* ix (1836e): 271–82.
Zampieri, Fabio. "Medicine, Evolution, and Natural Selection: An Historical Overview." *The Quarterly Review of Biology* 84 (2009): 333–55.
"Zoological Society of London, Meeting of Council." 1829–33. Archives of the Zoological Society of London: GB 0814 FAA.
Zoological Society of London. *Annual Report*.

CHAPTER 3

From Coordinated Campaigns to Watertight Compartments: Diseased Sheep and their Investigation in Britain, *c.*1880–1920

Abigail Woods

In the spring of 1881, diseased sheep in various parts of Scotland received a visit from a Mr Andrew Brotherston, taxidermist, gardener and plant collector from the border town of Kelso. He was accompanied by Professor Williams, principal of the New Edinburgh Veterinary College, Dr David Hamilton, an Edinburgh University pathologist, and Dr A.P. Aitken, a medical trained agricultural chemist. Assisted by local farmers, shepherds, landowners and a geologist, the men hunted down and tried to make sense of sheep suffering from the seasonally prevalent and geographically localized diseases known to farmers as 'braxy' or 'sickness', and 'louping ill' or 'trembling'.

Williams investigated the reported symptoms of louping ill, which ranged from swollen joints and navels to staggering, trembling, wasting, uncoordinated leaping or 'louping', and paralysis. He also conducted post-mortem examinations which identified pathological changes to sheep spinal cords. Hypothesizing that this tissue might contain a 'germ poison', Drs Hamilton and Aitken used mutton broth to culture germs from it, and from the blood of a diseased sheep they killed for the purpose. Initially they were excited to find bacteria resembling those of 'chicken cholera', the recent subject of Louis Pasteur's first vaccine, but these soon died out. Unable to locate any additional diseased sheep, they made no further progress. Meanwhile, Brotherston examined the physical features and vegetation of sheep pastures. He suspected that disease might be caused by ergot fungus, which he found on 23 types

A. Woods et al., *Animals and the Shaping of Modern Medicine*, Medicine and Biomedical Sciences in Modern History,
https://doi.org/10.1007/978-3-319-64337-3_3

of grass, but when they were fed to sheep, nothing happened. The men also explored popular hypotheses implicating climate, altitude, geology, soil type and blood-sucking ticks that inhabited the herbage, but they reached no definitive conclusions. The enquiry ended in 1884 with the rather generic recommendations that to improve sheep health, farmers should provide additional fodder, improve the fertility of pastures and remove rank vegetation that provided cover for ticks.[1]

At the time this was the largest independent investigation into sheep health ever undertaken in Britain.[2] It fashioned sheep into scientific subjects and reshaped their lived experiences by simultaneously fragmenting them into their bodily constituents and situating them within their wider environments. Setting the scene for a succession of similar enquiries that took place over the next two decades, it was informed by the sheep's tendency to fall ill at particular times and in particular places, and brought a variety of scientific perspectives to bear on them.

Williams' participation is easily attributed to his veterinary professional interest in sick sheep. However, the other participants present something of a puzzle to historians. While Brotherston's efforts to identify plant species and their geographical distribution were typical of amateur botanists of the time, historians have not associated such activities with the promotion of British livestock health.[3] When attempting to explain medical interest in livestock, authors typically refer to the profession's interest in preventing diseases that spread from animals to humans.[4] However, there was no indication that braxy or louping ill spread in this way: shepherds had long consumed the meat of 'braxy sheep' without suffering harmful effects.[5] It was animal health, not human health, that drove these investigations. Sponsored and directed by the prestigious Highland and

[1]'Proceedings' (1882), 'Second Report' (1883), 'Braxy and Louping Ill' (1884).

[2]The government's 1865–1867 enquiry into cattle plague or rinderpest had looked at whether sheep were susceptible to the disease, but they were not the main focus of investigation. United Kingdom Parliament (1866). The imported, scheduled disease, sheep pox, had also been subjected to publicly funded investigations on its appearance in 1862. These aimed to determine the efficacy of vaccination. Marson and Simonds (1864).

[3]Allen (1976), Kohler (1976), Cittadino (2009). However, in colonial contexts, investigations into the effects of certain plants on livestock health have been noted. Brown (2007), Clayton (2008).

[4]Cassidy et al. (2017).

[5]The right to carcasses of fallen sheep comprised an 'allowance in kind' for Highland shepherds. They were generally permitted a set number each year for consumption. United Kingdom Parliament (1900).

Agricultural Society (HAS), their history reveals that in late nineteenth-century Britain, diseased sheep were not perceived as the specifically veterinary problems that historians have assumed them to be. Rather, they appealed to, and forged connections between, experts in human medicine, veterinary medicine and the natural world.

After introducing sheep, and the manner in which they were farmed, the first part of this chapter seeks to explain their positioning at the hub of this eclectic research network. It will document the investigations performed, and how sheep influenced and were affected by them. It will reveal that while sheep played multiple roles within the research network, their investigation was underpinned by farmers' perceptions of them as products of place. On account of this perception, sheep were studied primarily in farmed environments, where they proved capable of making a difference to scientific enquiries. The remainder of the chapter explores how this mode of investigation changed in the early twentieth century, when investigators reconceptualized diseased sheep as hosts and transmitters of infection, decoupled them from their farmed environments, and promoted their investigation in laboratories in the hope of making them more amenable to human control. In the process, medical men and practical farmers became distanced from the scientific study of sheep, sheep lost influence over investigations, and veterinarians sought to capture sheep for themselves. This history therefore demonstrates how sheep first integrated, and then contributed to the disciplinary compartmentalization of experts in their diseases.

The shifting approach to diseased sheep was informed by the institutionalization, disciplinary specialization, and growth of state funding for agricultural research.[6] These changes are well documented by historians. However, in failing to award equal attention to the earlier mode of research,[7] and to recognize sheep as key shapers and participants,[8] authors offer a rather

---

[6] Olby (1991), Vernon (1997), Kraft (2004), Woods (2013).

[7] One of the few accounts of agricultural research in later nineteenth-century Britain is Brassley (1995). This overlooks investigations conducted by agricultural societies, and analyses British research in comparison with that pursued simultaneously in Germany and subsequently in Britain. The conclusion—that British research 'failed'—is not helpful in understanding its significance and pursuit at the time.

[8] In fact very few historians have elected to foreground sheep. They include: Crosby (1972), Ryder (1983), Melville (1994), Butler (2006), Franklin (2007), Ritvo (2010), Woods (2015), Armstrong (2016). Philosopher Vinciane Despret reflects on why ethologists have not found sheep interesting—a question that may have some bearing on why historians have not elected to study them (Despret 2006).

teleological, anthropocentric version of events, which overlooks the fact that sick sheep were once subjects of medicine and natural history as well as veterinary medicine. This point is also overlooked in histories of British medicine and veterinary medicine, which have little to say about diseased sheep in Britain except in regard to the zoonotic disease, anthrax.[9]

In shifting the historical focus from sheep diseases to diseased sheep, this chapter reinstates sheep as actors and brings them from the margins to the centre of enquiry. Like the other chapters in the volume, it relies on the material-semiotic traces they left on the historical record.[10] These traces document what humans did to sheep in order to enhance their performance as producers of meat, wool, profit and scientific knowledge. They survive in accounts of farming practices, geographies and landscapes; in the disease narratives of farmers and landowners; in reports of investigations performed by diverse scientific experts; and in government reports and statistics. They demonstrate the evolving relationships between sheep, humans and other non-human actors such as the farmed environment, microbes and parasites.[11] As Mol and Law have demonstrated for Cumbrian sheep during the British 2001 foot-and-mouth disease epidemic, it is through such relationships that sheep act, and are in turn acted on, with often unintended consequences for all parties. Following these authors, this chapter will reveal the ways in which sheep made a difference to human history, even though they did not control or set out intentionally to change it.[12] It will also develop new perspectives on the nature of, and relationships between, human medicine, veterinary medicine and the life sciences in Britain c.1900, and reflect, in conclusion, on the implications of these findings both historically and for the present-day agenda known as One Health (OH).[13]

---

[9] Accounts of anthrax include: Jones (2010), Stark (2013), Wall (2013). Sheep diseases have, however, been studied in colonial contexts owing to the significance of sheep to their economies. See Brown (2003, 2007), Clayton (2008), Peden (2010). Two important accounts of sheep as participants in other aspects of medicine are Schlich and Schlünder (2009), Kirk and Ramsden (2017).

[10] Haraway (2004), Haraway (2008), Benson (2011), Cassidy et al. (2017).

[11] Just as the exclusion of animals from history is a deliberate choice, so, too, is the elevation of sheep in this chapter. It would be equally possible to centre this history on a different non-human actor, as Chapter 5 does in its history of *Echinococcus granulosus*, a tapeworm that infected sheep.

[12] Law and Mol (2008).

[13] Zinsstag et al. (2011). See also Chapter 6.

3.1 Coordinated Campaigns

In mid-nineteenth-century Britain, mutton and wool prices were buoyant and sheep farming boomed. Much of the agricultural land in Scotland was devoted to this activity, especially on large commercial farms created by landlords' appropriation and enclosure of common land. Two breeds of sheep dominated: Cheviot and Blackface. Originating on the Cheviot Hills that straddled Northumberland and the Scottish borders, Cheviot sheep were perceived as an adaptable, hardy and easily maintained breed that contributed more than any other to the prosperity of Scottish farmers. They produced excellent mutton and a higher grade of wool than the Blackface, and therefore gained in popularity against them, until a series of bad winters around 1860 demonstrated the superior hardiness of Blackface sheep on hills and moorland. Said to possess 'wonderful individuality, no two being exactly alike', the semi-wild Blackface sheep were thought to add beauty to the Scottish landscapes.[14] They won respect for their stamina, maternal instincts and ability to survive on meagre pasture, which they sought out by digging through winter snowdrifts. They were also renowned for their excellent mutton. Like the Cheviot, they were sometimes crossed with lowland Border Leicester sheep to produce a larger, meatier carcass. Efforts to improve both breeds were under way. Their hill grazing land was also subject to improvement through drainage and the periodic burning of heather, which encouraged the growth of young grasses.[15]

These sheep were left to 'go at large over their walk'.[16] Having a deep knowledge of their location or 'heaf', they did not wander. Typically they swept down from the hills at dawn to graze—'taking no more off the grass than is required for future growth'—then moved back slowly by evening, having enriched the soil through their manure.[17] Guided and monitored by shepherds, they lived outdoors all year round, being gathered together at intervals for clipping, branding, chemical treatments to kill parasites, and selection for sale or breeding. While commentators acknowledged the great variability of these practices, they distinguished

[14] Usher (1875) p. 8.

[15] Reid and Kemp (1871), Usher (1875), Archibald (1880) pp. 110–22, Hart (1956), Carlyle (1979).

[16] Usher (1875) p. 15.

[17] Reid and Kemp (1871) p. 84.

hill farming from the mixed sheep farming systems that prevailed in Southern England. There, sheep provided not only meat and wool, but also fertility to fields that were rotated annually between fodder, barley, seeds and wheat production. They came from rapidly growing and early maturing lowland breeds which varied by locality and were perceived as gentler and less hardy than the hill breeds.[18]

British sheep production reached its zenith in the 1870s, when the population peaked at around 28 million. Subsequently, the rapid expansion of grain imports from the North American prairies undermined the viability of mixed farming, while imports from Australia, New Zealand and South Africa depressed British mutton and wool prices. Reportedly, Scottish mountain pastures were deteriorating, forcing farmers to reduce sheep stocking densities.[19] Difficulties were compounded by weather and disease. In the damp autumns of 1879–1881, millions of sheep died of liver rot, a long-recognized yet poorly understood parasitic disease associated with low-lying and poorly drained pastures. In the bad winter of 1879–1880, many sheep in the Highlands were lost, and others survived only through costly hand feeding.[20] Meanwhile, the diseases known as braxy and louping ill appeared to increase in prevalence and distribution. Braxy caused numerous sheep to die suddenly in the autumn. Louping ill was a frequently fatal disease of the spring. They occurred particularly in parts of the Scottish Borders and Highlands, and, like liver rot, were associated with particular tracts of land. Climate, soils, vegetation, the lie of the land and tick parasites were all implicated.[21] These challenges highlighted a tension inherent in sheep farming: breeds renowned for their hardiness and thought to be perfectly adapted to their local environments turned out to be vulnerable to the conditions in which they lived. While supposedly easy to manage, their health was actually rather difficult to maintain.

Sheep disease and death contributed to a deepening depression in British agriculture, which lasted until the First World War. The costs inflicted attracted the attention of several agricultural societies.

[18] Reid and Kemp (1871), Usher (1875), Archibald (1880), Hart (1956), Carlyle (1979).

[19] Latham (1883).

[20] Archibald (1880), Reinhard (1957) pp. 220–1, Symon (1959) pp. 192–3, Carlyle (1979).

[21] 'Second Report' (1883).

The most prominent were the HAS and its English equivalent, the Royal Agricultural Society of England (RASE). These had thousands of members, and were headed by aristocratic landowners and breeders of valuable pedigree stock. Founded at a time when universities and the state had little to do with agriculture, they provided crucial leadership in agricultural research, education, and the dissemination of knowledge and practice. They published journals, ran essay competitions, offered consultancy services to members, and appointed committees of enquiry into agricultural problems of the day.[22] During the 1880s, diseased sheep began to feature more prominently in their activities. These animals also attracted the attention of the Duke of Northumberland, one of Britain's wealthiest landowners, who owned vast tracts of diseased land on the Scottish borders.

As shown in Table 3.1, these parties dominated British research on diseased sheep during the late nineteenth century.[23] They initiated, coordinated and sponsored research, and appointed renowned experts or society consultants to conduct it. They discussed findings in their meetings and published them in their journals. When, in 1901, the government's Board of Agriculture (BA) agreed to appoint a Committee of Enquiry into braxy and louping ill, it was at the behest of these parties, and in response to their promise to provide facilities and expenses.[24] Most of these enquiries were directed towards braxy and louping ill. The findings varied considerably, and with the exception of Thomas's work on liver fluke—which identified the mollusc *Limnaea truncatula* as the intermediate host[25]—they did not make lasting contributions to science, medicine or agriculture. Nevertheless, their analysis offers important insights into how agricultural research was practised in Britain prior to the rise of state-sponsored, university-based enquiry, and the influence that sheep exerted over it.

The diverse qualifications and positions of the investigators listed in Table 3.1 reveals the broadly distributed nature of expertise in sick sheep in late nineteenth-century Britain. Veterinarians were acknowledged

---

22 Davidson (1984), Goddard (1998), Brassley (2000), Goddard (2000).

23 There were also smaller-scale enquiries conducted by local farming organizations such as the Teviotdale Farmers Club, but space does not permit their discussion here.

24 Board of Agriculture (1900).

25 Reinhard (1957) pp. 220–7.

Table 3.1 British research into diseased sheep, 1880–1901

Date	*Sponsor*	*Disease focus*	*Investigator*	*Position/qualifications*
1880–1882	RASE	Liver rot	George Rolleston	Professor of Anatomy and Physiology, Oxford University
			A.P. Thomas[a]	Demonstrator in Biology, Oxford University Museum.
1881–1884	HAS	Louping ill Braxy	Andrew Brotherston[b]	Amateur Botanist
			Prof. W.O. Williams	Principal, New Edinburgh Veterinary College; HAS Vet Consultant
			Dr A.P. Aitken	HAS Consulting Chemist
			Dr David Hamilton	Pathologist, Edinburgh University
1893	Duke of Northumberland	Louping ill	Dr Emmanuel Klein[c]	Bacteriologist, Brown Institute of Comparative Pathology, London
1894	RASE	Louping ill	Prof. John McFadyean[d]	Principal, Royal Veterinary College, London
1894–1897	HAS	Louping ill Braxy	Prof. W.O. Williams[e]	Principal, New Edinburgh Veterinary College; HAS Vet Consultant
1896–1897	Northumberland County Council, BA	Louping ill	Alexander Meek[f]	Lecturer in Veterinary Anatomy and Farm Hygiene, Durham College of Science
			Robert Grieg-Smith	Lecturer in Agricultural Chemistry, Durham College of Science
1899	Duke of Northumberland	Louping ill	E.H. Wheler[g]	Amateur entomologist; Land Agent to Duke of Northumberland
1901	HAS	Louping ill	Prof. David Hamilton[h]	Professor of Pathology, Aberdeen University

(continued)

Table 3.1 (continued)

Date	*Sponsor*	*Disease focus*	*Investigator*	*Position/qualifications*
1901–1907	BA Committee of Enquiry	Louping ill, braxy	Prof. David Hamilton[i]	Professor of Pathology, Aberdeen University
			E.H. Wheler	Amateur entomologist; Land Agent to Duke of Northumberland
			J. McI. McCall	Veterinary Officer, BA
			R.B. Grieg	Lecturer, Durham College of Science

[a]Thomas (1882, 1883).
[b]'Proceedings' (1882), 'Second Report' (1883), 'Braxy and Louping Ill' (1884).
[c]Klein (1893).
[d]McFadyean (1894, 1900).
[e]Williams (1897).
[f]United Kingdom Parliament (1896), Greig-Smith and Meek (1897a, 1897b).
[g]Wheler (1899).
[h]Hamilton (1902).
[i]United Kingdom Parliament (1906a, 1906b, 1906c).

experts, who worked as agricultural society consultants, and helped to make and implement government policy for the control of contagious animal diseases. However, they were not the only ones. Many farmers believed that their shepherds knew more about sick sheep and so summoned vets infrequently to their farms.[26] They also consulted country medical practitioners about the health of their stock.[27] Wider medical interest is revealed by commentaries on sheep diseases that appeared in the medical press.[28] Doctors investigated these diseases in private farm-based research programmes, in their capacities as appointees to government committees of enquiry, and as public health doctors who worked to prevent animal challenges to human health.[29] For example, Dr David Hamilton, the key medical participant in braxy and louping ill research, studied sick sheep during hiking holidays in the Highlands. Reportedly 'on the news of an animal dying from braxy he would take to the hill with the shepherds'. He also conducted enquiries into cattle diseases on behalf of the HAS.[30]

Other expert participants in sheep disease investigations included amateur natural historians, and professional life scientists who occupied recently established university posts in biology and agriculture. Their involvement reflected the importance that the farmers who sponsored and promoted these investigations placed on the environment as a contributor to sheep disease. Farming discussions frequently referred to the health implications of geology, soil, vegetation, season, temperature, wind direction, the lie of the land, and the presence of parasitic ticks and flukes that fed off sheep bodies and whose existence was, in turn, shaped by the characteristics of the soil, season and vegetation.[31]

Similar factors were commonly invoked in discussions of human health, particularly within colonial contexts.[32] However, they had special

[26] Armatage (1894).

[27] Tellor (1879).

[28] For example: Hutchinson (1877), 'The Report of the Departmental Committee' (1906), 'The Pathology of Louping-Ill and Braxy' (1906). Hutchinson's interest in sheep helps to explain his keenness to promote the zoo-based investigation of disease under the Pathological Society of London, as described in Chapter 2.

[29] Hutchinson (1877), Worboys (1991), Bresalier et al. (2015).

[30] 'Obituary' (1909).

[31] 'Proceedings' (1882), 'Second Report' (1883).

[32] Harrison (2000), Rupke (2000).

resonance for sheep because of how farmers perceived them, as essentially defined by their environments. Farmers attributed the existence of so many different sheep breeds to the influence of different locations, such that 'every description of soil and climate has its own variety of sheep'. As outlined above, they celebrated and valued sheep adaptations to environments, and witnessed on a daily basis how these environments both shaped and were shaped by sheep bodies and habits.[33] They perceived both bodies and environments to be highly variable: even within a single farm, no two stretches of grazing were alike, while in any flock, sheep exhibited a range of characters and physical needs.[34] The farmers and shepherds who knew their lands and flocks therefore had privileged insights into sheep health. These provided a crucial stimulus, a jumping-off point and an ongoing guide to scientists' investigations. While farmers did not write scientific reports, their disease experiences and opinions were frequently reported within them, and they were often thanked by scientists for providing information, advice, sheep bodies and facilities for investigation.[35]

Owing to their different backgrounds, experiences and skills, investigators viewed sheep in different ways and adopted different approaches to their diseases.[36] Brotherston, the amateur botanist, approached sheep as grazing animals, and sought to identify the type and health of the grasses they consumed.[37] Zoologist A.P. Thomas, and amateur entomologist E.G. Wheler, saw sheep as hosts for parasites whose life cycles, habits and environments they studied.[38] Doctors, veterinarians and the Durham College team approached sheep as harbourers of microbes and used bacteriological methods to try to determine the identities

[33] Reid and Kemp (1871), Scott (1886).

[34] Scott (1886).

[35] For example: 'Proceedings' (1882), 'Second Report' (1883), McFadyean (1894), Williams (1897), United Kingdom Parliament (1906a). The authority awarded to farmers' opinions, and their input into scientific investigations, was characteristic of livestock disease enquiries in this period. Woods (2009).

[36] Mol and Law describe an analogous process in reference to the 2001 foot-and-mouth disease epidemic, whereby sheep were defined differently by different actors, and in sometimes incompatible ways. They refer to its various framings as 'sheep multiple.' Law and Mol (2008).

[37] Brotherston (1882).

[38] Thomas (1882), Wheler (1899).

and routes of microbial transmission.[39] These men could not agree on whether the exciting cause of louping ill was a fungus, a bacterium or a tick-borne poison, or on its relationships to exposure, weather, nutrition and parasitic burdens. However, all concurred with their farming sponsors in viewing diseased sheep as essentially problems of place.

Some of these investigators emphasized the direct impact of farmed environments on sheep constitutions, others their indirect effects on the exciting agents of disease. They also noted how sheep had shaped the very environments that were undermining their health. Their grazing behaviours had damaged the fertility and composition of pastures, which their bodies had contaminated by shedding ticks and bacteria. Therefore to improve sheep health it was necessary to protect bodies from environments, and environments from bodies. Some experts recommended burning, draining or top-dressing pastures, supplementary feeding for sheep, and grazing cattle alongside them to distribute manure and discourage the rank grasses that supported ticks.[40] Others called for the isolation of newly sick and dead sheep to prevent ticks and bacteria from leaving their bodies. They attempted to protect sheep from environmental threats by dipping them in chemicals, moving them between pastures, drenching them with borax powers, or force-feeding them sulphur with oats.[41] These interventions impacted on the lived experiences of sheep and disrupted their abilities to 'go at large over their walk'. While occasionally farmers reported good effects, evidence suggests that the demographics of sheep disease did not change significantly during the later nineteenth century.

As problems of place, it made sense to investigate sick sheep within the environments that were so integral to their health. Researchers therefore based themselves on working farms, which they identified via agricultural society connections or by posting advertisements in newspapers. With the permission of their hosts—most frequently the Duke of Northumberland and his tenant farmers—they transformed fields into test sites, and farm buildings into hospital wards, isolation pens, post-mortem rooms and

---

39 Klein (1893), McFadyean (1894), Greig-Smith and Meek (1897a), United Kingdom Parliament (1906a).

40 Brotherston (1882), 'Second Report' (1883), Williams (1897).

41 'Second Report' (1883), Klein (1893), McFadyean (1894), Williams (1897), Greig-Smith and Meek (1897a, 1897b), Wheler (1899).

experimental laboratories.[42] The result was a curious hybrid, a place for producing meat, wool and scientific knowledge, which cannot be described adequately using standard historical categories of the 'field', 'laboratory' or even the 'field station' or 'model farm'.[43] There, sheep became subjects of commercialized production and medicalized investigation at the same time, their identities continually in flux.

Published reports reveal that in the investigation of braxy and louping ill, most investigators built individualized relationships with their sheep subjects, presenting each as a 'case' or 'experiment' whose features they described in turn.[44] This convention persisted even when several sheep were subjected to the same interventions. It can be explained partly by the very variable responses of sheep bodies to disease and experiment. While farmers attributed such variability to the differences between sheep, investigators suspected that the 'disease' under investigation was in fact several diseases.[45] In their efforts to disentangle and make sense of diseased sheep, they fashioned them into patients, pathological specimens and experimental material. They kept sheep patients in individual pens and monitored their individual signs and symptoms of disease. Through natural death or purposeful killing, they then transformed these patients into pathological specimens, observing their organs, tissues and bodily fluids with the naked eye and under the microscope. They also tried to culture bacteria from parts of sheep bodies, and to reproduce disease by injecting bacteria and bodily fluids into other healthy sheep, which functioned as experimental animals. To elucidate the contributions of plant fungus and ticks to sheep diseases, investigators experimented on farmed sheep, muzzling some to prevent grazing, and covering others in substances to repel ticks. Untouched sheep functioned as experimental controls. All were monitored and the state of their health compared.[46]

These activities informed other scientific work that was performed in geographically distant laboratories, stables and post-mortem rooms,

---

[42] Klein (1893), Williams (1897), United Kingdom Parliament (1906a).

[43] DeBont (2015), Kohler and Vetter (2016). For a contemporary analysis of the farm as a scientific site, see Henke (2000).

[44] For example: McFadyean (1894), United Kingdom Parliament (1906a).

[45] 'Proceedings' (1882), McFadyean (1894).

[46] 'Proceedings' (1882), Klein (1893), McFadyean (1894), Greig-Smith and Meek (1897b), Williams (1897) pp. 282–7, Wheler (1899) pp. 641–4, United Kingdom Parliament (1906a).

where investigators continued to refashion and probe the relationships between live sheep, dead sheep, parasites and microorganisms, which they transported from farms by road and rail. Sheep thereby connected rural farms and urban sites of scientific enquiry, and refashioned the activities of both.[47] Just as farms became laboratories, so laboratories became farms, dedicated to nurturing sheep bacteria and ticks through their life cycles—bacteria on nutrient media, and ticks in glass tubes that contained sand and damp moss. Scientists observed the appearance and behaviour of these organisms. Then, by exposure or injection, they inserted them into the bodies of experimental sheep and other animals that stood in for them—rabbits, guinea pigs, calves and occasionally monkeys. The findings informed their actions on returning to the field.[48]

It was not only the geographies but also the economies of science and agriculture that were closely intertwined. Farmers contributed to the costs of scientific enquiries via their subscriptions to agricultural societies and by making special donations.[49] They supplied labour for scientific investigations, and sheep subjects. To maintain these sheep, scientists purchased fodder, litter and the services of attendants, and paid the costs of carriage. When investigations were completed, sheep that had not been dismembered were—like the dead zoo animals examined in Chapter 2—transformed into commercial objects. As knackers' meat and wool, their sale helped to offset the costs of their purchase and maintenance.[50] As a culture medium for bacteria, their bodies also contributed to the development of an oral drench, which Hamilton trialled on farms and then sold as a preventive against louping ill and braxy. Farmers were enthusiastic purchasers, perhaps because the method resembled a folk remedy for louping ill, whereby sheep were drenched with the dung of pigs fed on pasture that was covered with sheep manure.[51] Illness

[47] Latour (1983).

[48] 'Proceedings' (1882), Klein (1893), McFadyean (1894), Greig-Smith and Meek (1897b), Williams (1897) pp. 282–7, Wheler (1899) pp. 641–4, United Kingdom Parliament (1906a).

[49] The HAS's 1881–1884 enquiry cost £400. Half of this sum was raised by subscription from farmers in the affected districts. 'Meeting, Board of Directors' (1882) p. 9.

[50] Williams (1897) pp. 282–7, Wheler (1899) pp. 641–4, Hamilton (1902), 'Louping Ill and Braxy' (1906).

[51] Board of Agriculture (1906). Hamilton conceded that there could be a scientific explanation for the reported success of this folk remedy. Hamilton (1909) pp. 475–6.

prevented Hamilton from performing a statistical analysis of the effects of the drench, and all data was lost on his death in 1909. However, subsequent trials suggested that he had considerably overstated its benefits, and its use was discontinued.[52]

In the course of these investigations, diseased sheep were refashioned not only physically but also conceptually, as investigators first used knowledge of other similar diseases to try to make sense of them, and then used the new knowledge created to make deductions about other puzzling health problems. Their investigations comprised another strand of the historically overlooked form of 'comparative pathology' described in Chapter 2. Pre-dating and continuing alongside the germ theory-inspired version, which probed the bacterial connections between human and animal diseases,[53] this field drew strength from existing ideas about the biological similarities between species, which allowed insights to be drawn through analogical reasoning.[54] Brotherston's suspicion that plant fungi were implicated in louping ill was informed by the analogy of ergot, a fungus found on rye, whose consumption was known to cause premature labour and nervous symptoms in humans and livestock.[55] In highlighting the role of ticks, Wheler drew analogies with the North American disease known as Texas fever, whose 1893 investigation by Smith and Kilbourne had established the principle of tick-borne infection.[56] Williams, Klein and the Durham College team drew analogies with anthrax, a high-profile and widely investigated disease that spread via spores insheep fleeces and the soil.[57]

By contrast, Hamilton claimed that louping ill and braxy exhibited an entirely new pathological phenomenon. He believed that the bacteria which caused them were always present in sheep's intestines but only became pathogenic under certain conditions. By applying this finding to other diseases, he hoped to shed 'new light on the pathology of many of the contagious and infectious diseases of man and lower animals'.[58]

52 Board of Agriculture (1908–12).

53 Wilkinson (1992), Hardy (2003).

54 This method found particular application within the field of comparative anatomy, as described in Chapter 2.

55 Armatage (1872), Plowright (1886) p. 197.

56 Wheler (1899), Farley (1989).

57 'Proceedings' (1882), Klein (1893), Greig-Smith and Meek (1897b).

58 United Kingdom Parliament (1906a) p. 5.

As possible analogies, he suggested several puzzling human diseases such as chlorosis, pernicious anaemia, a type of tetanus, chorea, epilepsy, insanity and cirrhosis of the liver.[59] Although later disproved, this idea generated medical interest at the time,[60] especially from longstanding advocate of comparative medicine, Clifford Allbutt, regius professor of physic at Cambridge University, who lauded the connections that Hamilton had drawn between animal and human health.[61]

Sheep were not passive participants in these enquiries. Their positioning at the hub of the research network that their diseases had brought into existence, and the primacy of farmers in that network, granted them many opportunities to influence its activities. Their tendency to fall sick in certain seasons, locations and circumstances informed farmers' encounters with, and understandings of them, which in turn shaped the work of scientists who relied on farmers to supply information, sheep bodies, funds and facilities for disease investigations.[62] Sheep also shaped investigations directly through their unremarked upon compliance with, and more obvious resistance to, scientists' efforts to make sense of them. This resistance took various forms. Sometimes their failure to fall sick in the anticipated times and places limited the course of scientific enquiry. Aitken and Hamilton had to abandon their 1881 enquiries on the Isle of Skye because only one diseased sheep could be found. McFadyean was disappointed to locate only 15 sheep during his 1894 visit to Northumberland, while Hamilton had to extend the duration of his BA enquiry by several years owing to the unpredictability of sheep sickness.[63] Sheep parasites proved equally unpredictable scientific subjects. In 1897, Williams blamed recent improvements in pasture for the non-appearance of ticks on a farm he had selected for experiment.[64] The implications for Thomas's work on liver rot were more serious. He set out to test suspicions that a certain snail was the intermediate host, but in 1881 it was nowhere to be found, even in places where it had existed

---

[59] Hamilton (1906).

[60] 'The Report of the Departmental Committee' (1906), 'The Pathology of Louping-ill and Braxy' (1906), Richardson (1909).

[61] Allbutt (1906).

[62] United Kingdom Parliament (1906a) pp. 5–12, 31–61.

[63] 'Proceedings' (1882), McFadyean (1894), United Kingdom Parliament (1906a).

[64] Williams (1897) pp. 282–7.

the previous year. In forcing Thomas to delay his enquiries until 1882, the snail enabled his rival in Leipzig, Rudolph Leuckart, to claim priority for its discovery.[65]

Sheep could disrupt scientists' plans in other ways. Those suffering from braxy often died suddenly, preventing investigation of their signs and symptoms in life.[66] Efforts to define louping ill were impeded by the great variety of symptoms and pathologies exhibited by sheep sufferers.[67] Hamilton eventually identified a whole class of sheep diseases whose symptoms, pathologies and causes overlapped with louping ill and braxy, and affected other species as well.[68] Diseased sheep often resisted the application of bacteriological techniques. Their bodily fluids would not transmit louping ill when conveyed orally or by injection. Nor would sick sheep infect healthy ones that were stabled with them.[69] Responses to tick infestation were equally ambiguous: some sick sheep exhibited few ticks; healthy ones were often covered in them.[70] Williams brought ticks from the Highlands to Edinburgh in order to determine how experimental sheep responded to them, but tick and sheep failed to bond.[71] Likewise, in Durham, Meek and Grieg-Smith carefully nurtured ticks through their life stages in the laboratory, only to find that their larvae formed just a brief attachment to the noses of experimental mice.[72] In these various ways, the non-human participants in sheep diseases influenced human attempts to make sense of them.

3.2 Research Reconfigurations

As outlined above, most investigations into diseased sheep in the period 1880–1901 were sponsored and directed by agriculturalists, whose concern for the agricultural economy, and vision of diseased sheep as environmental products and shapers, led them to appoint experts working

[65] Thomas (1882), Reinhard (1957) pp. 220–7.

[66] 'Proceedings' (1882) p. 46.

[67] 'Proceedings' (1882), McFadyean (1894).

[68] United Kingdom Parliament (1906c).

[69] United Kingdom Parliament (1906a, 1906b).

[70] 'Second Report' (1883) pp. 176–7.

[71] Williams (1897) pp. 282–7.

[72] Greig-Smith and Meek (1897a) p. 257.

across various fields of enquiry, whose methods and approaches were influenced by them and their sheep. Subsequently, however, the research network was reconfigured, as were its underpinning ideas, approaches and implications for sheep. This was the result of a gradual and uneven process of change that began with the 1889 formation of a government BA, and accelerated following the passage of the 1909 Development Act, which awarded substantial state funding for agricultural research and distributed it via a Development Commission (DC).

Formed in response to the agricultural depression, the BA and DC largely displaced the agricultural societies as sponsors of sheep disease research. Together with the concurrent expansion of civic universities, the BA's support for agricultural education encouraged the institutionalization, specialization and professionalization of sciences allied to agriculture, including the overlapping fields of agricultural zoology, economic biology (which promoted the practical applications of biology to agriculture) and entomology (the study of mites, ticks and insects).[73] The BA also provided funds for committees to enquire into the sheep diseases, scab (1903) and abortion (1905–1913), and supported additional investigations by its Veterinary Department. In 1908 it funded the expansion of the department's small, run-down laboratory into an 8-acre facility containing laboratories, post-mortem rooms, accommodation for livestock and experimental animals, and an experimental sheep dip.[74] Further expansion was supported by the DC, which channelled funds into selected fields of enquiry pursued within nominated institutions. Agricultural zoology and animal pathology were key beneficiaries.[75]

Table 3.2 outlines the main investigations into sheep diseases that took place during the first two decades of the twentieth century. It reveals that state funding permitted more extensive, longer-term investigations into a wider range of sheep diseases than before. The vets, John McFadyean and his son-in-law, Stewart Stockman, mounted an extensive, collaborative programme of research[76] that went beyond braxy

[73] Kraft (2004), Clark (2009).

[74] Stockman (1907), United Kingdom Parliament. Annual Reports (1910) p. 15. For more on the shifting modes and politics of state-sponsored veterinary research in this period, see Woods (2013).

[75] Anon (1967) pp. 62–8, Olby (1991).

[76] United Kingdom Parliament (1920) pp. 70–95.

Table 3.2 British research into diseased sheep, 1902–1920

Date	*Sponsor*	*Disease focus*	*Investigator*	*Position/ qualifications*
1901–1903	BA	Parasitic diseases of sheep	F.V. Theobald[a]	Lecturer in Zoology and Economic Entomology, Wye College of Agriculture
1903–1904	BA Committee of Enquiry	Sheep scab	Thomas Winter[b] and others	Professor of Agriculture, Bangor University
1905–1913	BA Committee of Enquiry	Epizootic abortion in cattle and sheep	John McFadyean	Principal, Royal Veterinary College; RASE Consulting Vet
			Stewart Stockman	Government Chief Veterinary Officer; Director of Government Vet Laboratory
			Dr G.H.F. Nuttall[c]	Lecturer in Bacteriology and Preventive Medicine, Cambridge University
1904, 1909	HAS	Sheep maggot flies	R. Stewart MacDougall[d]	Lecturer in Economic Entomology, Edinburgh University; Consulting Zoologist to HAS
1906–1920	Cambridge University (Quick bequest)	Sheep ticks	Dr G.H.F. Nuttall[e] (C.W. Warburton)	Quick Professor of Biology, (Lecturer in Agricultural Zoology; Consulting Zoologist to the RASE)
from 1907	BA, DC	Sheep scab Johne's Louping ill	Stewart Stockman[f]	Government Chief Veterinary Officer; Director of Government Vet Laboratory
from 1911	DC	Scrapie Johne's	John McFadyean[g]	Principal, Royal Veterinary College; RASE Consulting Vet

(continued)

Table 3.2 (continued)

Date	*Sponsor*	*Disease focus*	*Investigator*	*Position/qualifications*
1912–1919	HAS, East of Scotland College of Agriculture, BAS, DC	Louping ill Braxy Yellows Scrapie	Dr J.P. McGowan[h] (Theodore Rettie)	Medical Bacteriologist, Royal College of Physicians Edinburgh (Department of Zoology, Edinburgh University)

[a]Theobald (1901, 1903).
[b]United Kingdom Parliament (1905a, 1905b).
[c]United Kingdom Parliament (1914a).
[d]MacDougall (1904, 1909).
[e]Nuttall et al. (1908).
[f]Stockman (1910, 1911, 1913, 1916, 1918, 1919). See also United Kingdom Parliament. Annual Reports (1906–1920), passim
[g]McFadyean and Sheather (1913), McFadyean (1917).
[h]McGowan and Rettie (1913), McGowan (1914, 1915, 1916, 1919).

and louping ill to include sheep scab,[77] scrapie[78] and Johne's disease.[79] Zoologists and entomologists such as F.V. Theobald, C. Warburton and Dr G.H.F. Nuttall (who lectured in bacteriology and preventive medicine before benefiting from the Quick bequest, which funded his post and research as professor of biology at Cambridge University[80]) incorporated the ticks, mites and flies responsible for sheep diseases into wider studies of insects relevant to human, animal and plant health.[81] Further stimulus for their investigations was provided by the emergence, and promotion by the government's Colonial Office of tropical medicine as a specialism dedicated to diseases spread by insect vectors.[82] British agriculture and tropical medicine therefore shaped each other in ways that merit further historical elucidation.[83]

State-funded researchers possessed much more autonomy than under the previous, agriculturally-dominated regime. Those who were appointed to BA committees of enquiry were allowed to pursue their own lines of investigation into the diseases selected. Those funded by the DC were awarded considerable 'latitude and elasticity' owing to its perceived difficulty in predicting whether research would have the desired practical impacts.[84] Many researchers maintained close links with agriculture—for example, by providing consultancy services to societies. However, farmers were no longer their prime audiences or suppliers of information. Their creation of societies such as the Association of Economic Biologists, and their foundation of, and publication within, new scientific journals (e.g. *Parasitology*, *Journal of Agricultural Science*, *Journal of Economic Biology* and *Journal of Comparative Pathology and*

[77] This was understood to be an irritating and highly contagious skin disease caused by a mite. It impacted severely on sheep welfare, wool and meat production, and was notifiable by law.

[78] An obscure, chronic disease that caused wasting and itching.

[79] A chronic wasting disease that occasionally affected sheep but mainly cattle.

[80] Graham-Smith and Keilin (1939).

[81] F.V. Theobald was best known for his description of the 21,000 mosquitos gathered by colonial officials at the request of Colonial Secretary Joseph Chamberlain (Theobald (1901–1910)). In collaboration with Warburton and others, Nuttall wrote the definitive manual on ticks. He also conducted investigations into tick-borne diseases of dogs and livestock in the tropics. Clark (2009), Cox (2009).

[82] Worboys (1976), Farley (1989), Brown (2005).

[83] Kraft (2004), Clark (2009).

[84] United Kingdom Parliament (1912–1913a) p. 8.

Therapeutics) illustrate the emergence of professionalized, self-referential scientific communities for whom diseased sheep were not simply agricultural problems but also problems for science, whose solution promised personal and professional advancement.

Not all experts benefited equally from the new research landscape. Those located outside formal research institutions, such as amateur natural historians, were unable to tap DC funds and consequently became distanced from professional science.[85] Those working outside the areas prioritized by the DC, such as medical men working in medical institutions, could only compete for the small quantity of funds left over after nominated institutions had received their share.[86] The state's involvement therefore encouraged the separation of amateur from professional science, and of fields dedicated to animals and animal health (veterinary medicine and zoology) from those primarily concerned with humans.[87]

English agricultural societies were generally content to cede their leadership of agricultural research to scientists and the state. However, the Scottish societies, which had done the most to promote diseased sheep research, were unhappy that virtually all of the institutions supported by the DC were in England. The DC defended itself on the grounds that only institutions with a strong track record merited research funding, and that 'what may be called pure research is not a local matter, and consequently the proper division of effort is not by geographical districts'.[88] This did not satisfy the Scots, whose perceptions of sheep and their diseases were deeply localized. They also fumed over the BA's reluctance to cede control of livestock disease research to a new Board of Agriculture for Scotland (BAS, established in 1911).[89] The HAS and the East of Scotland College of Agriculture therefore decided to sponsor (with limited support from the BAS and the DC) their own enquiries into diseased sheep. Their appointment of the Scottish medical bacteriologist and farmer's son, Dr J.P. McGowan, to conduct these enquiries reveals continuing faith in medical expertise in sick sheep.

---

[85] Johnson (2016).

[86] 'Advances from the Development Fund' (1913).

[87] Kraft (2004).

[88] United Kingdom Parliament (1912–1913a) p. 7.

[89] Board of Agriculture (1912).

Working with the Edinburgh zoologist, Theodore Rettie, McGowan began in 1912 to investigate louping ill, which he saw as analogous to poliomyelitis in humans. He moved on to braxy (which he attributed to the same bacteria as louping ill), a type of jaundice he thought analogous to human cholera, and the obscure disease known as scrapie which was reportedly increasing in prevalence. His enquiries proceeded along established lines. Continuing to view diseased sheep as problems of place, he considered the local influences of season, pasture, weather patterns and landscape on their bodies. Working at the Edinburgh Lunacy Board's farm in Linlithgowshire, on private farms and in his laboratory at the Royal College of Physicians, Edinburgh, he examined sheep clinically in life and by post-mortem after death, and conducted bacteriological experiments on their bodily tissues and fluids. Sheep both facilitated and impeded his enquiries in the ways outlined above. Landowners and farmers provided crucial assistance 'in obtaining information regarding the occurrence of the disease, in procuring diseased animals for observation, and in other ways'.[90] His recommendations focused on the improvement of pasture, and the management of sheep grazing and breeding.[91]

In contrast, this approach was rarely adopted by the beneficiaries of BA and DC funding. Departing from the received view of sick sheep as products and shapers of unhealthy environments, they focused instead on sheep relationships with other infected and infective bodies. Believing that environments were unimportant, they sidelined the farmers and natural historians who knew about them, ignored the local specificities of vegetation, topography and sheep, and considered climate only in its effects on bacteria and parasites. They pursued their enquiries by extracting sheep and their infective agents, physically and conceptually from their specific farms of origin, and refashioning them within laboratories into generic subjects of investigation, which they hoped would produce universal knowledge of disease more readily than the locally specific sheep of the field.

Zoologists and entomologists investigated different stages in the life cycles of parasitic mites and ticks by 'farming' them in glass tubes and incubators, and working out how changes in temperature and moisture

[90] McGowan (1914).

[91] McGowan (1915, 1916).

influenced their development.[92] Within their separate institutions, vets replicated some of these enquiries and also worked on bacteria. They continued to fashion diseased sheep into patients, pathological specimens and experimental subjects in efforts to determine the identities and effects of infective agents, and how sheep bodies influenced their capacity to grow, reproduce and transmit. Drawing on his prior experience as principal veterinary officer to the Transvaal, Stockman devised new analogies for louping ill: the tick-borne protozoal cattle disease known as East Coast Fever, which ravaged Southern Africa in the early years of the century, and a milder equivalent known as redwater, which he had identified in Britain.[93] Recommendations focused on preventing the transmission of infection by controlling sheep movements between farms, removing them from tick-infested pastures and submerging them periodically in chemical dips—which occasionally killed sheep in addition to their parasites.[94]

These shifts in the ideas and locations of sheep disease research followed wider, well-documented trends in science and medicine. The period witnessed an uneven move from general environmental understandings to specific models of disease causation, which directed attention towards infectious agents invading susceptible bodies and away from the spaces they inhabited.[95] Concurrently, the scientific drive for greater control over natural phenomena encouraged the formation of laboratories and experimental stations, and downgraded the field as a site for constructing credible scientific knowledge.[96] These developments did not impact automatically on investigations into diseased sheep; rather, their effects were mediated by the changing capacity of sheep and their farmers to shape the course of scientific investigation.

As shown earlier, the late nineteenth-century farmers who sponsored and participated in sheep disease research (and by extension, the sheep whose habits and bodies moulded their views) had encouraged scientists to view diseased sheep as problems of place, and to study

[92] Theobald (1903), United Kingdom Parliament (1905b) pp. 23–36, Nuttall et al. (1908).

[93] Stockman (1911b), Stockman (1916), Cranefield (1991).

[94] Stockman (1910), McFadyean and Sheather (1913), Stockman and Berry (1913), Stockman (1916), McFadyean (1917), Stockman (1918), Stockman (1919).

[95] Worboys (2009).

[96] Kohler (2002).

them in their local environments with the aid of experts like themselves who understood these animals and landscapes. However, the shift from agricultural to state funding loosened the personal, geographical and economic ties that linked the commercial production of sheep to the scientific production of knowledge about their diseases. No longer answerable to agricultural sponsors or tied to their visions of disease, scientists were free to follow emerging scientific trends. The facilities supplied by state-funded scientific institutions meant that they no longer depended on farmers and their sheep for insights and bodies. They relied on labour supplied by technicians, not farm workers, and attempted to create their own research material by the deliberate infection of experimental sheep, or by fashioning other animal species into experimental models that could stand in for them.

There is little evidence to suggest that these changes in how diseased sheep were conceptualized and investigated brought more substantial benefits to sheep, science and agriculture than the former, agriculturally dominated regime. Investigators remained puzzled by the aetiologies of braxy and louping ill, sheep scab remained prevalent, and scrapie proved impossible to unravel. It was not until the interwar period that British scientists began to make headway against some of these diseases and to develop successful methods of managing them in the field.[97] One possible reason for this lack of progress is that sheep did not wholly support scientists' conceptions of them as infecting and infective agents, or comply with efforts to transform them from locally specific to generic laboratory sheep. Stockman tried in vain to locate in ticks and sheep blood cells the microscopic protozoon that he believed—from the analogies of East Coast Fever and redwater—to be the cause of louping ill. Nor could he induce disease by inoculating healthy sheep with the bodily fluids of sick ones, or with emulsions made from up to a thousand tick eggs. Consequently, he was unable to determine experimentally whether particular sheep possessed immunity to infection. Their resistance to his experimental manipulations forced him to return literally to the field, where he transformed experimental sheep into farmed sheep and vice versa, by collecting spontaneously sick sheep for his experiments, and depositing experimental sheep to test their immunity to natural infection.[98]

---

[97] Anon (1925), Anon (1965) pp. 62–8, Angus (1990).

[98] Stockman (1916), Stockman (1918). The cause of louping ill was later identified as a tick-borne virus.

Sheep also thwarted McFadyean's laboratory-based efforts to transmit scrapie experimentally and culture its causal agent, but farmers' secrecy concerning the presence of disease made it difficult for him to gather naturally infected sheep from farms.[99] Sheep abortion, too, posed challenges to veterinary researchers. They found it difficult to maintain causal bacteria in vitro, but sheep would only accept the infection when pregnant, and their physiologically restricted breeding seasons confined investigations to particular times of year.[100] Zoologists likewise relied on visits to the field to acquire new parasites for their investigations, while Stockman was forced to gather ticks from the bodies of dying farmed sheep because the ticks he nurtured in his laboratory would not reveal through experiment whether they contained the infective agent of louping ill.[101]

These investigations proved to scientists that it was not so easy to ignore the local circumstances, sheep and infective agents of the field in favour of those nurtured and manipulated within the laboratory. Unexpectedly, inhabitants of the laboratory's generic spaces sometimes proved more unpredictable than those found on locally specific farms. This may explain why Stockman embarked on efforts to recreate the natural conditions of the field in his laboratory. In one experiment he tried to mimic farm-based encounters between sheep and scab mites by tying wool and scurf from infected sheep into the fleeces of healthy ones.[102] He also fashioned pill boxes into cages for female mites and tied them to the skin of sheep to allow them to feed.[103] To test the tick's ability to acquire and transmit infection, he farmed them within his laboratory and actively encouraged them, at different stages in their life cycles, to fix onto and feed off sheep as they would in the field. He enclosed sheep ears and scrotums in cotton bags in order to capture the ticks for examination when they dropped off after eating their fill.[104] Following

[99] McFadyean (1917), United Kingdom Parliament (1920) pp. 77–9. The cause of scrapie remained contentious for decades and was eventually identified as a prion, a highly unconventional agent.

[100] Skirrow (2006).

[101] Stockman (1916) p. 259.

[102] Stockman (1910).

[103] Stockman and Berry (1913).

[104] Stockman (1911).

Latour, historians would typically interpret such activities as attempts to build authority for the laboratory, by inverting the power relationships between humans and disease agents that operated in the field.[105] In this context, however, when sheep and their infective agents had already demonstrated their capacity within the laboratory to subvert the power of humans, Stockman's work could be regarded as an acknowledgement of their agency, and the need to find space for its operation in the laboratory.[106] In these ways, sheep, their parasites and microorganisms made a difference to research practices, and maintained the permeability of emerging boundaries between the laboratory and the field.

3.3 Watertight Compartments

The final section of this chapter takes a more intimate look at some of the disciplinary politics of diseased sheep research in early twentieth-century Britain. As shown above, the growth of state funding in this period led to the narrowing of earlier eclectic perspectives on sick sheep, promoted the research of vets and zoologists over that of doctors and natural historians, and distanced practical farmers from the scientific study of sheep. For veterinary researchers, Stewart Stockman and John McFadyean, these changes did not go far enough. Keen to achieve the status of prime experts in animal health, they sought to capture sick sheep for themselves by awarding them a new role as vehicles for veterinary professional ambitions.

These vets were not the first to try to advance the profession's status. Earlier efforts, stretching back to the 1820s, had been impeded by internecine strife within the profession, its competitors' demonstrable effectiveness in the management and investigation of animal disease, and its inferior social and scientific status relative to human medicine.[107] However, John McFadyean had made some headway in attempts to create a distinctive veterinary research tradition. He had trained also as a doctor in order to gain a more advanced scientific education than that provided to vets, and proceeded to apply his skills in work performed at the Royal Veterinary College's Research Institute in Animal Pathology,

---

105 Latour (1983).

106 This interpretation is supported by Law and Mol (2008).

107 Worboys (1991), Woods (2007), Woods and Matthews (2010).

which was founded in 1892 with the support of the RASE. In 1888 he established the *Journal of Comparative Pathology and Therapeutics* (*JCPT*), which he used as a mouthpiece for his opinions and to publicize the results of his research.[108] His papers on louping ill, which appeared in *JCPT* in 1894 and 1900, were highly critical of other researchers. He condemned Dr Klein's 'failure to recognise that the name [louping ill] covers a variety of diseases' and declared the conclusions of Edinburgh vet, Professor Williams to be 'quite untrustworthy'.[109] He also claimed that other investigators' views about the causes of louping ill were simply 'theories' based on 'scraps of evidence', whereas what diseased sheep really required was 'painstaking reinvestigation at the hands of a competent pathologist'.[110]

By the early twentieth century, McFadyean and his son-in-law Stockman—who was appointed government chief veterinary officer in 1905—dominated the veterinary research scene. They ran laboratories that benefited considerably from public funding, and were knighted for their services in 1905 and 1913, respectively. However, the future was far from secure. In 1912, BA discussions about veterinary research generated proposals to divert funds and resources from Stockman's and McFadyean's institutions to Cambridge University, where medical and agricultural researchers were keen to investigate intransigent livestock diseases that Stockman had been unable to elucidate. A merger between The Royal Veterinary College, the medically run Brown Institute of Comparative Pathology, and London University was mooted, and the BAS was agitating for its own programme of animal disease research in Scotland.[111] One of the ways in which Stockman and McFadyean sought to counter these threats and elevate the status of their profession was through the physical and rhetorical manipulation of sick sheep.

---

[108] Pattison (1981).

[109] McFadyean (1894), McFadyean (1900). McFadyean's antipathy to Williams was partly political. As principal of the Dick College of Veterinary Medicine, Edinburgh, Williams had been asked by the governors to resign his post in 1893. He left to create a New Edinburgh Veterinary College, and took most of the students, museum specimens and library with him. McFadyean entered the Dick in 1874, and eventually married the daughter of Thomas Walley, who had worked under Williams and succeeded him as principal. Warwick and MacDonald (2003).

[110] McFadyean (1900).

[111] Board of Agriculture (1912), Hall (1913), 'Animal Diseases' (1914), United Kingdom Parliament (1914b) p. 441.

One of their strategies was to assert ownership of as many sheep diseases as possible, and to use Stockman's annual reports to Parliament and McFadyean's *JCPT* to publicize their investigations in progress. This enabled them to claim authority over sheep through long association with them, and to deny others the resources they needed to investigate sheep diseases. When Dr Frederick Twort, medical bacteriologist and director of the Brown Institute of Comparative Pathology in London, sought DC funds to continue his work on culturing the bacterium of Johne's disease and developing a vaccine, McFadyean engineered a rejection on the grounds that research was already under way in his laboratory.[112] When, in 1915, medical bacteriologist J.P. McGowan published the results of his investigations into scrapie, McFadyean dismissed them because the enquiry had only lasted 18 months, whereas his own research had begun seven years previously.[113]

Another veterinary strategy was to emphasize not only the duration but also the nature of their relationships with sick sheep. While they made no claims to an affective bond with sheep, the men argued repeatedly that their clinical experience, pathological knowledge, and epidemiological investigations had enabled them to develop intimate understandings of sheep bodies, sheep parasites, and, crucially, of the interactions between them. By making a distinction between their relationships with sheep and those built by zoologists, who were primarily interested in sheep parasites, they sought to differentiate and promote veterinary expertise.

This strategy is evident in veterinary responses to sheep scab, a disease caused by a highly contagious infective mite that lived in the skin and induced severe itching, loss of wool and loss of condition. In the late nineteenth century, scab was eradicated from New Zealand and Australia with the aid of regular, compulsory dipping of sheep in chemicals that killed the mite. In response to British agriculturalists' call for similar measures, in 1903 the government established a committee to consider the merits of dipping in relation to the practical conditions of sheep farming and the life history of the scab mite.[114] Composed of experts drawn from medicine, chemistry, biology, agriculture and veterinary

[112] 'Reports on Applications' (1911), Ingram and Twort (1913).

[113] McGowan (1914), McFadyean (1917), McFadyean (1918).

[114] 'Mr Long' (1898), Wallace (1900), Kirkwood (1986), Fisher (1998).

medicine, it oversaw dipping experiments conducted by Professor Winter, professor of agriculture at Bangor University. Expert witnesses included the zoologists F.V. Theobald and C. Warburton, who had performed independent investigations of the mite's life cycle and habits (Table 3.2).[115] On the strength of the committee's recommendations, in 1907 the government made annual sheep dipping compulsory, but this had little impact on the incidence or distribution of scab.[116]

Stockman believed that the foundations of this policy were insecure. The circumstances of the outbreaks that he had investigated—as required under law—led him to query 'the generally accepted facts regarding the epizootiology of scab', which derived from entomologists' 'somewhat academic' studies of parasite life cycles. He claimed that what was really needed was 'the study of the various habits of a parasite under actual conditions'.[117] McFadyean concurred. He claimed that Winter had conducted too few experiments and failed to take into account the sheep's clinical condition when assessing the effects of dipping.[118] Such criticisms implied that these researchers' relationships with diseased sheep were too superficial to generate authoritative knowledge.

Stockman made similar criticisms of zoologists' investigations into the ticks that were implicated in louping ill. Arguing that 'the study of the life-history of a parasite by entomologists is often limited to the cycle of its development', which 'does not by any means complete our knowledge of them', he called for observations of 'their habits, which, from the economic point of view, are of as much interest as their developmental cycle'.[119] By 'habits' he meant how parasites lived in relation to sheep, and acted to cause disease in them. While he believed that entomologists had their uses, particularly when working under veterinary direction,[120] the study of parasite habits was, for him, a pathological not a zoological problem, which could only be solved by veterinarians. When, in 1911, the Edinburgh zoologist, Theodore Rettie, bid for DC funds to investigate louping ill, Stockman objected 'on principle' because Rettie had 'no medical qualifications and proposed to do a path-

115 United Kingdom Parliament (1905a, 1905b).

116 Anon (1965) pp. 164–8.

117 United Kingdom Parliament. Annual Reports (1910) p. 11.

118 Editorial (1904) pp. 233–40.

119 Stockman (1911b).

120 United Kingdom Parliament (1912–1913b) p. 41.

ological experiment'. He was overruled by the BA's zoological advisor, S. MacDougall, on the grounds that sheep with louping ill were probably infected by ticks, which were Rettie's 'special province' as a zoologist.[121] Stockman retaliated by adding louping ill to the list of diseases that he was investigating. He also spoke out against Cambridge biology professor G.H.F. Nuttall, who claimed that a drug known as tryptanblue might be effective in the treatment of certain tick-borne animal diseases. Stockman objected because Nuttall had failed to conduct extensive trials on animals in the field.[122]

Medical bacteriologists were similarly accused of focusing on disease agents in isolation from sheep, instead of devoting attention to what they did 'in the body under different conditions'.[123] McGowan's research on scrapie, which implicated a parasite in the muscles known as sarcocystis, was a case in point. Although his own research on the disease had been unproductive, McFadyean rejected McGowan's conclusions as 'unproved and improbable', and his recommendations as based on inadequate experience.[124] Having spent considerable time consulting farmers and studying scrapie in the field, McGowan resisted this attempt to portray him as an abstract, laboratory-bound, out-of-touch theoretician. He accused McFadyean of dogmatism, a lack of evidence, and a failure to understand farming terminology and practice.[125] McFadyean maintained the attack, accusing McGowan of 'meagre' evidence and of failing to investigate the transmission of disease between sheep. As a parting shot, he claimed that McGowan would only do harm by delaying investigations along 'the only lines likely to yield satisfactory results'[126]—by which he meant, veterinary lines.

Veterinary attempts to set distance between their lengthy, meaningful interspecies relationships, and zoologists' and medical researchers' abstract focus on singular disease agents, were highly rhetorical. While there were some differences in their methods, objectives and relationships with research subjects, there was also considerable overlap. Stockman,

121 'Reports on Applications' (1911).

122 Nuttall and Hadwen (1909a), Nuttall and Hadwen (1909b), Stockman (1909).

123 United Kingdom Parliament (1912–1913b) p.41.

124 McFadyean (1917) p. 112.

125 McGowan (1918).

126 McFadyean (1918) p. 299.

too, studied parasites in the laboratory, in isolation from sheep hosts, and with the aid of 'artificial' incubation.[127] Nuttall and McGowan built close relationships with sheep as well as their parasites and bacteria, and sought to determine the relationships between them.[128] Investigations aimed at controlling disease were not the special province of veterinarians. McGowan was answerable to his agricultural patrons, who wished to promote sheep farming, while Theobald was a founder of the Association of Economic Biologists, which promoted the value of economic biology to practical agriculture.[129] Nuttall and Warburton studied the economic and medical significance of ticks as well as their life cycles, and Nuttall often commented on the economic importance of parasites and their relationship to disease in humans and animals.[130]

It was no coincidence that the people whom Stockman and McFadyean criticized or sought to exclude from diseased sheep research were investigating the same diseases as them, in association with institutions that stood to gain from the diversion of power and funds away from their own—the BAS, the Brown Institute and Cambridge University. Ultimately, this diversion did not occur. The Royal Veterinary College remained autonomous and in London; power to conduct disease research remained vested in the BA in London; and the foundation of a chair in comparative pathology at Cambridge University did not materialize until 1926, in isolation from veterinary research and teaching. However, these outcomes occurred not because of, but in spite of the relationships that Stockman and McFadyean built with their sheep. In fact, the sheep's role as carrier of professional ambitions was not particularly successful because it did not deter non-veterinarians from studying their diseases, or change wider perceptions of those researchers' abilities relative to those of vets. Parasitic causes of sheep diseases continued to attract attention from scientists who identified increasingly as 'parasitologists',[131] and McGowan continued to work on livestock diseases for Scottish agriculturalists and subsequently at an agricultural research institution, the Rowett Institute in Aberdeen.[132]

---

[127] United Kingdom Parliament. Annual Reports (1912–1913) pp. 22–9.

[128] Nuttall and Hadwen (1909a, 1909b), McGowan (1914).

[129] Collinge (1907), Kraft (2004).

[130] Nuttall et al. (1908), Nuttall (1914), Nuttall (1918), Kraft (2004).

[131] Worboys (1976), Cox (2009).

[132] Smith (1999).

Nevertheless, Stockman's and McFadyean's attempts to establish hierarchical relationships between disciplines on the basis of the relationships that their researchers built with sick sheep had some lasting effects. Although, for some years to come, diseased sheep and other livestock remained shared objects of concern for investigators in veterinary medicine, human medicine and the life sciences, the investigations that were performed on them were not shared but proceeded along parallel tracks. The veterinary fashioning of sheep into vehicles for their professional ambitions prevented the development of integrated research campaigns and constructive cross-disciplinary conversations. If the state funding of agricultural research had already fractured investigations coordinated by agricultural societies into disciplinary compartments, then it was the vets who made those compartments 'watertight'[133] through their antipathy to other researchers. Well beyond the period examined in this chapter, any institutional or state attempts to promote non-veterinary perspectives on sick livestock prompted a fierce backlash from veterinary leaders, who continued to assert their profession's unique possession of knowledge arising from their special relationships with animals.[134]

3.4 Conclusion

In outlining the structures, knowledge-practices and social configurations of agricultural research in Britain around the turn of the twentieth century, this chapter has highlighted the transition from scientifically eclectic, small-scale investigations that were funded and coordinated by farmers for farmers, to more substantial, state-funded enquiries that were performed by autonomous scientists. In treating the research of both periods symmetrically, and demonstrating the capacity of sheep to make a difference to scientific investigations, it highlights the inadequacy of existing historical accounts, which confine their attention to human actors and publicly funded research programmes.

Against a backdrop of rising international competition and falling meat and wool prices, it was the sheep's tendency to fall ill and die that prompted late nineteenth-century agricultural societies to commission enquiries into the causes and management of their diseases.

---

[133] 'Watertight compartments' was an actors' term that referred specifically to the separation of veterinary from human medicine. Allbutt (1906), McFadyean (1923) p. 253.

[134] Editorial (1931), Angus (1990), Woods (2004).

Subsequently, as contributors to the deepening depression in agriculture, their continuing deaths encouraged the state to assume some responsibility for this activity. Throughout, sheep exerted influence over how and where research was practised, and by whom. In the earlier period, the symptoms they suffered, and the geography and seasonality of their diseases, reinforced agricultural sponsors' perceptions of them as products of place, and led to their positioning at the hub of research networks populated by experts in their bodies and environments. Their tendency to fall ill at particular times and in particular places shaped the questions that these experts asked of them, and led to their investigation on farms. State-funded researchers in the early twentieth century paid less heed to the farmed environment and conducted narrower, discipline-specific, laboratory-based enquiries that were underpinned by their different perceptions of sheep as hosts and transmitters of infection. However, their non-human subjects forced them to return intermittently to the field. Throughout, the sheep's variable responses to both disease and scientific investigations generated a host of conflicting claims about their diseases. Their acknowledged importance as research subjects also encouraged ambitious veterinarians to enrol them in a campaign for professional advancement, which drew strength from the lengthy and intimate relationships that vets claimed to have developed with them.

In the course of these activities, sheep built relationships between diverse human and non-human actors including: scientific experts and the state; the microbes, parasites and environments implicated in sheep diseases; the human and animal victims of analogous diseases that helped to shed light on sheep; and the multiple species of experimental animals that acted as sheep proxies. Through these relationships, sheep were awarded new roles as patients, pathological specimens, experimental material, culture media, victims and shapers of their environments, subjects of field trials, hosts and transmitters of infection, food for parasites, points of comparison with other species, and commercial products. Made and remade in the course of scientific enquiries, the sheep's identity was in a constant state of flux. Their lived experiences also changed. As scientific subjects, sheep underwent clinical monitoring and treatment, feeding trials, dipping, experimental inoculations, parasitic infections, and premature, purposeful deaths. This had ramifications for farmed sheep, which were treated by dipping, drenching, dosing, isolation, managed grazing and restricted breeding in efforts to promote their health.

In these ways, sheep and scientific research were co-constituted. Two aspects of this process merit further note. First is the power of sheep to make a difference to research structures, practices and participants. This is an important issue for animal studies scholars because while they accept that, in theory, animals gain the capacity to inadvertently change history by entering into relationships with humans, it is the historically contingent nature of those relationships that determines the scope and effects of their influence.[135] This analysis has shown that in enquiries run by farmers for farmers, sheep made a considerable difference to how, where and by whom research was conducted. However, when state funding freed scientists from their obligations to agricultural sponsors, and endowed new laboratories for the pursuit of scientific enquiry, scientists sought to make sheep and their infective agents answerable to them. Their efforts were not entirely successful. As we have seen, sheep retained some of their power to frustrate and to require scientists to return to the field. There is little evidence to suggest that (in this period at least) this mode of investigation was more scientifically productive than that which it replaced. Nevertheless, the extraction of sheep—and scientific enquiries—from their local farmed environments did reduce their power to shape science, and indicates how the rise of modern, institutionalized, publicly funded research regimes elevated the authority of scientists at the expense of animals and their owners.

Second, this study reveals the capacity of sick sheep to shape the relationships between different fields of scientific enquiry. While historians of science and medicine have tended to view sheep as veterinary subjects and relegate them to the field of veterinary history, this chapter has shown that, in the late nineteenth century, sick sheep also attracted attention from—and therefore merit insertion within the histories of—human medicine, natural history and zoology, which came together to create the multifaceted domain of 'agricultural science'. It has also demonstrated how the position of sheep at the intersection of these fields changed during the early twentieth century as structural changes in university research and teaching, the growth and distribution of public funds for agricultural research, and the changing knowledge-practices of sheep investigations promoted professional zoology at the expense of amateur natural history, and veterinary research at the expense of

[135] Law and Mol (2008), Pearson and Weismantel (2010), Nance (2015) p. 3.

medicine. Ambitious vets then worked to consolidate these boundaries and elevate their own perspectives in a bid for recognition as supreme experts in sheep health. This historical study therefore offers important insights into disciplinary boundaries in the making, the ways in which sick sheep first brought together, and then contributed to the drawing apart of, human medicine, veterinary medicine and the life sciences. Its findings suggest that when deciding what constitutes the history of 'medicine', 'veterinary medicine' or 'the life sciences', historians need to seek out these fields' historical identities and relationships, which the history of animals—as key points of connection and disconnection—has a unique capacity to illuminate.

The historical forging of disciplinary identities and relationships is also an important issue for the present-day agenda known as OH. As described in Chapter 6, since 2000, OH has gained increasing international prominence in health research, policy and discourse. Its advocates argue that because many of today's most pressing health problems lie at the interface of human, animal and environmental health, they can only be managed effectively by breaking down traditional disciplinary silos and developing more collaborative ways of working. They often turn to history in attempts to build authority for this approach.[136] However, in the belief that its benefits are universal and self-evident, they tend to pluck historical figures out of their contexts and celebrate their OH achievements without considering the circumstances that made it possible or desirable for individuals to work in this way. Their celebration of John McFadyean as a figurehead for OH when he actually contributed to the early twentieth-century demise of this way of working flags up the problems associated with this approach to history.[137]

Late nineteenth-century research on sick sheep could, in retrospect, be described as OH because it cut across and drew connections between different fields of enquiry. As we have seen, this approach derived from the broadly distributed nature of expertise in sick sheep, and the leading role of agricultural societies, which selected from this pool of experts, and directed enquiries with agricultural ends in mind. Its subsequent fracturing was the result of institutional, funding and disciplinary changes, and the manoeuvrings of McFadyean and Stockman, which

[136] For example: Zinsstag et al. (2011).

[137] For example: Day (2008), Monath et al. (2010).

produced structures, career paths and disciplinary rivalries that privileged discipline-specific over problem-based approaches. Practical farmers, medical researchers and natural historians were marginalized, and vets grew more interested in exerting authority over zoologists than in working with them towards the improvement of sheep health. Sheep ceased to be subjects of OH not because they ceased to be pressing and costly problems for agriculture but because scientific investigators no longer had the will or the capacity to address them as such. If OH today is to move from 'rhetoric to reality', it is these sorts of dynamics and contexts that its advocates need to engage with, rather than simply urging scientists repeatedly to recognize the logic of a OH approach.[138]

Bibliography

"Advances from the Development Fund." 1913. British National Archives: D 2/8.

Allbutt, Clifford. "Comparative Medicine." *The Times*, June 5, 1906: 9.

Allen, David. *The Naturalist in Britain: A Social History.* London: Penguin, 1976.

Angus, K. *A History of the Animal Diseases Research Association.* Edinburgh: ADRA, 1990.

"Animal Diseases – Demand for Research." *The Times*, May 4, 1914: 4.

Anon. "Animal Pathology and Physiology." *The Lancet* 206 (1925): 343.

Anon. *Animal Health, a Centenary 1865–1965.* London: HMSO, 1965.

Anon. "The Central Veterinary Laboratory, Weybridge, 1917–1967." *Veterinary Record* 81 (1967): 62–8.

Archibald, David. "On the Cheviot Breed of Sheep." *Transactions of the Highland and Agricultural Society* VII (1880): 110–22.

Armatage, George. "On Abortion and Premature Labour in Mares, Cows, and Ewes." *Transactions of the Highland and Agricultural Society* IV (1872): 173-9.

Armatage, George. *The Sheep: Its Varieties and Management in Health and Disease.* London: F. Warne & Co, 1894.

Armstrong, Phillip. *Sheep.* London: Reaktion, 2016.

Benson, Etienne. "Animal Writes: Historiography, Disciplinarity, and the Animal Trace." In *Making Animal Meaning*, edited by L. Kalof and G.M. Montgomery, 3–16. East Lansing, MI: Michigan State University Press, 2011.

[138] Okello et al. (2011), Hueston et al. (2013).

Board of Agriculture. "Correspondence - Braxy and Louping Ill." 1900–01. British National Archives: MAF 35/246.

Board of Agriculture. "Correspondence - Departmental Committee, Interim Report. Louping Ill and Braxy." 1906–12. British National Archives: MAF 35/247.

Board of Agriculture. "Correspondence - Veterinary Education and Research." 1912. British National Archives: MAF 33/47.

Brassley, Paul. "Agricultural Research in Britain, 1850–1914: Failure, Success and Development." *Annals of Science* 52 (1995): 465–80.

Brassley, Paul. "Agricultural Science and Education." In *The Agrarian History of England and Wales, volume 7*, edited by E.J.T. Collins and J. Thirsk, 594–649. Cambridge: Cambridge University Press, 2000.

"Braxy and Louping Ill: Report by Committee." *Transactions of the Highland and Agricultural Society* XVI (1884): 300–3.

Bresalier, Michael, Angela Cassidy and Abigail Woods. "One Health in History." In *One Health: The Theory and Practice of Integrated Health Approaches*, edited by J. Zinsstag, E. Schelling, D. Waltner-Toews, M. Whittaker and M. Tanner, 1–15. Wallingford: CABI, 2015.

Brotherston, A. "Report on the Flora of Upper Teviotdale in Connection to its Relation to 'Louping Ill' in Sheep." *Transactions of the Highland and Agricultural Society* XIV (1882): 43–5.

Brown, Karen. "Political Entomology: The Insectile Challenge to Agricultural Development in the Cape Colony, 1895-1910." *Journal of Southern African Studies* 29 (2003): 529–49.

Brown, Karen. "Tropical Medicine and Animal Diseases: Onderstepoort and the Development of Veterinary Science in South Africa 1908–1950." *Journal of Southern African Studies* 31 (2005): 513–29.

Brown, Karen. "Poisonous Plants, Pastoral Knowledge and Perceptions of Environmental Change in South Africa, c.1880–1940." *Environment and History* 13 (2007): 307–32.

Butler, Alan. *Sheep.* Winchester: O Books, 2006.

Carlyle, W.J. "The Changing Distribution of Breeds of Sheep in Scotland, 1795–1965." *Agricultural History Review* 27 (1979): 19–29.

Cassidy, Angela, Rachel Mason Dentinger, Kathryn Schoefert and Abigail Woods. "Animal Roles and Traces in the History of Medicine." In Animal Agents: the Non-Human in the History of Science, edited by Amanda Rees. *BJHS Themes* 2 (2017): 11–33.

Cittadino, Eugene. "Botany." In *The Cambridge History of Science, volume 6: Modern Biological and Earth Sciences*, edited by Peter Bowler and John Pickstone, 225–42. Cambridge: Cambridge University Press, 2009.

Clark, John. *Bugs and the Victorians.* London: Yale University Press, 2009.

Clayton, N. "'Poorly Co-ordinated Structures for Public Science that Failed us in the Past'? Applying Science to Agriculture: A New Zealand Case Study." *Agricultural History* 82 (2008): 445–67.

Collinge, W. "The Application of Economic Biology to Agriculture." *Journal of Economic Biology* 3 (1907): 96–106.

Cox, F.E. "George Henry Falkiner Nuttall and the Origins of Parasitology." *Parasitology* 136 (2009): 1389–94.

Cranefield, Paul. *Science and Empire: East Coast Fever in Rhodesia and the Transvaal.* Cambridge: Cambridge University Press, 1991.

Crosby, A. *The Columbian Exchange: Biological and Cultural Consequences of 1492.* Westport, Conn.: Greenwood Publishing Company, 1972.

Davidson, James. *The Royal Highland and Agricultural Society of Scotland, A Short History: 1784–1984.* Ingliston: Blackwood Pillans and Wilson, 1984.

Day, M.J. "One Health and the Legacy of John McFadyean." *Journal of Comparative Pathology* 139 (2008): 151–3.

De Bont, R.F.J. *Stations in the Field: A History of Place-based Animal Research, 1870–1930.* London: University of Chicago Press, 2015.

Despret, Vinciane. "Sheep Do Have Opinions." In *Making Things Public. Atmospheres of Democracy*, edited by B. Latour and P. Weibel, 360–70. Cambridge: M.I.T. Press, 2006.

Editorial. "The Prevention and Treatment of Sheep Scab." *Journal of Comparative Pathology and Therapeutics* 17 (1904): 233–40.

Editorial. "Agricultural Research Council." *Veterinary Record* 43 (1931): 761–2.

Farley, John. "Parasites and the Germ Theory of Disease." *Milbank Quarterly* 67 (1989): S1, 50–68.

Fisher, John. "Technical and Institutional Innovation in Nineteenth Century Australian Pastoralism: The Eradication of Psoroptic Mange in Australia." *Journal of the Royal Australian Historical Society* 84 (1998): 38–55.

Franklin, Sarah. *Dolly Mixtures: The Remaking of Genealogy.* Durham, NC: Duke University Press, 2007.

Fudge, Erica, "Ruminations 1: The History of Animals' (2006). Accessed February 19, 2017. https://networks.h-net.org/node/16560/pages/32226/history-animals-erica-fudge.

Goddard, Nicholas. *Harvests of Change: The Royal Agricultural Society of England 1838–1988.* London: Quiller, 1998.

Goddard, Nicholas. "Agricultural Institutions: Societies, Associations and the Press." In *The Agrarian History of England and Wales, volume 7*, edited by E.J.T. Collins and J. Thirsk, 650–92. Cambridge: Cambridge University Press, 2000.

Graham-Smith, G.S. and D. Keilin. "George Henry Falkiner Nuttall. 1862–1937." *Biographical Memoirs of Fellows of the Royal Society* 2 (1939): 493–9.

Greig-Smith, R. and A. Meek. "Investigation into the Cause of Louping Ill." *Veterinarian* 70 (1897a): 249–62.

Greig-Smith, R. and A. Meek. "On Louping Ill and its Connection with the Tick." *Veterinarian* 70 (1897b): 698–709.

Hall, Daniel. "Memo." 1913. British National Archives: D4/91.

Hamilton, D.J. "On Braxy." *Transactions of the Highland and Agricultural Society* XIV (1902): 314–47.

Hamilton, David. "On the Alimentary Canal as a Source of Contagion." In *Studies in Pathology*, edited by W. Bulloch, 1–38. Aberdeen: University of Aberdeen, 1906.

Hamilton, D.J. "Evidence to Royal Commission on Vivisection." *British Medical Journal* I (1909): 475–6.

Haraway, Donna. *When Species Meet.* Minneapolis: University of Minnesota Press, 2008.

Hardy, Anne. "Animals, Disease and Man: Making Connections." *Perspectives in Biology and Medicine* 46 (2003): 200–15.

Harrison, Mark. "Differences of Degree: Representations of India in British Medical Topography, 1820-c.1870." *Medical History* 44 (2000): S20, 51–69.

Hart, J.F. "The Changing Distribution of Sheep in Britain." *Economic Geography* 32 (1956): 260–74.

Henke, C. "Making a Place for Science: The Field Trial." *Social Studies of Science.* 30 (2000): 483–511.

Hueston, W., J. Appert, T. Denny et al. "Assessing Global Adoption of One Health Approaches." *Ecohealth* 10 (2013): 228–33.

Hutchinson, Jonathan. "A Report on Certain Causes of Death in Ewes During and After Parturition, with Notes on the "Navel-Ill" in Lambs." *Transactions of the Obstetrical Society of London* 18 (1877): 88–109.

Ingram, G.A. and F.A. Twort. *A Monograph on Johne's Disease.* London: Bailliere, Tindall and Cox, 1913.

Johnson, K. "The Natural Historian." In *A Companion to the History of Science*, edited by B. Lightman, 84–96. Chichester: Wiley Blackwell, 2016.

Jones, Susan. *Death in a Small Package: A Short History of Anthrax.* Baltimore: John Hopkins University Press, 2010.

Kirk, Robert and Edmund Ramsden. "Working Across Species Down on the Farm: Howard S Liddell and the Development of Comparative Psychopathology, c.1923 to 1962." *History and Philosophy of the Life Sciences* (2017): forthcoming.

Kirkwood, A.C. "History, Biology and Control of Sheep Scab." *Parasitology Today* 2 (1986): 302–7.

Klein, E. "On the Etiology and Pathology of Louping-ill." *Journal of the Royal Agricultural Society of England* 4 (1893): 625–36.

Kohler, R. and J. Vetter. "The Field." In *A Companion to the History of Science*, edited by B. Lightman, 282–95. Chichester: Wiley Blackwell, 2016.

Kohler, Robert. *Landscapes and Labscapes: Exploring the Lab-Field Border in Biology*. Chicago: Chicago University Press, 2002.

Kohler, Robert. *All Creatures: Naturalists, Collectors, and Biodiversity, 1850–1950*. Princeton: Princeton University Press, 2006.

Kraft, Alison. "Pragmatism, Patronage and Politics in English Biology: The Rise and Fall of Economic Biology 1904–1920." *Journal of the History of Biology* 37 (2004): 213–58.

Latham, Patrick. "The Deterioration of Mountain Pastures and Suggestions for their Improvement." *Transactions of the Highland and Agricultural Society* XV (1883): 111–30.

Latour, Bruno. "Give Me a Laboratory and I Will Raise the World." In *Science Observed: Perspectives on the Social Study of Science*, edited by Karin D. Knorr-Cetina and Michael Mulkay, 141–70. London: Sage, 1983.

Latour, Bruno. *The Pasteurization of France*. Translated by Alan Sheridan and John Law. London: Harvard University Press, 1988.

Law, John, and Annemarie Mol. "The Actor-Enacted: Cumbrian Sheep in 2001." In *Material Agency: Towards a Non-Anthropocentric Approach*, edited by Carl Knappett and Lambros Malafouris, 57–77. London: Springer, 2008.

"Louping Ill and Braxy. Account of Committee Expenditure 1906–1912." British National Archives: MAF 35/247.

MacDougall, R.S. "The Sheep Maggot Fly." *Transactions of the Highland and Agricultural Society* XVI (1904): 128–43.

MacDougall, R.S. "Sheep Maggot and Related Flies, their Classification, Life History and Habits." *Transactions of the Highland and Agricultural Society* XXI (1909): 135–74.

McGowan, J.P. *Investigation into the Disease of Sheep called 'Scrapie.'* Edinburgh: Blackwood, 1914.

McGowan, J.P. "Braxy." *Transactions of the Highland and Agricultural Society* XXVII (1915): 54–141.

McGowan, J.P. *Louping Ill*. Edinburgh: Blackwood, 1916.

McGowan, J.P. "Scrapie." *Journal of Comparative Pathology and Therapeutics* 31 (1918): 278–90.

McGowan, J.P. "Cholera of the Sheep (Jaundice; Yellows or Yellowses)." *The Lancet* 194 (1919): 426–9.

McGowan, J.P. and T. Rettie. "Poliomyelitis in Sheep suffering from Loupin' Ill." *Journal of Pathology and Bacteriology* 18 (1913): 47–51.

McFadyean, John. "Louping-Ill in Sheep." *Journal of the Royal Agricultural Society of England* 7 (1894): 547–60.

McFadyean, John. "The Aetiology of Louping-Ill." *Journal of Comparative Pathology and Therapeutics* 13 (1900): 145–54.

McFadyean, John. "Scrapie." *Journal of Comparative Pathology and Therapeutics* 30 (1917): 102–31.

McFadyean, John. "Sarcosporidia as the Cause of Scrapie." *Journal of Comparative Pathology and Therapeutics* 31 (1918): 290–9.

McFadyean, John. "Review of the Progress of Veterinary Science in Great Britain during the Past One Hundred Years." *Journal of Comparative Pathology and Therapeutics* 36 (1923): 243–55.

McFadyean, J. and A.L. Sheather. "Johne's Disease: The Experimental Transmission of the Disease to Cattle, Sheep, and Goats." *Journal of Comparative Pathology and Therapeutics* 26 (1913): 62–94.

Marson, James and Professor Simonds. *Report of Experiments as to Vaccination of Sheep, and Influence of Vaccination in Preventing Sheep-pox.* London: Her Majesty's Stationary Office, 1864.

"Meeting, Board of Directors." *Transactions of the Highland and Agricultural Society* XIV (1882): 9.

Melville, Elinor G.K. *A Plague of Sheep: Environmental Consequences of the Conquest of Mexico.* Cambridge: Cambridge University Press, 1994.

Monath, T.P., L.H. Kahn and B. Kaplan. "Introduction: One Health Perspective." *ILAR Journal* 51 (2010): 193–8.

"Mr Long and the Sheep Breeders Association." *The Times,* April 27, 1898: 14.

Nance, Susan. "Introduction." In *The Historical Animal,* edited by Susan Nance, 1–18. New York: Syracuse University Press, 2015.

Nuttall, G.H.F. "'Tick Paralysis' in Man and Animals." *Parasitology* 7 (1914): 95–104.

Nuttall, G.H.F. "The Pathological Effects of Phthirus Pubis." *Parasitology* 10 (1918): 375–82.

Nuttall, G.H.F. and S. Hadwen. "The Successful Drug Treatment of Canine Piroplasmosis, Together with Observations upon the Effect of Drugs on Piroplasma Canis." *Parasitology* 2 (1909a): 156–91, 229–35.

Nuttall, G.H.F., and S. Hadwen. "The Drug Treatment of Piroplasmosis in Cattle." *Parasitology* 2 (1909b): 236–66.

Nuttall, G.H.F., C. Warburton, W.F. Cooper and L.E. Robinson. *Ticks, A Monograph of the Ixodoidea. Part I.* Cambridge: Cambridge University Press, 1908.

"Obituary, D.J. Hamilton." *The Lancet* 173 (1909): 730–1.

Okello, A., E.P. Gibbs and A. Vandersmissen. "One Health and the Neglected Zoonoses: Turning Rhetoric into Reality." *Veterinary Record* 169 (2011): 281–5.

Olby, Robert. "Social Imperialism and State Support for Agricultural Research in Edwardian Britain." *Annals of Science* 48 (1991): 509–26.

Pattison, Iain. *John McFadyean: Founder of Modern Veterinary Research.* London: JA Allen, 1981.

Pearson, S.J. and M. Weismantel. "Does 'The Animal' Exist? Toward a Theory of Social Life with Animals." In *Beastly Natures: Animals, Humans and the Study of History*, edited by Dorothee Brantz, 17–39. London: University of Virginia Press, 2010.

Peden, R. "Sheep Breeding in Colonial Canterbury (New Zealand): A Practical Response to the Challenges of Disease and Economic Change, 1850–1914." In *Healing the Herds: Disease, Livestock Economies and the Globalization of Veterinary Medicine*, edited by K. Brown and D. Gilfoyle, 215–31. Athens: Ohio University Press, 2010.

Plowright, Charles. "Some Remarks upon Ergot." *British Medical Journal* 1 (1886): 197.

"Proceedings at General Meetings: Louping Ill and Braxy." *Transactions of the Highland and Agricultural Society* XIV (1882): 39–46.

Reid, William, and James Kemp. *Sheep: Their History, Management, Diseases, and National Value.* Edinburgh: Nimmo and Elliot, 1871.

Reinhard, E.G. "Landmarks of Parasitology I. The Discovery of the Life Cycle of the Liver Fluke." *Experimental Parasitology* 6 (1957): 208–32.

"Reports on Applications for Advances from the Development Fund." 1911. British National Archives: D 2/4.

Richardson, W.G. "Tetanus Occurring after Surgical Operations." *British Medical Journal* 1 (1909): 948–51.

Ritvo, Harriet. "Counting Sheep in the English Lake District: Rare Breeds, Local Knowledge, and Environmental History." In *Beastly Natures: Animals, Humans, and the Study of History*, edited by Dorothee Brantz, 264–80. University of Virginia Press, 2010.

Rupke, N. (ed.). *Medical Geography in Historical Perspective.* London: Wellcome Trust Centre for the History of Medicine at UCL, 2000.

Ryder, M.L. *Sheep and Man.* London: Gerald Duckworth & Co, 1983.

Schlich, Thomas and Martina Schlünder. "The Emergence of 'Implant-Pets' and 'Bone-Sheep': Animals as New Biomedical Objects in Orthopedic Surgery (1960s–2010)." *History and Philosophy of the Life Sciences* 31 (2009): 433–66.

Scott, Charles. *The Practice of Sheep-Farming.* Edinburgh: T.C. Jack, 1886.

"Second Report by Special Committee on Braxy and Louping Ill." *Transactions of the Highland and Agricultural Society* XV (1883): 176–201.

Skirrow, M. "John McFadyean and the Centenary of the First Isolation of Campylobacter Species." *Clinical Infectious Diseases* 43 (2006): 1213–7.

Smith, David. "The Use of 'Team Work' in the Practical Management of Research in the Inter-War Period: John Boyd Orr at the Rowett Research Institute." *Minerva* 37 (1999): 259–80.

Stark, James. *The Making of Modern Anthrax, 1875–1920.* London: Pickering and Chatto, 2013.

Stockman, Stewart. "Permanent Laboratory." October 25, 1907. British National Archives: MAF 35/578.

Stockman, Stewart. "The Treatment of Redwater in Cattle (Bovine Piroplasmosis) with Trypanblue." *Journal of Comparative Pathology and Therapeutics* 22 (1909): 321–40.

Stockman, Stewart. "Some Points on the Epizootiology of Sheep Scab in Relation to Eradication." *Journal of Comparative Pathology and Therapeutics* 23 (1910): 303–14.

Stockman, Stewart. "Johne's Disease in Sheep." *Journal of Comparative Pathology and Therapeutics* 24 (1911a): 66–9.

Stockman, Stewart. "The Habits of British Ticks found on Sheep and Cattle." *Journal of Comparative Pathology and Therapeutics* 24 (1911b): 229–37.

Stockman, Stewart. "Scrapie: An Obscure Disease of Sheep." *Journal of Comparative Pathology and Therapeutics* 26 (1913): 317–27.

Stockman, S. and A.H. Berry. "The Psoroptes Community Ovis." *Journal of Comparative Pathology and Therapeutics* 26 (1913): 45–50.

Stockman, Stewart. "Louping-ill." *Journal of Comparative Pathology and Therapeutics* 29 (1916): 244–64.

Stockman, Stewart. "Louping-ill." *Journal of Comparative Pathology and Therapeutics* 31 (1918): 137–93.

Stockman, Stewart. "Louping-Ill: Duration of the Infectivity of the Ticks." *Journal of Comparative Pathology and Therapeutics* 32 (1919): 283–5.

Symon, J.A. *Scottish Farming, Past and Present.* Edinburgh: Oliver and Boyd, 1959.

Tellor, Lloyd V. *The Diseases of Live Stock and their Most Efficient Remedies.* London: Baillière and Co, 1879.

"The Report of the Departmental Committee." *The Lancet* 168 (1906): 232–3.

"The Pathology of Louping-Ill and Braxy." *British Medical Journal* 1 (1906): 1472–4.

Theobald, F.V. *Diptera, A Monograph of the Culicidae of the World.* British Museum: London, 1901–1910.

Theobald, F.V. "The Parasitic Diseases of Sheep." *Livestock Journal*, November 8, 1901: 576.

Theobald, F.V. "Sheep Scab." *Journal of the Land Agent's Society* II (1903): 150–66.

Thomas, A.P. "The Rot in Sheep, or the Life-History of the Liver-Fluke." *Nature* 26 (1882): 606–8.

Thomas, A.P. "The Natural History of the Liver Fluke and the Prevention of Rot." *Journal of the Royal Agricultural Society of England* xix (1883): 276–305.

United Kingdom Parliament. Third Report of the Commissioners Appointed to Inquire into the Origin and Nature, &c. of the Cattle Plague; with an Appendix, Vol. XXII:321, Cd.3656. London: The Stationary Office, 1866.

United Kingdom Parliament. Report on Distribution of Grants for Agricultural Education in Great Britain, 1895–96, Appendix, Vol. LXVII.585, C.8228. London: The Stationary Office, 1896.

United Kingdom Parliament. Report on Wages and Earnings of Agricultural Labourers in United Kingdom, Vol. LXXXII.557, C.346. London: The Stationary Office, 1900.

United Kingdom Parliament. Report of the Departmental Committee Appointed by the Board of Agriculture and Fisheries to Investigate Experimentally and to Report upon Certain Questions Connected with the Dipping and Treatment of Sheep, Vol. XXI:1, Cd. 2258. London: The Stationary Office, 1905a.

United Kingdom Parliament. Minutes of Evidence taken before the Departmental Committee Appointed by the Board of Agriculture and Fisheries to Investigate Experimentally and to Report upon Certain Questions Connected with the Dipping and Treatment of Sheep, with Appendices, Vol. XXI:27, Cd. 2259. London: The Stationary Office, 1905b.

United Kingdom Parliament. Report of the Departmental Committee Appointed by the Board of Agriculture to Inquire into the Aetiology, Pathology, and Morbid Anatomy and Other Matters Connected with the Diseases of Sheep known as Louping-ill and Braxy, Part 1. Vol. XXIV:519, Cd. 2932. London: The Stationary Office, 1906a.

United Kingdom Parliament. Report of the Departmental Committee Appointed by the Board of Agriculture to Inquire into the Aetiology, Pathology, and Morbid Anatomy and Other Matters Connected with the Diseases of Sheep known as Louping-ill and Braxy, Part 2. Vol. XXIV:555, Cd. 2933. London: The Stationary Office, 1906b.

United Kingdom Parliament. Report of the Departmental Committee Appointed by the Board of Agriculture to Inquire into the Aetiology, Pathology, and Morbid Anatomy and Other Matters Connected with the Diseases of Sheep known as Louping-ill and Braxy, Part 3. Vol. XXIV:921, Cd. 2934. London: The Stationary Office, 1906c.

United Kingdom Parliament. Development Commission. Second Report of the Development Commissioners, Vol. XVII.837. London: The Stationary Office, 1912–13a.

United Kingdom Parliament. Minutes of Evidence taken before the Departmental Committee Appointed by the President of the Board of Agriculture and Fisheries to Inquire into the Requirements of the Public Services with Regard to Officers Possessing Veterinary Qualifications; with Appendices and Index, Vol. XLVIII:267, Cd.6652. London: The Stationary Office, 1912–13b.

United Kingdom Parliament. Report of the Departmental Committee of the Board of Agriculture Appointed to Enquire into Epizootic Abortion.

Appendix to part III – Abortion in Sheep, Vol. XII.101, Cd. 7157. London: The Stationary Office, 1914a.

United Kingdom Parliament. Second Report of the Board of Agriculture for Scotland, Vol. XII.897, Cd. 7434. London: The Stationary Office, 1914b.

United Kingdom Parliament. Development Commission. Fourth Report of the Development Commissioners, Vol. XXV.I. London: The Stationary Office, 1916.

United Kingdom Parliament. Development Commission. Tenth Report of the Development Commissioners, Vol. XIII.901. London: The Stationary Office, 1920.

United Kingdom Parliament. Annual Reports of Proceedings under the Diseases of Animals Acts. London: The Stationary Office, 1900–20.

Usher, John. *Border Breeds of Sheep.* Kelso: J. & J.H. Rutherfurd, 1875.

Vernon, Keith. "Science for the Farmer? Agricultural Research in England 1909–1936." *Twentieth Century British History* 8 (1997): 310–33.

Wall, Rosemary. *Bacteriology in Britain, 1880-1939.* London: Pickering and Chatto, 2013.

Wallace, Professor. "Scab in Sheep: Suggestions for its Eradication." *Transactions of the Highland and Agricultural Society* 12 (1900): 117–36.

Warwick, Colin and Alastair Macdonald. "The New Veterinary College, Edinburgh, 1873 to 1904." *Veterinary Record* 153 (2003): 380–6.

Wheler, E.G. "Louping-Ill and the Grass Ticks." *Journal of the Royal Agricultural Society of England* 10 (1899): 626–44.

Wilkinson, Lise. *Animals and Disease: An Introduction to the History of Comparative Medicine.* Cambridge: Cambridge University Press, 1992.

Williams, W.O. "Louping Ill." *Transactions of the Highland and Agricultural Society* IX (1897): 278–90.

Woods, Abigail. *A Manufactured Plague: The History of Foot and Mouth Disease in Britain, 1839–2001.* London: Earthscan, 2004.

Woods, Abigail. "'Partnership' in Action: Contagious Abortion and the Governance of Livestock Disease in Britain, 1885–1921." *Minerva* 47 (2009): 195–217.

Woods, Abigail. "From Practical Men to Scientific Experts: British Veterinary Surgeons and the Development of Government Scientific Expertise, c1878–1919." *History of Science* li (2013): 457–80.

Woods, Abigail. "From One Medicine to Two: The Evolving Relationship between Human and Veterinary Medicine in England, 1791–1835." *Bulletin of the History of Medicine* 91 (2017), 494–523.

Woods, Abigail and Stephen Matthews. "'Little, If At All, Removed from the Illiterate Farrier or Cow-Leech': The English Veterinary Surgeon, c.1860–85, and the Campaign for Veterinary Reform." *Medical History* 54 (2010): 29–54.

Woods, Rebecca. “From Colonial Animal to Imperial Edible: Building an Empire of Sheep in New Zealand, ca. 1880–1900.” *Comparative Studies of South Asia, Africa and the Middle East* 35 (2015): 117–36.

Worboys, M. “The Emergence of Tropical Medicine: A Study in the Establishment of a Scientific Specialty.” In *Perspectives on the Emergence of Scientific Disciplines*, edited by Gerard Lemaine et al., 75–98. The Hague: Mouton, 1976.

Worboys, M. “Germ Theories of Disease and British Veterinary Medicine.” *Medical History* 35 (1991): 308–27.

Worboys, M. “Public and Environmental Health.” In *The Cambridge History of Science, Volume 6: Modern Biological and Earth Sciences*, edited by Peter Bowler and John Pickstone, 141–64. Cambridge: Cambridge University Press, 2009.

Zinsstag, J., E. Schelling, D. Waltner-Toews and M. Tannera. “From ‘One Medicine’ to ‘One Health’ and Systemic Approaches to Health and Well-being.” *Preventive Veterinary Medicine* 101 (2011): 148–56.

CHAPTER 4

From Healthy Cows to Healthy Humans: Integrated Approaches to World Hunger, *c.*1930–1965

Michael Bresalier

From 1945, Zebu cattle living on the Indian subcontinent were exhaustively identified, enumerated and evaluated by officials working for the newly created Food and Agriculture Organization (FAO) of the United Nations (UN). These indigenous, humped-backed cattle (*Bos indicus*) provided crucial sources of draught power, food and income to the area's human inhabitants. Surveying them was a lengthy and painstaking process that took seven years to complete. It was disrupted by political events such as the Partition of India, the creation of Pakistan and the end of British rule in 1947, which impacted on the provision of agricultural services and the presence of technical experts able to attend to the Zebu. It was made more difficult by the Zebu themselves. Numbering more than 100 million in India alone (which held nearly half of the world's population), their living conditions, locations and roles within agrarian systems varied greatly, as did their physical state. Investigators identified at least twenty eight distinct breeds, whose diverse sizes, shapes and productive capacities reflected their adaptation to particular climates and environments. Many were burdened by chronic infections, parasites and malnutrition, which undermined their health and limited their ability to fulfil their human-designated roles.[1]

The Zebu attracted attention at this time as a result of the findings of the FAO's first *World Food Survey*. Reporting in 1946, it anticipated

[1] Joshi and Phillips (1953).

A. Woods et al., *Animals and the Shaping of Modern Medicine*, Medicine and Biomedical Sciences in Modern History, https://doi.org/10.1007/978-3-319-64337-3_4

a growing food crisis across much of the world: production was below pre-war levels, famine had just devastated Bengal and millions of people were unable to meet their basic calorie requirements. With the world's population predicted to increase exponentially, the situation would only deteriorate.[2] The Zebu survey formed one facet of the FAO's response. It sought to identify those cattle with the greatest potential to develop more productive bodies, and to enrol them in a campaign to combat human hunger. This extended beyond India to Latin America, Africa and much of Asia, and enlisted not only cattle but also buffalo, chickens, pigs and other animals. However, the recognized importance of milk for child growth and development, and the vitamin, mineral and protein deficiencies that it helped to address, meant that cattle played a central role.

This role was not entirely new. The twin challenges of improving human nutrition through increased milk consumption, and developing agriculture through improvements in livestock health and production, had preoccupied nations, colonies and the League of Nations during the interwar years, culminating in calls to 'marry food and agriculture'.[3] However, it was only after the war, under the aegis of the FAO and the World Health Organization (WHO), that these two agendas became truly integrated. In framing healthy, productive cattle as essential to the production of healthy, well-nourished humans, these organizations encouraged experts in human and veterinary medicine to transcend the institutional and disciplinary boundaries that had grown to separate them,[4] and to forge new relationships with each other, and with the human and bovine subjects whose bodies they sought to transform.

Taking the interwar period as its jumping-off point, this chapter explores and accounts for these previously undocumented post-war developments. In revealing the centrality of cattle to the international campaign to feed the world, it adds a crucial zoological strand to the existing historiography on world hunger, and demonstrates the importance of a cross-cutting approach to domains of science and policy that historians typically study in isolation from each other. Existing accounts of world hunger adopt two distinct approaches. Some historians have examined how it was framed as a problem of overpopulation, and have

[2]FAO (1946).

[3]Amrith and Clavin (2013), Way (2013).

[4]On the emergence of these boundaries, see Chapter 3.

explored neo-Malthusian efforts by American philanthropists such as the Ford Foundation, and UN experts such as Julian Huxley, to manage the crisis by controlling human fertility.[5] Others have examined approaches to hunger as a problem of agricultural development, and interrogate the alliances between the Rockefeller Foundation, the US government and the FAO that resulted in efforts to modernize food production through seed-and-soil science and hybrid crops, culminating in the so-called 'Green Revolution'.[6] In these accounts and in the burgeoning literature on international health organizations,[7] livestock hardly feature.[8] Relegated to histories of development, they are viewed largely in terms of their ability to promote economic growth and destroy the environment.[9] When their influence over human health is considered, it is primarily as hosts and transmitters of infectious diseases to humans.[10]

However, as this chapter demonstrates, livestock attracted attention for other reasons. Post-war experts from across the UN and its allied agencies viewed them not only as threats to human health but also as potential contributors to it, suppliers of highly nutritious foodstuffs that would benefit human health and strength.[11] This role was not disconnected from that of disease transmitter because many of the zoonotic infections that animals conveyed to humans undermined their own health and productivity. However, as we shall see, international efforts to promote cattle as sources of meat and milk focused not only on the prevention of their diseases but also—in line with the WHO's definition of human health as 'a state of complete physical, mental, and social well-being and not merely the absence of disease or infirmity'—on improving their feeding, breeding, husbandry and general health.[12] The unproductive bodies of developing world cows therefore shaped and were produced by the post-war

---

[5] For example: Connelly (2003, 2006, 2008), Bashford (2014).

[6] For example: Marglin (1996), Perkins (1997), Cullather (2004, 2010).

[7] For example: Borowy (2009), Borowy et al. (2016) and other papers in this special issue.

[8] Veterinary contributions to the post-Second World War campaign to feed the world are, however, mentioned briefly by Jones (2003) pp. 96–100.

[9] Steinfeld et al. (2006), Hodge (2007), Weis (2013).

[10] Hardy (2003b). For other references, see Appendix: Annotated Bibliography of Animals in the History of Medicine.

[11] Wiley (2011).

[12] WHO (1946) p. 100. For a general discussion see Staples (2006) pp. 132–6.

international campaign against world hunger, which brought experts and activities that historians have tended to regard as 'veterinary' in character into the realms of human health and medicine.[13]

In recounting the history of that campaign, and its bovine subjects and shapers, this chapter draws on the traces that cows left on the historical record.[14] As subjects of investigation by experts in animal pathology, nutrition and physiology, cattle frequently feature within their scientific literatures. They also appear in the statistical surveys and documents of the FAO, WHO and allied agencies. As producers of vitamins, fats and proteins for human consumption, they left indirect traces on the bodies of their human consumers, and in scientific and documents dedicated to human health and nutrition.[15] By analysing these traces, the people and circumstances that gave rise to them, and the methods used to create them, this chapter sheds new light on the people, organizations and agendas that drove the interlinked creation of healthy cattle and healthy humans in the post-war international arena.

The first section will explore the parallel development during the interwar period of scientific literatures and policy agendas that granted two distinctive roles to cows. In human health and nutrition, new knowledge of vitamins and trace elements led experts to regard cows as important sources of human food, and to promote the consumption of their milk.[16] In agriculture and veterinary medicine, scientific advances and the deepening agricultural depression led experts to view cows as key sources of farming income, and to attempt improvements to their health and productivity. In colonial and international settings, links formed between these two agendas, resulted in calls for the 'marriage of food and agriculture'. The second section will relate how, in wartime and the immediate post-war era, these links were concretized by food shortages and the identification of 'protein malnutrition' as a key problem in the developing world, such that world hunger came to be viewed as a problem of unproductive cattle, whose health and nutrition had a direct bearing on the health and nutrition of their human consumers. The third section outlines how the FAO and the WHO responded to this problem by creating

[13] Orland (2004).

[14] Benson (2011).

[15] Wiley (2014).

[16] Valenze (2011).

new structures within which different types of expert came together to plan the creation of new bovine bodies and new experts capable of bringing them into being. It also touches on the consequences of these plans for the cows that helped to shape them.

4.1 Cows in Interwar Medicine and Agriculture

The interwar period witnessed a new consciousness about the centrality of foods produced by animals to the nourishment of humans. By the 1930s, patterns of food consumption in most of the industrial world had shifted from grain-based to animal-based diets—the so-called 'nutrition transition'.[17] Meat, milk and other livestock products gained pride of place on the tables of all classes, becoming integral to national cultures, tastes and identities.[18] Their significance to human health and nutrition was increasingly recognized. In the later nineteenth century, early nutrition scientists had regarded animals as crucial sources of calories and protein, whose meat and milk could help to repair muscles and ensure the efficient functioning of the human motor.[19] During the early twentieth century, as nutrition science expanded, gained institutional expression and won new sources of public funding, the evaluation of animal foods shifted to focus on newly identified components—amino acids, minerals and vitamins—which scientists deemed essential for normal physiological growth, development and function. In 1918 the American biochemist and nutrition scientist E.V. McCollum heralded this as the 'newer knowledge of nutrition'.[20] Despite early controversies, this new knowledge was eventually accepted as nutritional fact, generating a Nobel Prize for the discoverers of vitamins, Christiaan Eijkman and Sir Frederick Gowland Hopkins.[21]

A number of nutritional scientists sought to translate the findings of experimental research into practical knowledge that could guide medical and public health professionals, policy-makers and the public.[22] Ranking

---

[17] Popkin (1993), Grigg (1995), Otter (2012).

[18] Knapp (1997), Cantor and Bonah (2010).

[19] Rabinbach (1990) pp. 120–45.

[20] MCollum (1918).

[21] Smith and Nicolson (1989), Smith (1997), Carpenter (2003), Gratzer (2005), Vernon (2007).

[22] Barona (2010).

foods according to their nutritional value, they concluded that those derived from animals were the best for humans.[23] Their laboratory and field studies showed that milk, meat, eggs and fish not only provided high-quality proteins—with the best combination of essential amino acids—but also other micronutrients, notably vitamins A and D, which were identified as especially important for infants, children, and pregnant and lactating women. In this evaluation, milk was awarded pride of place and defined as a 'protective food'.[24] The dairy cow therefore became an essential contributor to the health and efficiency of human bodies.[25] For McCollum, 'the consumption of milk and its products form[ed] the greatest factor for the protection of mankind',[26] while an enquiry by experts associated with the League of Nations characterized it as the best and most readily available 'protective food', 'the nearest approach we possess to a perfect and complete food'.[27]

In shifting attention from the quantity to quality of food intake, the newer knowledge of nutrition reframed understandings of an adequate diet, its cost and its relationship to health. It also led to the identification of 'malnutrition' as a new medical problem caused by inadequate dietary intake of vitamins, amino acids or minerals, and characterized by suboptimal growth, health and productivity.[28] Scientific investigations revealed that malnutrition could be rectified by adding bovine bodily products to human diets. They stimulated significant improvements in human growth and efficiency, lowered the incidence of deficiency diseases such as rickets, and helped to reduce maternal mortality. Dietary surveys conducted in 1930s Britain, where economic depression had devastated industrial heartlands, suggested that a fifth of all children were chronically malnourished. Read alongside scientists' calculations of the cost of a nutritious diet, this finding stimulated criticisms of a government that repeatedly asserted the adequacy of its responses to poverty. It also encouraged efforts to increase the consumption of 'protective foods' such as milk.[29] In Britain and the

---

[23] McCollum (1918) pp. 69–83.

[24] Ibid. p. 82.

[25] On McCollum's work see Valenze (2011) pp. 238–50.

[26] McCollum (1918) p. 67.

[27] League of Nations (1937) p. 87.

[28] For accounts of this development, see Vernon (2007), Barona (2012).

[29] Mayhew (1988), Smith (1997), Barona (2008), Barona (2012).

USA, policies were introduced to provide daily milk for schoolchildren.[30] There was also a movement to encourage pasteurization as a means of improving the quality and public appeal of milk, which was often produced in unhygienic conditions and contaminated with germs that caused scarlet fever and tuberculosis in humans.[31]

John Boyd Orr, a medically trained nutrition scientist who headed the Rowett Institute of Animal Nutrition in Aberdeen, was at the forefront of British nutritional research, dietary surveys and the political campaign to promote government action.[32] He also helped to establish malnutrition as a colonial problem. With the head of the Kenyan Medical Department, John Gilks, he surveyed the diet and health of different tribes, finding differences in the health and physique of populations that consumed animal-based diets compared with grain- and vegetable-based diets. Similar observations had been made by Robert McCarrison in India, and were subsequently confirmed and elaborated there by W. Akyroyd, and by other colonial investigators working in West Africa, the Middle East and Kenya, where field studies were impeded by the Maasai migrating to fulfil their cows' need for water.[33]

In the Gold Coast (present-day Ghana), the Jamaican-born British paediatrician Cicely Williams, working for the Colonial Medical Service, identified a new form of malnutrition that she attributed to 'some amino or protein deficiency'.[34] Found in infants who had been breast-fed by malnourished mothers and weaned on maize porridge, it led to severe bloating, loss of hair, blotched skin, wasting, diarrhoea and oedema. She named it with the native Ga term, 'kwashiorkor'.[35] The condition was also identified by investigators working in other parts of colonial Africa, though they used different terms for it.[36] In drawing medical attention away from the tropical diseases that had lent medical definition to

---

[30] Welshman (1997), DuPuis (2002), Atkins (2005).

[31] Atkins (1992), Waddington (2004).

[32] Orr (1936), Pemberton and White (2000), Vernon (2007).

[33] Worboys (1988), Arnold (1994), Weindling (1995), Vernon (2007). The colonial agendas which drove this work, and which contributed to the health problems identified, have been investigated and critiqued. See Brantley (1997).

[34] Williams (1933, 1935).

[35] Stanton (2001).

[36] Trowell (1940, 1949).

these regions since the later nineteenth century,[37] these discoveries suggested that the prime animal shapers of human health were not the parasitic animals that transmitted tropical diseases but the bovine animals that supplied nutrition to humans. They also fuelled concerns that low-level production and consumption of bovine bodies was holding back economic development in Africa, and could threaten global security by prompting a Malthusian crisis in India and mass migration to the West.[38]

These investigations awarded cattle the role of food producers for undernourished humans. However, other experts awarded them a different role—as resources for agricultural and economic development that suffered health and nutritional problems of their own. This bovine role became increasingly important during the interwar depression. British dairy farming won many new converts in this period because the perishability of milk afforded protection from the flood of cheap food imports that depressed the prices of other products. By 1930–1931, dairy cows supplied 27% of the gross agricultural produce of England and Wales and were farmed by three-quarters of the members of the National Farmers' Union. However, the large volume of domestic milk production resulted in low prices, particularly in summer when cows tended to calve. British efforts to address this issue focused on expanding the market for milk, through its provision to schoolchildren, and with the aid of a national Milk Marketing Board.[39] There were also research and policy initiatives that aimed to make production more efficient by improving the health, nutrition and breeding of dairy cows, whose bodies were reportedly deteriorating as farmers adopted cost-saving measures to ride out the depression.[40]

As subjects of scientific investigation, British cattle were distributed between the 'watertight compartments' whose formation was described in Chapter 3. The policy of channelling public funds for agricultural research into selected fields and institutions, and the hostility expressed by veterinarians towards disease investigations performed by non-veterinarians, meant that the breeding of cows was investigated at Cambridge University, their nutrition at Cambridge and the Rowett Institute in

[37] Worboys (1988).

[38] Hutchinson (2002), Tilley (2011), Amrith and Clavin (2013).

[39] Atkins (2005).

[40] DeJager (1993), Vernon (1997), Woods (2007), Woods (2010).

Aberdeen, aspects of dairying at University College Reading, and cow health at the Royal Veterinary College and State Veterinary Laboratory. In these various locations, researchers worked to promote the development and application of rational breeding practices, to apply the new knowledge of nutrition to bovine diets, and to counteract diseases such as brucellosis and tuberculosis which undermined cattle (re)production.[41] Their research programmes—which impacted on the bodies, behaviours and lived experiences of cows owned by Britain's more progressive farmers—were quite separate from those concerned with human health and nutrition, which took place in medical schools and in research institutions supported by the publicly funded Medical Research Council (MRC).[42] This separation was reflected in policy: health matters were dealt with by the Ministry of Health and farming matters by the Ministry of Agriculture. Where connections were inescapable, as with the management of zoonotic diseases such as bovine tuberculosis, which spread via milk to humans and was a major focus of concern in this period, they were characterized by conflict owing to very different framings of the problem by experts and officials concerned with human and animal health.[43]

As director of the Rowett Institute and a member of the MRC's Nutrition Committee, who conducted research on the mineral content of livestock pastures and the nutritional content of human diets, Orr was one of the few individuals to transcend these institutional, disciplinary and species boundaries and approach cows as simultaneously medical and agricultural problems.[44] As a qualified doctor, his research on bovine nutrition perpetuated longstanding zoological traditions in medicine, as outlined in Chapters 2 and 3. This work proceeded in tandem with his concern for human nutrition, and may even have enabled it, by allowing him to draw analogies between the causes of malnutrition in animals and humans.[45]

---

[41] Woods (2007).

[42] DeJager (1993). From 1933 the MRC was headed by Edward Mellenby, who built on the zoo-based investigations of John Bland Sutton, as described in Chapter 1, to cement the link between rickets and vitamin D. See Petty (1989).

[43] Waddington (2004), Hardy (2003).

[44] Valenze shows that McCollum also sought to transcend these boundaries in the USA. Valenze (2011).

[45] Orr (1966), Kay (1972), Smith (1999).

Orr also benefited from, and contributed to, the more fluid situation in colonial contexts where research and policy compartments were less watertight, enabling the cow's dual roles to be considered in tandem. As a member of the Research Committee of the Empire Marketing Board, he travelled and conducted dietary surveys throughout the empire. His survey on the health and nutrition of Kenyan humans followed on directly from a survey he conducted on the health and nutrition of Kenyan settlers' cattle, and was stimulated by co-investigator John Gilks' observation that the Kikuyu sometimes sought out the same substances as those contained within the special saltlicks that they encouraged their cattle to consume.[46] While the report of the cattle survey did not directly connect the health and feeding of cattle with that of humans, it did argue that 'a general improvement of agriculture and animal husbandry' would advance 'the health and working capacity of the native'.[47] In promoting the production and consumption of milk, it lent support to the Kenyan government's efforts to improve agriculture through the development of mixed farming, a method extrapolated from the British context, which received wider support in this period from colonial agricultural scientists alarmed by the ecological and economic consequences of arable monoculture and nomadic pastoralism.[48] Studies like Orr's and Gilks' strengthened the belief that relationships between humans, cows and the land needed to change, and that, by developing agriculture, they would advance human health, working capacity and, by extension, the colonial economy.[49]

The League of Nations took up these issues as part of its wider agenda of achieving global security through economic stability. Its 1931 publication *The Agricultural Crisis* studied the effects of the Great Depression on world agriculture, and identified lack of purchasing power as a key problem.[50] In 1932 it initiated enquiries (to which Orr contributed) into the impacts of depression on public health and nutrition. These integrated the dietary standards and recommendations drawn up by different

[46] Brantley (1997) p. 55.

[47] Gilks and Orr (1927), Orr and Gilks (1931).

[48] Hodge (2002), Hodge (2007).

[49] Hall (1936), Worboys (1988), Little (1991).

[50] League of Nations (1931).

governments and researchers, and placed the issue on the League Assembly's agenda.[51] In 1935, Frank McDougall, an Australian economist and expert on imperial trade, presented his analysis of these dual problems in a 15-page memo to the League of Nations. He outlined how, in the West, scientific advances had led to increases in agricultural production, but owing to plummeting prices, some farmers were disposing of surpluses by burning wheat or pouring milk down gutters. To support their farmers, some governments had introduced protectionist trading policies and agricultural subsidies, but this was preventing the distribution of nutritious food to the people who most needed it. The problem was not that the world had too much food but that, owing to flaws in pricing and marketing, it was not being consumed.[52]

The belief that fulfilling human nutritional needs would lift agriculture—and the world economy—out of depression generated calls to 'marry food and agriculture'.[53] MacDougall argued that this could be achieved through agricultural policies that promoted farm-based production, rationalised distribution, and greater consumption of nutritious foods. The principle won support from a League of Nations Mixed Committee, which was highly unusual in bringing together experts in public health, agriculture and economics. Its interim report, released in 1936, emphasized the need to increase the production and consumption of protective foods such as milk.[54] It argued that on account of the 'application of science to agriculture' there was already 'ample scope' to shift world agricultural production in this direction, so that with appropriate government support 'the real needs of each community for the health-giving foods may be correlated with the undoubted power of agriculture to produce all that is necessary for abundant health'.[55]

Among the obstacles to this shift, which the committee identified in its 1937 *Final Report*, were natural conditions—soil and climate—which limited what foods could be produced; the structure of agricultural

---

[51] Terroine (1936). For the development of League's nutritional policies see Borowy (2009) pp. 379–93.

[52] Burnet and Aykroyd (1935), Staples (2006) pp. 71–4, Borowy (2009) pp. 379–93, Amrith and Clavin (2013), Way (2013) pp. 153–73.

[53] Jachertz and Nützenadel (2011).

[54] League of Nations (1936), Way (2013) pp. 153–73.

[55] League of Nations (1936) p. 87.

holdings; lack of capital; the conservative outlooks of peasant farmers; the need for more scientific research and education; and the cleanliness, quality and safety of products such as milk. The *Report* also highlighted recent changes that were helping to address these problems. However, as in other discussions of interwar nutrition, the health, feeding and keeping of cows was hardly mentioned.[56] While commentators acknowledged cows as key participants in plans to feed the world, they did not draw direct associations between the bodily condition of cows and those of their human consumers. With the outbreak of war, however, this would begin to change.[57]

4.2 War and its Aftermath

Although looming hostilities prevented the translation of the Committee's findings into action, Orr took its lessons back to Britain, where heavy reliance upon imported food was undermined by war. In his 1940 volume *Feeding the People in Wartime*, and in advice that he and other nutrition scientists provided to the Ministry of Food about the development of a nutrition-based national food plan, he promoted the consumption of home-produced milk, vegetables and arable foods.[58] This advice had little influence on rationing policy but it did inform the creation of schemes that channelled protective foods such as milk to children, and pregnant and nursing women. Dairy cows served not only these groups but consumers in general, because a reduction in other, imported animal proteins enhanced human reliance on home-produced milk.[59] As vital suppliers of food, and key contributors to national defence, they were rewarded with privileged access to scarce supplies of imported feedstuffs. However, these supplies soon ran short, forcing farmers to utilize and grow different types of feed to which bovine bodies proved less responsive. Their reduced milk output could not be addressed by increasing cow numbers because there was nothing to feed them. The only solution was to increase the efficiency of production.

[56] League of Nations (1937) pp. 151–84.

[57] Collingham (2012) pp. 467–500.

[58] Orr and Lubbock (1940).

[59] Smith (2000).

To this end, scientists intensified their scrutiny of cows and their efforts to rectify deficiencies in their feeding, breeding and health.[60]

British veterinarians played an important part in this process. Their leaders—who included Thomas Dalling, head of the Government Veterinary Laboratory—won the attention of farmers and the state by estimating the enhanced quantity of milk that they could generate through a state-subsidized veterinary scheme for controlling certain diseases of dairy cows.[61] Significantly, the diseases targeted by this scheme were not the zoonotic conditions such as tuberculosis, which had acted as points of connection between interwar human and veterinary medicine, but those that impacted primarily on milk output and therefore human nutrition: mastitis, infertility, brucellosis and Johne's disease.[62] In winning support for their scheme, vets forged important connections between the health and productivity of bovine bodies and those of humans, and made their expertise relevant to both. Their interventions reshaped the bodies and lived experiences of cows. They subjected them to rectal examinations to assess and promote their reproductive performance, to udder manipulations aimed at evaluating their milk-producing capacity, and to vaccinations and drug treatments. They also branded unproductive cows as 'passengers' and recommended their culling.[63]

At the end of the war, similar connections between the health and productivity of bovine and human bodies were forged on the international stage as the newly formed FAO surveyed the state of global food and agriculture.[64] The FAO found that some areas devastated by the fighting lacked the human and animal resources they needed to produce sufficient food.[65] In other areas these resources existed but were not up to the task. The Zebu survey mentioned above was just one of several that revealed very large livestock populations but startlingly low levels

---

[60] Woods (2007).

[61] 'Sir Thomas Dalling' (2012).

[62] Woods (2010).

[63] Ibid. Although brucellosis was a zoonosis, its transmission to humans was infrequent and not widely recognized.

[64] FAO (1946, 1952). For the history of the FAO, see Phillips (1981), Staples (2006), Biswas (2008), Jachertz and Nützenadel (2011), Jachertz (2014).

[65] Dodd (1949), Phillips (1951), Hambidge (1955).

of animal protein consumption by humans.[66] Throughout the developing world, cows were failing to perform their human-designated roles as food producers. India held 250,000 million or a quarter of all cattle and water buffaloes in the world, but the average annual yield per milk animal was only 200 kg compared with 4000 kg in the Netherlands.[67] Whereas the average annual yield of an American beef cow was 75.6 kg, in Asia the figure was less than 12 kg. These unproductive bovine bodies caused particular alarm owing to unprecedented (and unexpected) population growth in the Far East, Africa and Latin America. Population experts predicted an impending collapse as human numbers outstripped food supplies. The FAO's first *World Food Survey* in 1946 estimated that two-thirds of the world's human population were hungry. Their findings added the threat of starvation to the persistent problem of malnutrition.[68] As the Cold War set in and decolonization began, fears grew that hungry people would join disaffected rebel groups or turn to communism.[69] In this context, cows were not only crucial sources of food but also political actors capable of influencing global security.

As the FAO's first director, Orr responded by attempting to implement earlier ideas of a marriage of food and agriculture.[70] He sought to create a World Food Board, which would centrally organize world food production according to actual needs rather than the market, with the ultimate aim of ensuring food as a basic human right. This radical vision never materialized, largely because of resistance from major agricultural powers. Instead it developed into a system for donating, disposing of or trading agricultural surpluses from the developed to the underdeveloped world through mechanisms such as the FAO's World Food Programme, the USA Food for Peace Programme, and the United Nations Children's Fund (UNICEF's) child health–milk initiatives.[71] On taking control in

---

66 Joshi et al. (1957).

67 Cattle estimates are from Phillips (1951) pp. 241–56. Yield estimates are from Sukhatme (1963) p. 12, Phillips (1963) pp. 254–55.

68 FAO (1946) pp. 6–7.

69 Perkins (1997) pp. 118–39, Cullather (2007) pp. 11–43, Robertson (2012) pp. 85–103.

70 Orr (1943), Orr (1948).

71 Staples (2006) pp. 84–96.

1949, Orr's successor, the American Norris E. Dodd, maintained this system of food redistribution. However, he also turned more directly to the problem of food production in the face of new evidence about the scope and severity of global undernutrition.[72] This evidence was gathered by a joint FAO/WHO Expert Committee on Nutrition. Formed in 1949, it was charged with determining and developing strategies to tackle the most pressing human nutritional problems.[73] It integrated the WHO's interest in improving human health and nutrition with the FAO's interest in improving the efficiency and equitability of food production, distribution and consumption.[74] At its first session in Geneva, it identified kwashiorkor as a key nutritional problem and target for international action.

Interest in this disease had grown considerably in the decade since Williams had identified it in the Gold Coast. Studies by medical researchers, including Hugh Trowell in East Africa, John Fleming Brock in South Africa, and the British physiologist and nutrition expert J.C. Waterlow in Central America, suggested that it potentially affected many parts of the world.[75] Unlike other forms of malnutrition, which were associated with vitamin deficiencies, it was linked to deficiencies of certain amino acids which were obtained from proteins found particularly in milk and meat. Its problematization therefore re-emphasized the cow's significance as a supplier of these products. The joint Committee recommended that kwashiorkor be adopted as the official term for malnutrition directly arising from milk protein deficiency, and that the FAO and the WHO support surveys to determine its prevalence in different parts of the world.[76]

The first survey was conducted in sub-Saharan Africa in 1950 by Brock (a Committee member and WHO consultant) and Marcel Autret (a biochemist and member of the FAO's Nutrition Division). Their 1952 report, *Kwashiorkor in Africa*, claimed that the condition was evident in every community they visited, except the Maasai and the Batussi

[72] Staples (2000).

[73] FAO/WHO (1949).

[74] For a history of the committee, see Barona (2012) pp. 263–94.

[75] FAO/WHO (1949) p. 15. For a full account see Ruxin (1996).

[76] FAO/WHO (1949) pp. 15–16.

(Tutsi) in Rwanda, who produced and consumed a large amount of cow's milk.[77] A second survey, conducted in 1953 by Autret and the Guatemalan pediatrician, Moisés Béhar showed that kwashiorkor was prevalent throughout Central America.[78] These studies confirmed the international scale of the problem. They also raised new questions about its specific nature and identity, for, while protein malnutrition was the key variable it was not unique to the condition, and was implicated in several other deficiency diseases, including marasmus and nutritional anaemia. Distinguishing kwashiorkor from these conditions was necessary to determine its prevalence and to develop programmes to tackle it. Following meetings in The Gambia and Jamaica, in late 1952 the joint Committee decided to redefine it as one of a number of conditions they brought together under the new category of 'protein malnutrition.'[79] While not entirely straightforward, this category expanded the focus of international concern, as illustrated by the claim made by one of its creators, J.C. Waterlow that 'we are concerned not only with the very sick and the dying, but perhaps much more with mild or chronic, so-called 'marginal', states in infants and … this is a far more important problem than acute kwashiokor.'[80]

The Third Report of the FAO/WHO Expert Committee on Nutrition, published in 1953, consolidated this change in focus. Protein malnutrition had become the single most important world health problem, the cause of an epidemic of deficiency diseases in underdeveloped countries, which severely burdened their populations, economies and healthcare systems.[81] The Committee was quite clear about the general causes of and solutions to protein malnutrition. First, *food supply* was a key determining factor: many underdeveloped countries were unable to meet the nutritional needs of their populations and particularly suffered from 'low production' of milk, meat, fish and eggs. Therefore, the 'first and essential step' in tackling protein malnutrition was to ensure that 'the right kinds of food' were available 'all the time'. Second, *population growth* had exacerbated the problem. Partly resulting from improvements in public health, it had spurred increasing production of starchy foods,

---

[77] Brock and Autret (1952).

[78] Autret and Béhar (1954).

[79] Waterlow (1955) p. 3. See Carpenter (1986, 1994).

[80] Waterlow (1955) p. 3.

[81] FAO/WHO (1953).

which satisfied the immediate needs of the growing numbers of hungry people but not their protein requirements.[82] Therefore agriculture in underdeveloped countries needed to be transformed to meet these requirements, with a focus on generating more animal proteins, particularly from the bodies of cows. The unique importance of milk proteins (and, by extension, cows) was emphasized at a second conference on protein malnutrition in Princeton in 1955, which proposed milk as a reference protein for determining the amino acid requirements for infants and young children.[83] These developments opened up new avenues for linking human nutrition to livestock bodies. World hunger was being bound up with world cattle populations. As the key means of rectifying protein malnutrition, cows were becoming more important to human health and nutrition than ever before.

Curiously, these connections have been largely overlooked in historical accounts of the growing hegemony of protein malnutrition in world hunger campaigns spearheaded by the FAO, the WHO and UNICEF in the 1950s and 1960s.[84] Considerable attention has been paid to the work of the Protein Advisory Group (PAG), created in 1955, which brought together nutrition experts from the three main UN agencies and various academic and research institutions.[85] PAG played a leading role in identifying a growing 'protein crisis' across the world and in characterizing it in terms of a widening 'protein gap' between regions with adequate per capita supplies and those without—most of Africa, Asia and large parts of Latin America. Along with fixing world attention on protein malnutrition, PAG also promoted particular solutions to the problem.[86] The best known were its efforts to develop and market 'new protein foods' synthetically derived from plants, algae and petroleum products.[87] Criticisms both before and after pointed out that these efforts directed large financial investments to first-world scientists, institutions and industries, but did little to foster agricultural and economic development in hungry countries, and ultimately failed to redress the chronic problem of

---

[82] FAO/WHO (1953) pp. 8–9, 25–27.

[83] Waterlow and Stephen (1957).

[84] Carpenter (1986, 1994), Newman (1995), Ruxin (1996).

[85] Ruxin (2000).

[86] Ruxin (1996) pp. 156–8.

[87] For example, Altschul (1976).

inadequate protein supplies.[88] While such criticisms were well founded, it is important to note that these schemes represented only a small fraction of international efforts. Far greater importance was placed on improving 'traditional' sources of animal protein, particularly cows.[89]

4.3 Healthy Cows, Healthy Humans

By the mid-1950s, international experts had reached a consensus that the developing world required more animal food, particularly the vitamin- and protein-rich foods derived from bovine bodies.[90] Ralph Wesley Phillips, an American specialist in animal husbandry and breeding, who oversaw the Zebu study and became the first director of the FAO's Department of Agriculture, recognized that 'there are many areas in the world where human needs for animal protein are not adequately met'. Highlighting the 'striking variation' in food availability in underdeveloped and developed regions, he aimed to address the significant shortfalls in production in countries outside North America, Australia, New Zealand and Europe.[91] One way of achieving this goal was to increase livestock numbers. This had been a short-term strategy in post-war Europe but seemed less applicable on a global scale. The world livestock population was already large—roughly equivalent to the human population (soon to reach 3 billion), or double if domesticated fowl were included.[92] Although on average the protein that animals supplied seemed adequate, the highest levels of production and consumption were concentrated in the developed world, which contained less than 40% of the world's livestock but produced nearly 80% of its meat and eggs.[93] The problem elsewhere was not livestock numbers but productivity. In a review of world cattle for *Scientific American*, Phillips noted that 'the best zebu performances have been far below those of European breeds. In India a few well-handled Sahiwal cows have

[88] McClaren (1974), Tappan (2013).

[89] For example, see FAO (1957) pp. 19–20.

[90] Autret, who had carried out a study of kwashiorkor in Africa, declared that 'protein malnutrition is without doubt the main nutritional problem in the underdeveloped countries today'. FAO (1960) p. 1.

[91] Phillips (1951) p. 244.

[92] Phillips (1963b) p. 15. Phillips' figures were taken from FAO (1962).

[93] Pritchard (1966) p. 361.

produced somewhat more than 10,000 pounds of milk in a year. In the United States, Holsteins have produced as much as 40,000 pounds.'[94] If third-world animals could match the outputs of first-world animals, then threats of starvation and malnutrition could be averted.

Achieving this goal was far harder than adding numbers to existing stocks because it involved tackling the reasons why third-world animals were so unproductive. W. Ross Cockrill, a Scottish veterinarian who joined the FAO's Department of Agriculture in 1953 and later became assistant director of its Animal Production and Health Division (APHD), summed up the problem: 'multitudes of livestock which could be the genesis of alleviation of human hunger are themselves suffering from disease and malnutrition'.[95] For Cockrill, the state of bovine bodies was both analogous to, and a cause of, the condition of the human bodies they were supposed to be nourishing. Cows were frequently stunted and unproductive because they relied on deficient forage, grazing and pasture lands. They suffered from endemic infectious, parasitic, nutritional, metabolic and organic diseases that sometimes killed them but more usually reduced their growth and productivity.[96] The majority were produced by opportunistic matings rather than those planned to effect improvements in their bodies. Husbandry practices such as overstocking, or traditions which derived from the symbolic or economic value that humans placed on cows, further undermined their health and productivity. Consequently, as Cockrill later reflected, 'The world's livestock population which, if properly managed, could be the genesis of alleviation of human hunger and malnutrition, is itself in large part starved, diseased and parasitic upon the human race.'[97]

Efforts to address these problems were mounted by not only the FAO but also the WHO. Each formed a section that enrolled cows in the campaign against world hunger. Each positioned veterinarians and experts in animal science (which brought together genetics, nutrition and husbandry, and had developed into a taught discipline in US universities in the 1930s) as crucial to the improvement of bovine—and,

[94] Phillips (1958) p. 57.

[95] Cockrill (1964) p. 260.

[96] See, for example, Meyer (1953).

[97] Cockrill (1968) p. 12.

by extension, human—bodies.[98] This turn to veterinary expertise was stimulated not only by shifting perceptions of the relationships between bovine and human health but also by vets' wartime activities, which had demonstrated their capacity to serve human health as well as agriculture. As outlined above, vets claiming to be 'physician of the farm and the guarantor of the nation's food supply' had worked to improve British milk output for the benefit of consumers, while in the USA they had helped to ratchet up livestock production.[99] War had also granted vets opportunities to operate on the world stage, assisting in the relief and redevelopment of war-torn nations. Such activities elevated their status and encouraged a shift in professional identity, putting them in a strong position to join other experts in addressing the challenges of feeding the world. Their involvement fashioned the world's cows into veterinary subjects, and reinvigorated and expanded older veterinary public health agendas stretching back to the nineteenth century.[100]

The FAO's AHPD was one of the key institutional contexts for these developments.[101] From 1950 it was headed by the Australian Keith Kesteven, who had left livestock farming and breeding in the late 1930s to study veterinary science at the University of Sydney. During the war he had acted as veterinary advisor to the Australian armed forces.[102] Afterwards, as a member of the United Nations Relief and Rehabilitation Administration (UNRRA), he led efforts in China to redevelop its livestock industry and eradicate rinderpest. He built the APHD into an important body employing 32 specialists at headquarters in Rome and more than 300 in the field, where they helped some 60 different countries to plan livestock health and production programmes.[103] Most staff came from universities, institutes and agricultural departments of leading livestock-producing nations, with the USA, Britain, Denmark, Australia, New Zealand and Canada heavily represented. A few came from developing nations, particularly India and parts of Latin America, where veterinary and animal production services were fairly well established.

[98] Jones (2003) p. 99.

[99] Woods (2007).

[100] Koolmees (2000), Hardy (2003).

[101] Phillips (1981) pp. 102–7.

[102] 'The Gilruth Prize Citation' (1975).

[103] Keseteven (1966), Cockrill (1968).

A selection of staff were sent to member countries for specialist training in an aspect of animal or veterinary science.[104] By 1959 the division consisted of three branches focusing on production, health and dairy production. Each was dedicated to developing and applying forms of expertise that would bring the bodies of third-world livestock in line with those of the first-world.

The Dairy Branch grew out of the APHD's work in providing technical assistance in milk production and plant management for the Milk Conservation Programme.[105] This had been established by UNICEF in 1948 to distribute dried skimmed milk powder from major dairy-producing countries to war-ravaged and underfed countries across Europe, Asia and Africa.[106] The FAO supported the programme as a short-term solution to shortages of dairy foods, while also promoting the expansion and improvement of local milk production, with the long-term aim of enabling countries to become self-sufficient.[107] One means of achieving this goal was through technical and material assistance for dairy cooperatives.[108] From 1946 the FAO supported a dairy cooperative in the Anand district of Gujarat province outside Bombay, which broke an old monopoly, rooted in British colonial rule, that underpaid farmers and supplied substandard milk.[109] With FAO and bilateral support from Denmark and New Zealand, new dairy plants were built and new dairy technicians and veterinarians were trained to run them. The cooperative enabled small producers to pool and receive a reasonable price for relatively small quantities of milk. Their cows became subjects of shared veterinary animal husbandry services that aimed to enhance their productivity. The FAO viewed the cooperative as a key model for its approach to improving dairy production in the developing world.[110]

Technical support for dairy cooperatives relied on the expertise of the APHD's other branches. The Animal Production Branch focused on developing programmes that combined breeding, nutrition and

---

[104] Dalling (1957). For a study of Swedish input into this programme, see Bruno (2016).

[105] Phillips (1981) pp. 105–6.

[106] For UNICEF's milk programmes, see Gillespie (2003).

[107] Pederson (1967).

[108] For FAO work on cooperatives, see Simons (1976).

[109] The best historical account of the cooperative is Valenze (2011) pp. 238–50.

[110] Kesteven (1966) pp. 236–7, Cockrill (1968).

husbandry. From its inception, it concentrated on collecting information about 'animal genetic resources' through surveys of cattle breeds in different regions. The Zebu in India and Pakistan, and other breeds in Africa and Europe, were scrutinized and evaluated as a basis for advising governments and local breeders on 'how best to utilize their valuable animal genetic resources'.[111] Nutrition was also a key focus. One of the Division's first reports, *Nutritional Deficiencies in Livestock*, detailed the state of animal nutrition in much of the world, the variety of nutritional diseases that burdened livestock, and ways of improving their nutrition.[112] Building on almost a half-century of animal nutrition research in the USA,[113] the authors argued that just as with humans, poor animal diets led to poor growth and dietary deficiencies, and were a 'chief factor limiting production of meat, milk and eggs ... Tremendous quantities of the world's feeds are wasted in this type of feeding, resulting in large losses of human foods.' Not only was 'the vitamin A value of milk... entirely dependent upon the amount present in the feed', but 'underfeeding dairy cows results in the reduction of milk supply as much as 75%'.[114] Therefore, '*correcting dietary deficiencies in livestock rations will do much to increase the world's supply of meat, milk and eggs*'.[115] To address the problem, the American nutritionists who wrote the report placed particular emphasis on improving the quality of pastures through mixed farming and the application of fertilizers.

The APHD also had a Health Branch. Its activities were coordinated by vet Thomas Dalling, who had helped to lead the British veterinary profession's wartime efforts to connect bovine and human health. He had also advised UNRRA and the FAO on the post-war reconstruction of European veterinary services and livestock economies.[116] He was convinced that 'to improve the food supplies of protein origin for people in different parts of the world ... we must increase animal production; and if we can increase and can better the health of animals, then we will have gone quite a long way towards increasing that animal production.'[117]

[111] Phillips (1981) p. 105.

[112] Allman and Hamilton (1949).

[113] Olmstead and Rhode (2008) pp. 270–4.

[114] Allman and Hamilton (1949) p. 20.

[115] Ibid. p. 1, original italics.

[116] 'Sir Thomas Dalling' (2012).

[117] Dalling (1957) p. 238.

Certainly, the health of animals needed improving. Third-world cattle were burdened with all manner of disease: major epizootics such as rinderpest and foot-and-mouth disease were a constant threat to herds; scores of parasitic infections presented chronic problems across the world, rarely killing animals but seriously reducing their productive and reproductive abilities; finally there were the zoonoses, which undermined the health and strength of animals and the humans they infected.[118] Dalling's branch supported an exhaustive array of activities aimed at each of these types of disease. The most high-profile was its campaign to eradicate rinderpest, but its work on parasitic and zoonotic diseases was no less important.[119] The Branch provided veterinary expertise together with tools such as vaccines, antibiotics and diagnostics. By 1957 it had a field staff of more than 40 veterinarians, most of whom were highly experienced and had taken leave from established positions to be assigned to a particular country or region for a year or two.[120]

While each country presented its own needs, field veterinarians adopted a shared approach to planning veterinary programmes.[121] First, they worked with government officials to evaluate the nature and extent of existing veterinary services, including available laboratories, equipment and materials. Second, they helped formulate general programmes of disease control, which included prioritizing diseases according to their burden and available means of control. Third, they instructed local people in how to diagnose livestock diseases, prepare biological products (diagnostic tests, therapies and vaccines), and develop and deliver veterinary education. As Kesteven explained in 1961:

> [Control over animal diseases] can only be done by setting up veterinary services in the countries which now lack them, strengthening services in the other countries, and establishing effective international co-operation and co-ordination ... Only by such international effort will man be able to control and perhaps ultimately eradicate animal diseases.[122]

---

[118] Kesteven (1961a, 1961b).

[119] Kesteven (1963).

[120] Dalling (1957) p. 239.

[121] Shaw (1962), Kesteven (1963).

[122] Kesteven (1961a) p. 109.

In its efforts to create new experts capable of transforming unproductive bovine bodies into plentiful sources of human food, the FAO worked closely with the Veterinary Public Health (VPH) unit of the WHO, which was created in 1948 within its Division of Communicable Diseases.[123] It had been proposed by James Steele, who as chief of the United States Public Health Service's newly created Veterinary Division had overseen the 1945 creation of a specialized VPH programme at the US Communicable Diseases Centre.[124] A key proponent of bringing veterinary expertise into public health, who had a particular interest in zoonotic diseases, Steele envisioned that the WHO's unit would collect information on zoonoses, distribute data, provide seminars and consultancy services to physicians and veterinarians, conduct investigations, and promote research on the control or elimination of zoonoses. It would also cooperate with the national and international agencies responsible for animal and human health. The unit's first head was the American, Martin Kaplan, who had degrees in veterinary medicine and public health.[125] Having worked for the FAO and as a veterinary consultant for the UNRRA in Europe at the end of the war, he was convinced of the value of veterinary medicine for human health. His unit spelt out this aim in its working definition of VPH as: 'all the community efforts influencing and influenced by the veterinary medical arts and sciences applied to the prevention of diseases, protection of life and promotion of the well-being and efficiency of man'.[126]

The VPH unit forged close relations with other organizations that were similarly drawn to study and improve unproductive bovine bodies—the FAO, other UN agencies and the World Organisation for Animal Health—leading to collaborative programmes on zoonoses, meat hygiene and veterinary education, which drove the integration of veterinary with public health and agricultural services.[127] For example, Kaplan's unit worked in partnership with Dalling's Animal Health Branch under a Joint WHO/WHO Expert Committee on Zoonoses, which was established in 1950 in response to the World Health Assembly's identification of zoonotic diseases

[123] Kaplan (1953).

[124] Steele (1979) p. 6.

[125] Martin Kaplan (1976), Soulsby (2006).

[126] This definition came out of WHO/FAO (1951) p. 3.

[127] 'Veterinary Public Health' (1974) p. 108.

as key threats to human health in newly independent and developing agrarian nations.[128] The Committee was tasked with identifying zoonoses that were evident 'world problems' and for which effective control measures had already been developed.[129] Over the next decade, it agreed a standard definition of these diseases, which brought over 100 different infections under one general category, creating fertile terrain for veterinarians to expand their international role in human health.[130]

Perceptions of zoonotic disease threats had shifted significantly in the context of the world hunger campaign. Previously, the animals affected had been regarded as costly impediments to agricultural production, and as transmitters of infections to humans. However, their promotion as food sources for hungry humans led to the realization that, in addition, these animals produced less food for humans, thereby posing dual threats to human health. This was highlighted by one of the Committee's leading experts, the Swiss-American veterinary scientist Karl Meyer, in a technical paper on 'The Zoonoses in Their Relation to Rural Health' that he presented, on Kaplan's invitation, to the Seventh World Health Assembly:

> One need only to consider all of the adverse effects of the zoonoses to realize the urgency of control: loss of life, acute and chronic illness of inhabitants of rural areas, loss of life and impairment of productivity of farm animals with all of the social and economic implications, and loss of life and acute and chronic illness of city dwellers to whom the zoonoses may spread ... These infections unquestionably have far-reaching economic aspects; they may mean mere loss of profit or they may mean critical want. In some areas they preclude the raising of livestock altogether ... in others they make an already poverty-stricken group poorer still and deny food supply to undernourished populations. In their destruction of food supply alone they are major economic problems. Some of the diseases ... are detrimental to rural populations because of their direct effects on health of farm people, making habitation in rural areas impossible or hazardous; some are more important in their effect on the world's food supply.[131]

[128] FAO/WHO (1951).

[129] 'Veterinary Public Health' (1974) p. 108.

[130] WHO/FAO (1959).

[131] Meyer (1954) p. 4.

Pointing to the complex challenges that zoonoses posed, Meyer laid out an agenda for positioning veterinary public health as integral to their control. Tackling zoonoses in developing countries would require extensive technical assistance, close 'co-operation between physicians, health workers and veterinarians', and between veterinary and agricultural agencies. Kaplan's VPH unit sought to implement this agenda. It coordinated epidemiological studies and basic laboratory research on zoonoses, including the development and standardization of diagnostics, treatments and vaccines.[132] It invested in technical assistance to resource-poor countries that helped them to build or expand veterinary laboratory services, and to train local veterinarians and technicians in how to make and administer biological products for zoonotic disease control. As with Dalling's Animal Health Branch, veterinary education formed an important part of its strategy.[133]

In all of these efforts, international experts remained acutely aware of local contingencies. Kaplan was especially adamant about avoiding one-size-fits-all approaches (which many of his WHO colleagues were to take in campaigns against malaria and other human infections).[134] This approach probably stemmed partly from these experts' experiences of working in different countries, which alerted them to how specific environmental, cultural, agricultural and economic contexts shaped livestock health and production.[135] The results of their own surveys also revealed that cows came in many different shapes and sizes, with varying physiologies, genetic traits, nutritional needs and biological capacities. There was also great diversity in how they were bred and fed; the natural and built environments in which they were housed, milked and slaughtered; the ways in which they were managed; and the customs and cultures through which they were valued. Therefore, while the principles and aims of livestock improvement might have been universal in kind, in practice there was no single technological fix or magic bullet that could transform them into more efficient suppliers of protein. Programmes had to be modified according to the particular livestock bodies and cultures affected.

---

[132] Kaplan (1954).

[133] For example: FAO/WHO (1962, 1963).

[134] See especially Kaplan (1966).

[135] FAO/WHO (1951) p. 16.

Turning the aspirations of expert committees in Rome or Geneva into bovine bodily realities was made more difficult by the shortage of veterinarians and veterinary assistants: 'We estimate that there are about 1000 million cattle and buffalo in the world ... [But] there are not more than 200,000 qualified veterinarians to cope with this vast general practice and many fewer specialists in husbandry and nutrition.'[136] Moreover, most of these experts were based in developed countries. To overcome this problem, the FAO and WHO committees envisaged the creation of a new kind of veterinarian, which Cockrill referred to as the 'international veterinarian'. This was a trained professional who would be concerned not with the treatment of individual sick or injured animals, but with 'prophylactic, curative or management methods designed to apply collectively to national herds and flocks'.[137] The goal was to foster 'the healthy animal and the means by which it can live its life in a state of health and productivity'.[138] These aspirations reveal, once more, the perception of bovine bodies as analogous to humans, whose health was defined by the WHO in 1948 as 'a state of complete physical, mental, and social well-being and not merely the absence of disease or infirmity'.[139] The general strategies for creating these healthy bodies were also analogous: population and disease control were seen as first measures, which would lay the ground for others.

What this meant for many cows was, in the first instance, culling.[140] In countries such as India, overstocking and overpopulation were viewed by veterinary and livestock planners as the foremost obstacles to improvement.[141] Cattle competed for land with humans, and, as Indian agricultural policy promoted increases in crop production for human consumption, the production of cattle fodder declined, resulting in rising numbers of malnourished cattle.[142] The Indian statistician and influential director of the FAO's Statistics Department, P.V. Sukhatme, pushed for population control in both humans and cattle as key to India's

136 Cockrill (1967) p. 56.

137 Cockrill (1966) p. 9.

138 Cockrill (1964) p. 252.

139 WHO (1946) p. 100.

140 Hambidge (1955) p. 157.

141 Ibid. p. 166.

142 Ibid.

modernization, but the cow's sacred status protected it.[143] In other parts of Asia and in Africa, it was not so fortunate. Old, 'useless' and surplus young cows were slaughtered to improve stock quality, alleviating pressure on pastures, grazing lands and water supplies, and reducing competition with hungry humans for grains and other crops. Surviving cows—which were deemed potentially productive—had their bodies scrutinized by veterinary services, the exact nature of their examination and manipulation shaped by everything from available funding and technical assistance to whether they were owned by large dairies, cooperatives or subsistence farmers.

At the Anand dairy cooperative, a flagship initiative for the FAO and the WHO, the bodies and lives of cows were significantly transformed over a twenty year period.[144] These were mostly Gir cows, the most famous and widely used breed of Zebu dairy cattle in India.[145] When the project began in 1946, they were housed in 'villagers' dwellings or in filthy annexes', but by 1966 they had 'hard standing and comfortable quarters'.[146] Some 30 veterinarians monitored all aspects of their health. Their health and productive capacities were preserved by vaccination against rinderpest and brucellosis; regular monitoring for symptoms of foot-and-mouth disease and bovine tuberculosis; antibiotic treatments for bacterial infections such as mastitis and metritis (inflammation of the uterus); and antihelminthic treatments for chronic parasitic infections. Every village centre was supplied with a veterinary kit containing simple remedies and antiseptics, which was used by trained animal health assistants to treat minor infections and ailments.[147] Feeding had also become more regulated and routinized. No longer reliant on limited grazing and pastures, cows received fodder grown with added nitrogen to improve its nutritional quality, and a daily portion of a vitamin-enriched feed mix to improve the quality and quantity of their milk. A feed-mixing plant, supplied by OXFAM, processed 100 tons of this mix each day for the cooperative's dairy cows and buffalo. Cow genetics were also being modified. With FAO support, the cooperative built an artificial insemination

143 Sukhatme (1963) p. 3, Sukhatme (1966) p. 7.

144 Bellur (1990).

145 Gaur, Kaushik and Garg (2001). The dairy almost made extensive use of buffalo for dairy production.

146 Kesteven (1966) p. 336.

147 Cockrill (1968) pp. 10–12.

centre run by Vergehse Kurien, who had studied nuclear physics in the USA but returned to India in 1946 to manage the cooperative's dairy operations.[148] Trained by the FAO in veterinary and animal science, he worked with FAO experts to develop a breeding programme that would 'increase the genetic potential' of dairy cows and buffalo. Gir bulls were used to improve other native dairy cows, and cows were crossbred with high-yielding Friesian and Jersey cattle. These transformations in the material conditions and biological capacities of the cooperative's cows radically transformed their productivity. In 1946 they were producing between one and two thousand gallons of milk a day. By 1966 this had risen to 25,000 gallons a day.[149]

Kesteven and his colleagues regularly referred to the Anand cooperative as a successful example of how improving the general health of dairy cows could improve the production and supply of milk, leading, in turn, to improvements in human health and productivity.[150] Throughout the 1960s, the APHD vigorously pursued the development of dairy cooperatives as a crucial strategy for getting more protein out of animal bodies and into human bodies.[151] However, translating the local successes of Anand into other parts of India and beyond proved a formidable challenge.[152] The sheer variability of cow bodies and the contexts in which they lived generated equally variable sets of interventions, with varying implications for the lived experiences of cows, and the health and nutrition of their human consumers.

4.4 Conclusion

International concern with protein malnutrition reached its apex in the mid-1960s. Reports issued by the FAO, the WHO and other UN agencies warned of an 'impending protein crisis' in the developing world.[153] Increasing supplies of animal protein—particularly from milk and milk

---

[148] For an excellent account of Kurien's work, see Valenze (2011).

[149] Kesteven (1966) p. 336.

[150] It gave rise to what, by the 1980s, was being called India's 'white revolution'. Bellur et al. (1990).

[151] Simons (1976).

[152] Basu (2009).

[153] *Feeding the Expanding World Population* (1968).

products—lay at the heart of their recommendations and solutions.[154] The FAO's *Third World Food Survey*, issued as part of its Freedom From Hunger Campaign in 1962, concluded that, because in developing countries 'the level of animal protein intake is only one fifth of that in the more developed areas, world food supplies would have to rise by 50% by 1975'.[155] Two years later, the FAO characterized protein shortages as being 'at the heart of the world food problem'. While acknowledging that proteins could be derived from certain vegetable foods, its official view was that it was 'far easier to build satisfactory diets, particularly for these vulnerable groups, when good supplies of animal protein are available'. Meeting the challenge meant that 'much greater resources [had to] be expanded to increase production of such protein-rich foods as fish, meat, eggs and milk'.[156] Such increases could only be achieved by increasing the efficiency of livestock production: healthier, better-nourished cows were key to the creation of healthier, better-nourished humans.[157]

As we have seen, while nutrition experts trained in human medicine played vital roles in characterizing the nature and extent of the crisis, they did not work alone. The belief which emerged through and after the Second World War, that the state of human bodies was deeply dependent on, and also analogous to that of bovine bodies, resulted in a campaign against world hunger which integrated medical expertise with that of vets and animal scientists, under new institutional structures created by the FAO and the WHO. Veterinary and animal experts brought crucial knowledge and skills that derived from their own relationships with food animals. At one and the same time they highlighted the essential roles of animals *and* of animal experts in meeting the urgent and growing needs of a protein-hungry world. If, 'in a world where so many people go hungry, any menace to the health of man's food-yielding animals is a menace to the health of man himself,'[158] then, according to Kesteven and his colleagues, 'in the forces which are fighting protein lack, the veterinarian and the animal production specialist are [the] vanguard.'[159]

---

154 Phillips (1963).

155 FAO (1963) p. 9, FAO (1964a).

156 FAO (1964b) p. i.

157 FAO (1962), FAO (1967).

158 'Healthy Animals' (1964) p. 257.

159 FAO (1967) p. 8.

While experiments and fieldwork on livestock animals had been essential to the development of 'new nutritional knowledge' since the turn of the century, veterinary and animal production experts generated new understandings of the complex and intimate connections between animal health and nutrition, and human health and nutrition, and applied them to the production of more animal protein, especially cow's milk. Since the interwar period, nutritionists had pointed to the miraculous properties of milk in improving the health and efficiency of children, mothers and workers, in their own nations and in colonies stricken by kwashiorkor and other deficiency diseases. After 1945 they recognized and promoted its significance for both human health and the economic health of farmers and agrarian societies in the so-called developing world. Thus, milk, and the bovine bodies that created it, represented a *material site* in which veterinary and nutritional expertise could be integrated for a common purpose. With the formation of new international organizations, most notably the FAO and the WHO, and the making of protein malnutrition into a new field of international action, their formerly loose associations under the interwar 'marriage of agriculture and health' were transformed into institutionally embedded connections and incorporated into the international campaign to feed the world.

All of the human activities described in this chapter were inspired and shaped by cows, in their various roles as producers of food for humans, transmitters of infection to humans, victims of poor health and husbandry, and producers of agricultural profit. While, as we have seen, these roles could inspire quite different responses mounted by different groups of experts, under the campaign to feed the world they began to be considered together. The millions of cows identified in Asia, Africa and Latin America as diseased, malnourished, overpopulated and poorly bred were seen as a key reason why so many humans suffered ill health and poor nutrition: they did not produce enough food for humans and they could also transmit infections to them. It was in order to address these issues—and thereby enable cows to perform better as sources of human food as well as agricultural development—that WHO and FAO experts came together in the 1950s and 1960s to survey, evaluate and work out how to improve bovine bodies.

Yet, while part of the solution was to create new healthy cows by scientifically controlling their diseases, nutrition, breeding and management, doing so involved creating new animal experts—veterinarians, animal scientists, technicians and many more—along with an array of services, facilities, laboratories and clinics that would provide the infrastructure for their work. Therefore, in responding to, and reshaping perceived connections between bovine and human bodies, the incorporation of veterinary medicine and agricultural science into international health agendas had profound and far-reaching impacts. It changed the bodies, surroundings and lived experiences of cows, and brought them into new relationships with a new type of local expert and the facilities and technologies they employed. It also created new opportunities for vets and animal scientists to participate in, and shape, human health agendas. As the next two chapters will reveal, this context proved crucial to the development of self-conscious philosophies of One Medicine, and subsequently One Health.

Bibliography

Allman, Richard and T.S. Hamilton. *Nutritional Deficiencies in Livestock*. Washington: FAO, 1949.

Amrith, S. "Food and Welfare in India c.1900–1950." *Comparative Studies in Society and History* 50 (2008): 1010–35.

Amrith, S. and P. Clavin. "Feeding the World: Connecting Europe and Asia, 1930–1945." *Past & Present* 218 (2013): 29–50.

Arnold, David. "The 'Discovery' of Malnutrition and Diet in Colonial India." *The Indian Economic & Social History Review* 31 (1994): 1–26.

Altschul, A.M. (ed.). *New Protein Foods, Volume 2*. New York: Academic Press, 1976.

Atkins, Peter. "Fattening Children or Fattening Farmers? School Milk in Britain, 1921–1941." *The Economic History Review* 58 (2005): 57–78.

Atkins, Peter. "White Poison? The Social Consequences of Milk Consumption, 1850–1930." *Social History of Medicine* 5 (1992): 207–27.

Atkins, Peter. "The Pasteurisation of England." In *Food, Science, Policy and Regulation in the Twentieth Century: International and Comparative Perspectives*, edited by D.F. Smith and J. Phillips, 37–51. London: Routledge, 2000.

Autret. M. and M. Béhar. *Síndrome Policarencial Infantile (Kwashiorkor) and Its Prevention in Central America*. FAO Nutrition Studies No. 13. Rome: Food and Agriculture Organization, 1954.

Barona, J.L. *The Problem of Nutrition: Experimental Science, Public Health, and Economy in Europe, 1914–1945*. PIE: Peter Lang, 2010.

Barona, J.L. "Nutrition and Health. The International Context during the Interwar Crisis." *Social History of Medicine* 21 (2008): 87–105.

Barona, J.L. *From Hunger to Malnutrition: The Political Economy of Scientific Knowledge in Europe, 1818–1960*. PIE: Peter Lang: 2012.

Bashford, A. *Global Population: History, Geopolitics, and Life on Earth.* New York: Columbia University Press, 2014.

Basu, Pratyusha. "Success and Failure of Crossbred Cows in India: A Place-Based Approach to Rural Development." *Annals of the Association of American Geographers* 99 (2009): 746–766.

Bellur, V. et al. "The White Revolution: How Amul Brought Milk to India." *Long Range Planning* 23.6 (1990), 71–9.

Benson, E. "Animal Writes: Historiography, Disciplinarity, and the Animal Trace." In *Making Animal Meaning*, edited by L. Kalof and G.M. Montgomery, 3–16. East Lansing: Michigan State University Press, 2011.

Beveridge, W.I.B. "Economics of Animal Health." *Veterinary Record* 72 (1960): 810–5.

Biswas, M. *FAO: Its History and Achievements during the First Four Decades, 1945–1985.* Oxford: University of Oxford Press, 2008.

Borowy, I., J.H. Mills, Y-a. Zhang. "Introduction: International Health Organisations and their Histories." *Hygiea Internationalis* 13 (2016): 7–17.

Borowy, I. *Coming to Terms with World Health: The League of Nations Health Organisation 1921–46.* Frankfurt: Peter Lang: 2009.

Brantley, C. "Kikuyu-Maasai Nutrition and Colonial Science: The Orr and Gilks Study in Late 1920s Kenya Revisited." *The International Journal of African Historical Studies* 30 (1997): 49–86.

Brock J.F. and M. Autret. *Kwashiorkor in Africa.* WHO Monograph Series No. 8. Geneva: WHO, 1952.

Bruno, K. "Exporting Agrarian Expertise: Development Aid at the Swedish University of Agricultural Sciences and its Predecessors, 1950–2009." Ph.D thesis, University of Uppsala, 2016.

Burnet, E. and W. Aykroyd. "Nutrition and Public Health." *Bulletin of the Health Organization* iv (1935): 232–474.

Cantor, D. and C. Bonah. "Introduction." In *Meat, Medicine and Human Health in The Twentieth Century*, edited by D. Cantor and C. Bonah, 1–21. London: Chatto & Pickering, 2010.

Carpenter, K.J. "The History of Enthusiasm for Protein." *Journal of Nutrition* 116 (1986): 1364–70.

Carpenter, K.J. *Protein and Energy: A Study of Changing Ideas in Nutrition.* Cambridge: Cambridge University Press, 1994.

Carpenter, K.J. "A Short History of Nutritional Science: Part 3 (1912–1945)." *Journal of Nutrition* 133 (2003): 3023–32.

Cepede, M. "The Fight Against Hunger: Its History on the International Agenda." *Food Policy*, 9.4 (1984): 282–90.

Cockrill, W.R. "The Profession and the Science: International Trends in Veterinary Medicine." *Advances in Veterinary Science* 9 (1964): 251–325.

Cockrill, W.R. "The Role for Animals." Address: Canada. January 11, 1966. FAO AN/MISC/61/66.

Cockrill, W.R. "Patterns of Disease." *Veterinary Record* 78 (1966): 259–66.

Cockrill, W.R. "Of Husbandry and Health." In *World Protein Hunger: The Role of Animals*, edited by Anon, 53–6. FAO: Rome, 1967.

Cockrill, W.R. "Feeding Tomorrow's World." Address at University of Guelph. December 21, 1967. FAO AN/Misc/59.

Cockrill, W.R. "The FAO Veterinarian." Address, Ottawa, Canada. January 19, 1968. FAO AN/Misc/63/68: AN 101955.

Connelly, M. *Fatal Misconception: The Struggle to Control World Population*. Cambridge MA: Harvard University Press, 2008.

Connelly, M. "'To Inherit the Earth': Imagining World Population, from the Yellow Peril to the Population Bomb." *Journal of Global History* 1 (2006): 299–19.

Connelly, M. "Population Control is History: New Perspectives on the International Campaign to Limit Population Growth." *Comparative Studies in Society and History* 45 (2003): 122–47.

Cullather, N. *The Hungry World: America's Cold War Battle against Poverty in Asia*. Cambridge, Mass., 2010.

Cullather, N. "Miracles of Modernization: The Green Revolution and the Apotheosis of Technology." *Diplomatic History* 28 (2004): 227–54.

Collingham, L. *The Taste of War: World War II and the Battle for Food*. New York: Penguin, 2012.

Dalling, T. "The Food and Agriculture Organization of the United Nations." *Canadian Journal of Comparative Medicine* XXI (July 1957): 236–45.

Dalling, T. "The Economic Importance of the Health of Livestock in Milk Production, with Special Reference to the Eradication of Brucellosis and Tuberculosis." Appendix to Report on the FAO/UNICEF/WHO Training Course on Quality Control of Milk and Milk Products, 25–35. FAO: Rome, 1961.

Dejager, T. "Pure Science and Practical Interests: The Origins of the Agricultural Research Council, 1930–1937." *Minerva* 31 (1993): 129–50.

Dodd, N.E. "The Food and Agriculture Organization of the United Nations: Its History, Organization and Objectives." *Agricultural History* 23 (1949): 81–6.

Dupuis, M. *Nature Perfect Food: How Milk Became America's Drink*. New York University Press: New York, 2002.

FAO. *Proposals for a World Food Board and World Food Survey*. Combined Reprint, FAO: Washington, October 1, 1946.

FAO. *Second World Food Survey*. Rome: FAO, 1952.

FAO. *Millions Still Go Hungry*. FAO: Rome 1957.

FAO. *Symposium on Protein Malnutrition*. August 20–24, 1960.

FAO. *Production Yearbook, Volume 16*. FAO: Rome, 1962.

FAO. "The Livestock Industries in Underdeveloped Countries." In *State of Food and Agriculture*, authored by FAO, 129–57. FAO: Rome 1962.

FAO. *Third World Food Survey*. Freedom from Hunger Campaign, Basic Study No. 11, FAO: Rome, 1963.

FAO. "Protein Nutrition: Needs and Prospects." In *State of Food and Agriculture*, authored by FAO, 7–11, 98–132. FAO: Rome 1964a.

FAO. *Protein: At the Heart of the World Food Problem*. World Food Problems No. 5. FAO: Rome 1964b.

FAO. *World Protein Hunger: The Role for Animals*. Rome: FAO/Merck, 1967.

FAO. *Filling the Protein Gap*. FAO: Rome. 1969.

FAO/WHO Expert Committee on Nutrition. *Report of the First Session*. WHO Technical Report Series No. 16. WHO: Geneva, 1949.

FAO/WHO Expert Panel on Brucellosis. *First Report*. WHO TRS, No. 37, 1951.

FAO/WHO Expert Committee on Nutrition. *Report of the Third Session*. WHO Technical Report Series No. 72, WHO: Geneva, 1953.

FAO/WHO Report of the International Meeting on Veterinary Education. London, April 25–30, 1960. WHO Meeting Report, AN-1960/4.

FAO/WHO Expert Panel on Veterinary Education. *Report of the First Meeting*. FAO: Rome, 1962.

FAO/WHO Expert Panel on Veterinary Education. *Report of the Second Meeting* FAO: Rome, 1963.

Feeding the Expanding World Population: International Action to Avert the Impending Protein Crisis, Report to the Economic and Social Council of the Advisory Committee on the Application of Science and Technology to Development. New York: United Nations, 1968.

Gaur, G.K., S.N. Kaushik and R.C. Garg. "The Gir Cattle of India—Characteristics and Present Status." *Animal Genetic Resources Information*, 33 (2001): 21–30.

Gillespie, J. "International Organizations and the Problem of Child Health, 1945–1960." *Dynamis* 23 (2003): 115–42.

Gilks, J.L. and J. Boyd Orr. "The Nutritional Condition of the East African Native." *Lancet* 29 (1927): 561–2.

Grigg, D. "The Nutritional Transition in Western Europe." *Journal of Historical Geography*, 22 (1995): 247–61.

Gratzer, W. *Terrors of the Table: The Curious History of Nutrition*. New York: Oxford University Press, 2005.

Hall, A.D. *The Improvement of Native Agriculture in Relation to Population and Public Health*. Oxford: Oxford University Press, 1936.

Hambidge, G. *The Story of FAO*. New York: D. Van Nostrand Co., 1955.

Hardy, A. "Beriberi, Vitamin B1 and World Food Policy, 1925–1970." *Medical History* 39 (1995): 61–77.

Hardy, A. "Animals, Disease, and Man: Making Connections." *Perspectives in Biology and Medicine* 46 (2003a): 200–15.

Hardy, A. "Professional Advantage and Public Health: British Veterinarians and State Veterinary Services, 1865–1939." *Twentieth Century British History* 14 (2003b): 1–23.

"Healthy Animals—or Hungry Humans?" *WHO Chronicle* 18 (1964): 256–60.

Hodge, J.M. *Triumph of the Expert: Agrarian Doctrines and the Legacies of British Colonialism*. Athens: Ohio University Press, 2007.

Hodge, J.M. "Science, Development and Empire: The Colonial Advisory Council on Agriculture and Animal Health, 1929–43. *The Journal of Imperial and Commonwealth History* 30 (2002): 1–26.

Hutchinson, J.F. "Promoting Child Health in the 1920s: International Politics and the Limits of Humanitarianism." In *The Politics of the Healthy Life: An International Perspective*, edited by Esteban Rodríguez-Ocaña, 131–50. Sheffield: European Association for the History of Medicine and Health, 2002.

Jachertz, R. "To Keep Food Out of Politics: The UN Food and Agricultural Organization, 1945–1965." In *International Organizations and Development, 1945–1990*, edited by M. Frey et al., 76–101. Basingstoke: Palgrave, 2014.

Jones, S.D. *Valuing Animals: Veterinarians and Their Patients in Modern America*. Baltimore: Johns Hopkins University Press, 2003.

Jachertz, R. and A. Nützenadel. "Coping with Hunger? Visions of a Global Food System, 1930–1960." *Journal of Global History* 6 (2011): 99–119.

Joshi, N.R. and R.W. Phillips. *Zebu Cattle of India and Pakistan* Rome: FAO, 1953.

Joshi, N.R., E.A. McLaughlin and R.W. Phillips. *Types and Breeds of Africa Cattle*. Rome: FAO, 1957.

Kaplan, M. "The Concept of Veterinary Public Health and its Application in the World Health Organization." *WHO Chronicle* 7.9 (1953): 227–36.

Kaplan, M. "Zoonoses." *WHO Chronicle* 8.7–8 (1954): 231–4.

Kaplan, M. "Global Priorities in Animal Disease Control." *Annals of the New York Academy of Sciences* 70 (1958): 743–6.

Kaplan, M. "Social Effects of Animal Diseases in Developing Countries." *Bulletin of the Atomic Scientists* 22.9 (1966): 15–21.

Kaplan, M. "Curriculum Vitae. 1976" In *General Information on WHO or Joint Conferences on VPH, 1956–1980*. WHO Archives, Geneva: VH-348-1.

Kay. H.D. "John Boyd Orr." *Biographical Memoirs of the Royal Society* 18 (1972): 43–81.

Kesteven, K.V.L. "The Rising Threat from Animal Diseases." *Discovery* (1961a): 107–9.

Kesteven, K.V.L. "Epizootic Diseases which Threaten to Cause Famine in Large Areas of the World: The Necessity for International Veterinary Co-operation to Strengthen Preventive Medicine Services in all Countries." *British Veterinary Journal* 117 (1961b): 57–60.

Kesteven, K.V.L. "International Animal Health Problems." *Australian Veterinary Journal*, 39 (1963): 406.

Kesteven, K.V.L. "The Veterinarian and the World Food Problem." *Veterinary Record* 79 (1966): 332–7.

Kesteven, K.V.L. "Animals in the Service of Man." In *World Protein Hunger: The Role of Animals*, edited by Anon, 11–12. FAO: Rome, 1967.

Knapp, V.J. "The Democratization of Meat and Protein in late 18th and 19th Century Europe." *Journal of History* 59 (1997): 541–51.

Koolmees, P. "Veterinary Inspection and Food Hygiene in the Twentieth Century." In *Food Science, Policy and Regulation in the Twentieth Century*, edited by D. Smith and J. Phillips, 53–68. London: Routledge, 2000.

League of Nations, Economic Committee. *The Agricultural Crisis, Vol. 1.* Geneva: League of Nations, 1931.

League of Nations. *Interim Report of the Mixed Committee on the Problem of Nutrition.* Geneva: League of Nations, 1936.

League of Nations. *Final report of the Mixed Committee of the League of Nations on the Relation of Nutrition to Health, Agriculture and Economic Policy.* Geneva: League of Nations, 1937.

Little, M. "Imperialism, Colonialism and the New Science of Nutrition: The Tanganyika Experience, 1925–1945." *Social Science & Medicine*, 32 (1991): 11–14.

Marglin, S.A. "Farmers, Seedsmen, and Scientists: Systems of Agriculture and Systems of Knowledge." In *Decolonizing Knowledge: From Development to Dialogue*, edited by Frederique Appfel-Marglin and Stephen Marglin, 185–248. Oxford: Oxford University Press, 1996.

Mayhew, M. "The 1930s Nutrition Controversy." *Journal of Contemporary History* 23 (1988): 445–64.

Maclaren, D. "The Great Protein Fiasco." *Lancet* 304 (1974): 93–6.

McCollum, E.V. *The Newer Knowledge of Nutrition.* New York: Macmillan Co., 1918.

Meyer, K.F. "Animal Diseases and Human Welfare." In *Advances in Veterinary Science, Volume 1*, edited by C.A. Brandly and E.L. Jungherr, 1–48. New York: Academic Press, 1953.

Meyer, K.F. "The Zoonoses in their Relation to Rural Health." Seventh World Health Assembly. March 3, 1954. WHO Archives, Geneva: A7/Technical Discussion/3.

Newman, J.L. "From Definition, to Geography, to Action, to Reaction: The Case of Protein Malnutrition." *Annals of the Association of American Geographers* 85 (1995): 233–45.

Olmstead, Alan and Paul Rhode. *Creating Abundance: Biological Innovation and American Agricultural Development.* Cambridge: Cambridge University Press, 2008.

Orland, B. "Turbo-cows: Producing a Competitive Animal in the Nineteenth and Early Twentieth Centuries." In *Industrialising Organisms: Introducing Evolutionary History*, edited by S. Schrepfer and P. Scranton, 167–90. London: Routledge, 2004.

Orr, J.B. and J.L. Gilks. *Studies of Nutrition: The Physique and Health of Two African Tribes.* London: Medical Research Council, Special Report Series no. 155, 1931.

Orr, J.B. *Food, Health and Income. Report on a Survey of Adequacy of Diet in Relation to Income.* London: Macmillan & Co., 1936.

Orr, J.B. and David Lubbock. *Feeding People in Wartime.* London: Macmillan, 1940.

Orr J.B. *The Role of Food in Post-war Reconstruction.* Geneva: International Labour Organisation, 1943.

Orr, J.B. *Food: The Foundation of World Unity.* London: National Peace Council, 1948.

Orr, J.B. *As I Recall.* London: MacGibbon & Kee, 1966.

Otter, C. "The British Nutrition Transition and its Histories." *History Compass* 10/11 (2012): 812–25.

Pederson, H. "FAO and the Dairy Industry." In *World Protein Hunger: The Role for Animals*, edited by Anon., 21–23. Rome: FAO/Merck, 1967.

Pemberton, J. and J. White. "The Boyd Orr Survey of the Nutrition of Children in Britain, 1937–1939." *History Workshop Journal* 50 (2000): 205–29.

Perkins, J. *Geopolitics and the Green Revolution: Wheat, Genes and the Cold War.* Oxford: Oxford University Press, 1997.

Petty, C. "Primary Research and Public Health: The Prioritization of Nutrition Research in Inter-war Britain." In *Historical Perspectives on the Role of the MRC*, edited by J. Austoker and L. Bryder, 83–108. Oxford: Oxford University Press, 1989.

Phillips, R.W. "Expansion of Livestock Production in Relation to Human Needs." *Nutrition Abstracts and Reviews* 21 (1951): 241–56.

Phillips, R.W. "Cattle." *Scientific American* 198 (June 1958): 51–9.

Phillips, R.W. "Animal Products in the Diets of Present and Future World Populations." *Journal of Animal Science* 22 (1963a): 251–62.

Phillips, R.W. "Animal Agriculture in the Emerging Nations." In *Agricultural Sciences for the Developing Nations*, edited by A.H. Moseman, 15–32. New York: American Association for the Advancement of Science, 1963b.

Phillips, R.W. *FAO: Origins, Formation, Evolution, 1945–1981.* Rome: FAO, 1981.

Popkin, B.M. "Nutritional Patterns and Transitions." *Population and Development Review* 1 (1993): 138–57.

Pritchard, W.R. "Increasing Protein Foods through Improving Animal Health." *Proceedings of the National Academy of Sciences* 56 (1966): 360–9.

Rabinbach, A. *The Human Motor: Energy, Fatigue and the Origins of Modernity.* Berkeley: University of California Press, 1990.

Robertson, T. *The Malthusian Moment: Global Population Growth and the Birth of American Environmentalism.* New Jersey: Rutgers, 2012.

Ruxin, J. "Hunger Science and Politics: FAO, WHO and UNICEF Nutrition Policies, 1945–1978" (PhD diss, University of London, 1996).

Ruxin, J. "The United Nations Protein Advisory Group." In *Food Science, Policy and Regulation in the Twentieth Century: International and Comparative Perspectives,* edited by D.F. Smith and J. Phillips, 151–66. London: Routledge, 2000.

Shaw, J.C. "Problems of Increasing Animal Production." *Proceedings of the Nutrition Society* 21 (1962): 99–106.

Simons, W. "FAO's Industry Cooperative Programme." *Food Policy* 1.2 (1976): 173–4.

"Sir Thomas Dalling." In *Twentieth Century Veterinary Lives,* edited by Bruce Vivash Jones, 64–6. Cirencester: The Granville Press, 2012.

Smith, D.F. and M. Nicolson. "The 'Glasgow School' of Paton, Findlay and Cathcart: Conservative Thought in Chemical Physiology, Nutrition and Public Health." *Social Studies of Science* 19 (1989): 195–238.

Smith, D.F. "Nutrition Science and the Two World Wars." In *Nutrition in Britain: Science, Scientists and Politics in the Twentieth Century,* edited by D.F. Smith, 142–165. Routledge: London, 1997.

Smith, D.F. "The Use of 'Team Work' in the Practical Management of Research in the Inter-War Period: John Boyd Orr at the Rowett Research Institute." *Minerva* 37 (1999): 259–80.

Smith, D.F. "The Rise and Fall of the Scientific Food Committee." In *Food, Science, Policy and Regulation in the Twentieth Century: International and Comparative Perspectives,* edited by D.F. Smith and J. Phillips, 101–16. London: Routledge, 2000.

Soulsby, Lord. "Veterinary Public Health in a Global Economy: A Tribute to Martin Kaplan." University of Pennsylvania School of Veterinary Medicine, 2006. Accessed April 6, 2017. http://cal.vet.upenn.edu/projects/vphconf/kaplan.html.

Staples, A.L.S. *The Birth of Development. How the World Bank, Food and Agriculture Organization, and World Health Organization Changed the World, 1945–1965.* Kent: Ohio, 2006.

Staples, A.L.S. "Norris E. Dodd and the Connections between Domestic and International Agricultural Policy." *Agricultural History* 74 (2000): 393–403.

Stanton, J. "Listening to the Ga: Cicely Williams' Discovery of Kwashiorkor on the Gold Coast." in L. Conrad & A. Hardy (eds.), *Women and Modern Medicine* (Amsterdam: Rodopi, 2001), 149–171.

Steele, J.H. *Animal Disease and Human Health, Freedom from Hunger Campaign*. Basic Study, No. 3. Rome: FAO, 1962.

Steele, J.H. "International and World Developments in Veterinary Public Health with a Comment on Historical Developments." *International Journal of Zoonoses* 6 (1979), 1–32.

Steinfeld, H., P. Gerber, T. Wassenaar, V. Castel, M. Rosales and C. de Haan. *Livestock's Long Shadow: Environmental Issues and Options*. Rome: FAO, 2006.

Sukhatme, P.V. "The Phenomenon of Hunger as FAO Sees It." FAO Report No: 064074, 1963.

Sukhatme, P.V. "Control of Human and Cattle Populations: Food, Fodder and Nutrition Problems in India." *Commerce Annual*, December 1966. FAO WS/57042.

Terroine, E.F. "The Protein Component in the Human Diet." *League of Nations Quarterly Bulletin of the Health Organisation* 5.3 (1936): 427–92.

Tappan, J. "The True Fiasco: The Treatment and Prevention of Severe Acute Malnutrition in Uganda, 1950–74." In *Global Health in Africa: Historical Perspectives on Disease Control*, edited by T. Giles-Vernick and J.L.A Webb, 92–113, Athena: Ohio University Press, 2013.

Tilley, H. *Africa as a Living Laboratory: Empire, Development and the Problem of Scientific Knowledge, 1870–1950*, Chicago: University of Chicago Press, 2011.

Trentmann, F. "Coping with Shortage: The Problem of Food Security and Global Visions of Coordination, c.1890–1950." In *Food and Conflict in the Age of the Two World Wars*, edited by F. Trentmann, 13–48. Basingstoke: Palgrave, 2006.

Trowell, H.C. "Infantile Pellagra." *Transactions of the Royal Society of Tropical Medicine and Hygiene* 33.4 (1940): 398–404.

Trowell, H.C. "Malignant Malnutrition (Kwashiorkor)." *Transactions of the Royal Society of Tropical Medicine and Hygiene* 42.5 (1949): 417–41.

Valenze, D. *Milk: A Local and Global History*. New Haven: Yale University Press, 2011.

Vernon, J. *Hunger: A Modern History*. London, England: Harvard University Press, 2007.

Vernon, K. "Science for the Farmer? Agricultural Research in England 1909–36." *Twentieth Century British History* 8 (1997): 310–33.

"Veterinary Public Health: A Review of the WHO programme 1." *WHO Chronicle* 28.3 (1974): 103–12.

Waddington, K. "To Stamp Out 'So Terrible a Malady': Bovine Tuberculosis and Tuberculin Testing in Britain, 1890–1939." *Medical History* 48 (2004): 29–48.

Waterlow J.C. (ed.). *Protein Malnutrition*. Cambridge: Cambridge University Press, 1955.

Waterlow J.C. and J.M.L Stephen (eds). *Human Protein Requirements and Their Fulfillment in Practice.* New York: John Wright and Sons, 1957.

Weindling, P. "The Role of International Organizations in Setting Nutritional Standards in the 1920s and 1930s." In *The Science and Culture of Nutrition, 1840–1940*, edited by H. Kamminga and A. Cunningham, 48–74. Amsterdam: Rodopi, 1995.

Way, W. *A New Idea Each Morning: How Food and Agriculture Came Together in One International Organisation.* Canberra: ANU E Press, 2013.

Weis, T. *The Ecological Hoofprint: The Global Burden of Industrial Livestock.* London: Zed Books, 2013.

Welshman, J. "School Meals and Milk in England and Wales, 1906–45." *Medical History* 41 (1997): 6–29.

Whyte, R.O. *Land, Livestock and Human Nutrition in India.* New York: Praeger, 1968.

Wiley, A.S. "Milk for 'Growth': Global and Local Meanings of Milk Consumption in China, India, and the United States." *Food and Foodways* 19 (2011): 11–33.

Wiley, A.S. *Cultures of Milk: The Biology and Meaning of Dairy Products in the United States and India* Cambridge MA: Harvard University Press, 2014.

WHO. Constitution of the World Health Organization. *Official Records of the World Health Organization. No. 2. Summary of Proceedings, Minutes, and Final Acts of the International Conference.* Off. Rec. Wld Hlth Org, 1946.

WHO/FAO Expert Group on Zoonoses. "Report on the First Session." *WHO Tech Report Series* 40 (1951).

WHO/FAO Expert Group on Zoonoses. "Second Report." *WHO Tech Report Series* 169 (1959).

Williams, C.D. "A Nutritional Disease of Childhood Associated with a Maize Diet." *Archives of Diseases in Childhood* 8 (1933): 423–33.

Williams, C.D. "Kwashiorkor: A Nutritional Disease of Children Associated with Maize Diet." *The Lancet* 226 (1935): 1151–2.

Woods, A. "The Farm as Clinic: Veterinary Expertise and the Transformation of Dairy Farming, 1930–50." *Studies in History and Philosophy of Biological and Biomedical Sciences* 38 (2007): 462–87.

Woods, A. "Breeding Cows, Maximizing Milk: British Veterinarians and the Livestock Economy, 1930–50." In *Healing the Herds: Essays on Livestock Economies and the Globalization of Veterinary Medicine*, edited by K. Brown and D. Gilfoyle. 59–75. Athens: Ohio University Press, 2010.

Worboys, M. "The Discovery of Colonial Malnutrition Between the Wars." In *Imperial Medicine and Indigenous Societies*, edited by David Arnold, 208–25. Manchester: Manchester University Press, 1988.

CHAPTER 5

The Parasitological Pursuit: Crossing Species and Disciplinary Boundaries with Calvin W. Schwabe and the *Echinococcus* Tapeworm, 1956–1975

Rachel Mason Dentinger

In August 1964, on a sheep ranch in the San Joaquin valley in California, a five-year-old boy, known to us only as 'J.O.', leapt to the ground from the back of a flatbed truck. Though the 0.75-metre drop should have been trivial, J.O. fell to the ground in tears, collapsing in sudden abdominal pain. By evening he was admitted to the hospital with suspected appendicitis. Instead, doctors discovered that J.O.'s liver and lungs were strewn with cysts, varying in diameter from 2 to 10 cm. His leap had ruptured a cyst in his liver, causing pain and a subsequent reaction as its contents spread inside his body.[1]

The cysts that J.O.'s doctors removed that night were larval bodies of the tapeworm *Echinococcus granulosus*, which were bequeathed to him by one of the many dogs that lived on his family's ranch. His father, Salvador, like other sheep ranchers of Basque descent, kept a range of dogs: from his favourite, Blue, who was treated as a pet, to the sheepdogs Murico and Pancho, who were treated as workers.[2] As a child roaming the ranch, J.O. might have tussled with any of these dogs; and, for his part, the dog would have responded affectionately by licking the

[1] Araujo et al. (1975) p. 298.

[2] These are the names of dogs on the ranch in 1968, but they illustrate the importance granted to the dogs by the humans, including Araujo et al. (1975), which listed their names, ages and sexes.

A. Woods et al., *Animals and the Shaping of Modern Medicine*, Medicine and Biomedical Sciences in Modern History,
https://doi.org/10.1007/978-3-319-64337-3_5

child's face. Since the dog's faeces were likely teeming with the tapeworm's eggs, which he had picked up from eating the flesh of diseased sheep on the ranch, so too was his tongue. And in this commonplace domestic interaction, *E. granulosus* entered J.O.'s body.

The child's infection reached a crisis point at a time when parasitologists, physicians and epidemiologists were not yet convinced that *E. granulosus* was an endemic resident of the USA. Instead, many believed that this particular parasite was only an import, an infection that immigrants contracted prior to their arrival. However, cases like J.O.'s—infections in people who had been born in the USA and never travelled outside of it—belied this assumption.[3] The case of J.O. and a subsequent study of his family soon became part of a multifaceted investigation into *E. granulosus*, a large-scale study conducted by American veterinary epidemiologist Calvin W. Schwabe with the aim of understanding how the parasite could be transmitted and sustained in the USA, below the radar of the public health system.

A pivotal figure in this volume, Schwabe was one of the original formulators of One Medicine (OM), a later twentieth-century philosophy predicated on the idea that human and non-human health were intimately connected and therefore most effectively studied in tandem. As this chapter will demonstrate, this philosophy grew from, and was reflected in, his efforts to understand *E. granulosus* as a biological and a cultural phenomenon, through the application of scientific methods that together transgressed multiple disciplinary boundaries. His investigations into how the parasitic animal both shaped and was shaped by the relationships between other animals in the wild, on the farm and within the homes of Basque sheep farmers illuminate his multidisciplinary ethos, but also demonstrate his rootedness in a parasitological tradition that placed the parasite at the centre of the study, treating it as an animal as biologically interesting and important as its host. For Schwabe, the human, wild and domestic animals that *E. granulosus* infected were not victims but hosts, which interacted with their tapeworm partner in a number of ecologically complex ways.

This view of parasites *as animals* unsettled the prevailing dichotomy between humans and other animals, and between the biological study of animal life and the medical study of animals as shapers of human health. It drew on older traditions, those explored in Chapters 2 and 3, which were developed in the context of nineteenth-century zoology, natural history, and agricultural and veterinary research, and which

[3] On shifting assumptions about infection on US soil, see Brooks et al. (1959).

saw knowledge about animal and human bodies and diseases as mutually informative. But it also gained strength from post-Second-World-War efforts to promote international health, which, as described in Chapter 4, brought the health of humans and animals together in new and important ways. In tracking the parasite that drew Schwabe onward and led him between different species and domains, this chapter demonstrates both the continuity, and the continually evolving nature and circumstances, of cross-species approaches to health, showing how this was done, robustly and productively, through cross-disciplinary tools and alliances. It will follow Schwabe's lead in placing *E. granulosus* at the centre of historical analysis, and approaching it as an animal that merits historical investigation in its own right and for its own sake,[4] not simply on account of the threat that it posed to human health—which is the role most often awarded these organisms by medical practitioners and medical historians alike.[5]

In exploring how Schwabe studied, tracked and conceptualized the parasite, this chapter also throws new light on his life and work. As described in Chapter 6, the movement for OM which Schwabe spearheaded would not begin to gather momentum until the last decades of the century. However, from 1964, when Schwabe published his first monograph, *Veterinary Medicine and Human Health* (*VMHH*), he was building an argument and a body of practical recommendations for the joint practice of human–non-human medicine, which would become the basis of OM and its later incarnation, the twenty-first-century One Health (OH) movement, which adopted Schwabe as its figurehead.[6] When discussing his role as 'founding father' of OM and the field of veterinary epidemiology, commentators tend to focus attention mainly on the years following 1974, when Schwabe largely left the laboratory behind and launched a new epidemiological phase of his career, working as a global health advocate for the World Health Organization (WHO), and as an academic and administrative bridge between medical and veterinary training. This has elided important aspects of his earlier,

[4] Benson (2011) p. 5.

[5] For further reading on this role and others assigned to animals in the history of medicine, see Appendix: Annotated Bibliography of Animals in the History of Medicine.

[6] As discussed in Chapter 6, OM was renamed OH closer to the turn of the century, when a series of worrying zoonotic pandemics (e.g. SARS and avian influenza) vividly demonstrated just how intimate the human–non-human connection really is.

parasitological experience, which, as this chapter demonstrates, was crucial to his story and to the wider histories of OM and OH.

To begin, I reconstruct Schwabe's first decade of research on *E. granulosus* at the American University of Beirut (AUB), placing his work theoretically and practically in the disciplinary context of parasitology, showing how he drew from and elaborated on this tradition in order to understand the tapeworm, which was widespread among the human and non-human inhabitants of Beirut. Through this work, *E. granulosus* occupied multiple roles, far beyond that of the circumscribed 'infective agent'. It served as a point of comparison in understanding the biology of other animals,[7] as an ally in the pursuit of scientific knowledge in the laboratory,[8] and a symbiont with the ability to both respond adaptively to and shape its own environment—in this case, the bodies of the larger animals that hosted it, *and* the careers of the researchers whose lives' work revolved around it.

In the second section I show how the parasite drew Schwabe out of the laboratory and into the city, where its dynamic movement between the host populations of Beirut, including both human and non-human animals, intrigued and challenged parasitologists. Schwabe responded to the parasite's challenge by developing a new mode of parasitological pursuit, observing how biological and sociocultural factors interacted to provide new opportunities for *E. granulosus.* Finally, in the third section, I follow Schwabe as he transplanted this new culturally sensitive epidemiology to a new geography, moving from Beirut to California. At this point I return to the Basque sheep farm, where a new and as-yet-undetected epicentre of *E. granulosus* had developed. Schwabe, with his parasitological background, a methodological arsenal developed in Beirut, and his special sensitivity to the parasite that he had tracked for decades, quickly detected its presence and resumed his pursuit of it in this new environment. In this phase of his career, Schwabe adopted more epidemiological and programmatic emphases. Yet this period did not represent a dramatic divergence from his earlier work, and his commitment to *E. granulosus* persisted. Further, it is in this final transition that we see most vividly how each elaboration of his career—from laboratory to population, from Beirut to Kenya to California, from veterinary medicine to OM—took shape in response to the movement of this miniscule, parasitic animal.

---

[7]See Chapter 2.

[8]See Chapter 3.

5.1 Pursuing *Echinococcus* in Beirut: The Parasitology of Calvin W. Schwabe

In 1956, Calvin Schwabe moved his young family from Boston, Massachusetts, to Beirut, Lebanon. He had just completed his doctorate of science in parasitology and public health at Harvard University, as well as a postdoctoral fellowship, funded by the National Institutes of Health (NIH), investigating the physiology of a rodent parasite. His qualifications did not stop there: with a doctor of veterinary medicine, a master of public health and a master of science in zoology, Schwabe was well prepared for his new post as the associate professor of parasitology and chairman of the Department of Parasitology at AUB, where he would rapidly launch a research programme focused on the tapeworm parasite *E. granulosus*.[9]

Hoping to 'hit the ground running', Schwabe had already begun to consider possible research subjects before leaving Boston.[10] He knew that *E. granulosus*—which constituted a 'medical and economic problem on all inhabited continents'[11]—was widespread in Beirut and wielded a significant impact on human health. The life cycle of this parasite had already been worked out. It had a diminutive worm stage that lived mostly in

[9]MS in zoology from the University of Hawaii, 1950; DVM, Auburn University (Alabama), 1954; and MPH in tropical public health from Harvard, 1955. Schwabe (2004) p. 208. Schwabe later recalled that he had never once attended a class on parasitology *per se*. Schwabe (n.d.) pp. 153, 186. However, his sequence of degrees, in combination with his clinical, agricultural and laboratory research experience in parasitology, qualified him for this position. While a biology undergraduate at Virginia Polytechnic Institute, he became an 'Assistant in Parasitology' at the Virginia Agricultural Experimentation Station, an experience that he repeatedly referred to as the foundation of his parasitological training. Indeed, the importance of this undergraduate job to him is evident in that he continued to list it on his CV for the duration of his career. His Master's research project at the University of Hawaii focused on an agricultural parasite of chickens (Schwabe 1951, 1957). Then, from 1950 to 1953, while earning his DVM at Auburn, he worked again as a parasitologist, this time in a US Department of Agriculture laboratory. After leaving Auburn for Boston, he became a staff affiliate in parasitology and zoonoses at Angell Memorial Hospital. 'Curriculum Vitae' (n.d.).

[10]Schwabe (n.d.) pp. 212, 336.

[11]Schwabe (1964) p. 208.

the guts of canines (the 'definitive host').[12] Its eggs exited canine bodies via their faeces, to enter the bodies of humans and other animals that came into contact with it, such as livestock that grazed on faeces-contaminated pastures. Within the intestines of these 'intermediate hosts', the eggs hatched and a new larval stage penetrated the intestinal wall, travelled through the host's bloodstream and came to rest in any number of locations, particularly the lungs or the liver. There it integrated itself into the host's tissues and developed into a cyst, on whose sheltered interior a multitude of larval parasites thrived. Carnivores that gained access to these bodies consumed the larvae, and the cycle began again.

Cysts grew very slowly over the course of many years but could reach extreme sizes, containing several litres of fluid, 'swarming' with thousands of larvae.[13] Outside this restless vitality, however, cysts seemed remarkably benign. *E. granulosus* parasites appeared to work away unnervingly: rooting themselves tenaciously in the host's tissues, growing perpetually, and remaining entirely invisible to the outside observer. Australian *E. granulosus* researcher Harold Dew had observed in 1930 how the cyst 'merges gradually and intimately into the tissue of the host',[14] to the extent that 'there seems to be a perfect symbiosis between the parasite and the host tissues'.[15] As a result, cysts often went unnoticed by their hosts.

[12] *E. granulosus* is the smallest tapeworm; compared with the pork tapeworm, *Taenia solium*, which can reach a length of 7 metres, the maximum length of *E. granulosus* is 6 millimetres: Craig and Faust (1964) pp. 640, 657. Of 'the many parasites which infest man', prominent parasitologist and veterinary doctor T.W.M. Cameron claimed in 1927 (p. 547), 'none is more serious than the larval stage of tapeworm of the genus *Echinococcus*.' For other examples of claims that *E. granulosus* infection is the 'most serious' tapeworm infection, see Rausch (1952), Noble and Noble (1964) and Baer (1971).

[13] 'swarming with scolices' from Barnett (1939) p. 593.

[14] Dew (1930) p. 275.

[15] Dew (1958) p. 448. At the time, Dew wrote that 'symbiosis' might have been taken to mean merely that two different animals live together, with no connotation of benefit or cost in the relationship. This strict definition of 'symbiosis' subsumes a range of phenomena, from severely asymmetrical relationships (e.g. parasitism) to symmetrically beneficial relationships (e.g. mutualism). However, since its first invocation in 1877, the meaning of 'symbiosis' has often been confused and regarded by many as a synonym for 'mutualism'. (On the shifting definitions of 'symbiosis', see Sapp (1994), especially pp. 3–34). Taking this into consideration, in the context of a paper already focused on a parasitic organism, the inclusion of the word 'symbiosis', particularly as it was preceded by the word 'perfect', suggests that Dew saw the relationship between *Echinococcus* and its host as at the very least ambiguous, and not strictly deleterious to the host, despite the fact that he, as a surgeon, had seen his share of the damage that the cysts could do to the human body.

The abbreviated lives of sheep meant that few ever suffered symptoms of echinococcosis, although its presence was frequently revealed on the transformation of their bodies into meat.[16] In humans (which were only infected via definitive hosts, such as dogs, and not other intermediate hosts, such as sheep[17]), cysts were often discovered only when in the operating theatre for a different reason, or undergoing post-mortem examinations (after death by an entirely different cause). However, later in human life when cysts grew so large that they began to impinge on the functioning of an organ, or when—as in the case of J.O.—a cyst burst, the implications for human health were severe.

The life cycle and habits of *E. granulosus* suggested a wily and insidious parasite which managed simultaneously to present a health threat to humans and to perform the movements of a complex animal in its own right. It was seen as an animal that had its own ecological demands and outputs, and was capable of having tangible and intangible effects on its larger animal hosts—which constituted a responsive ecosystem for the equally responsive parasite, and through which it associated into a 'host–parasite biological unit'.[18] These features had already attracted the attention of a number of researchers. Following the disciplinary norms of parasitology, they had worked in the laboratory to probe the interactive relationships between *E. granulosus* and its human–animal hosts, and the participants' physiological and biochemical responses to that relationship. At AUB, during the 1930s, an earlier generation of parasitologists had attempted to induce immunity to infection in Lebanese populations

[16]For example, in 1852, T.H. Huxley was called in to London Zoo to examine the remains of a 'fine female zebra' who died of an accidentally broken neck, and whose liver had been revealed, on post-mortem examination, to be 'one mass of cysts, varying in size from a child's head downwards'. Nevertheless, the zebra itself 'had always appeared to be quite healthy, and it was in perfectly good condition.' Huxley (1898) p. 197. Veterinarians, doctors and parasitologists all marvelled at the appearance of these hosts, whom they could only ever describe as vigorous specimens: infected humans were most often 'well nourished and of an athletic physique', while non-human hosts, whether monkey or moose, were evidently 'in good health.' For the human patient, see Tenenbaum (1937); for the monkey, see Nelson and Rausch (1963); for the moose, see Rausch (1952).

[17]The definitive host is the one in which a parasite reaches sexual maturity. In intermediate hosts, the parasite passes through asexual larval stages.

[18]Baer (1971) p. 8. This was often taken to the extreme of assuming that evolutionarily older host–parasite relationships would be, as a rule, more benign—an assumption with staying power despite being debunked multiple times. Méthot (2012).

of sheep and dogs. Promising results were obtained, but as the immunization was only ever partial, and soon the researchers returned or emigrated to the USA, the programme lost energy.[19]

Schwabe revitalized this defunct AUB research programme through his parasitological practices. Between 1958 and 1965 he and his team published more than 15 papers on *E. granulosus*. They began by closely examining the interface between its cysts and the bodies of its hosts. Conceiving of *E. granulosus* as both responder to and shaper of its host environment, they addressed longstanding questions: Was it the agent of a dangerous infection or was it a peaceful symbiont? Was the cyst fundamentally inert or vitally alive? How did the parasite's ecosystem—the interior world of the host—affect its ability to thrive?[20]

Answering these questions required attention to the physiological mechanisms of the parasite. Schwabe and his team probed how cysts grew and how they exchanged fluids and gases with the interior host ecosystem.[21] Their tables of data reveal efforts to correlate the weight of the cyst with varying salt concentrations in its environment. These observations, and their prior conceptions of *E. granulosus* as an active animal, capable of responding to its environment and shaping it to suit its own needs, led them to conclude that the cyst was able to actively maintain its internal water level relative to the water in its environment, through its own 'behaviour' rather than as a result of passive diffusion across the membrane of the cyst.[22]

To conduct these enquiries, Schwabe needed to find ways of encouraging vigorous growth in his parasitic subject. Consequently, he sought new conditions and new host animals in the hope of finding—in the words of Webster and Cameron, writing in 1961—a way to 'maintain hydatid infections which grew rapidly and luxuriantly in animals which

[19] Because the widespread infection of dogs was recognized as the primary problem in Beirut, these AUB researchers had focused on the possibility of immunizing dogs against the parasite. For example: Turner et al. (1936). After multiple AUB parasitologists relocated or returned to the USA soon after these studies, *E. granulosus* research in Beirut dwindled.

[20] His team mainly comprised parasitologists whom Schwabe had either brought to AUB or worked hard to promote, and all of these launched successful research careers working with Schwabe during this period.

[21] For example: Farhan et al. (1959), Schwabe (1959) and Schwabe et al. (1959).

[22] For the table and reference to cyst's 'behaviour', see Schwabe (1959) p. 21.

could be kept conveniently in the laboratory'.[23] Paradoxically, therefore, although Schwabe, like earlier researchers, worked under the auspices of disease prevention, funded and motivated through the desire of governmental agencies and corporations striving to control and prevent parasitic infection in humans and livestock,[24] his actual research sought to stimulate their 'rapid' and 'luxuriant' growth in the laboratory. Parasitologists thereby became parasites' allies: their experimental protocols provided material resources for the parasites' success, while the parasites became dependent on their efforts for their survival.

This approach can also be seen in efforts to test the survival and vitality of larvae in response to different hosts, which was a common parasitological practice. *E. granulosus* researchers found a great deal of variation in patterns of response. For example, they found that cysts from a sheep could easily infect mice and rabbits, but rarely rats; part of their task was then seeking the factors that made such cross-infection more or less successful.[25] For his part, Schwabe collected cysts from a human brain and coaxed them back to life in a 'secondary' mouse host—a form of cross-infection that had proved exceedingly difficult in the past. Cutting open the mouse's abdomen, he discovered and photographed enormous clusters of cysts. Micrographs of cyst cross-sections showed the parasitic larvae multiplying on its interior.[26] These findings made visible the extent to which the parasite had altered the interior cellular landscape of the host. They laid bare the processes that usually happen beyond the sensory and analytical reach of medical scientists. Through such work—which constituted a type of human–non-human 'co-evolutionary process'—*E. granulosus* was transferred experimentally from one animal body to another, and gained access to new host species and a form of immortality.[27] In return, Schwabe gained an enriched

---

[23] Webster and Cameron (1961) p. 877.

[24] For example: Schwabe (1959).

[25] From Australia to France, in centres of vigorous *Echinococcus* research, parasitologists paired studies of the minute chemical properties of the hydatid cyst wall with experiments attempting to pass those same cysts from humans to pigs, or to transfer cysts between rabbits, squirrels, mice and gerbils. Others found that cysts from sheep could infect mice and rabbits, while rats resisted infection; conversely, cysts from horses could infect mice and rats, while rabbits were resistant. All of these cases are reported in Webster and Cameron (1961) p. 878.

[26] Schwabe et al. (1959) pp. 31–4.

[27] Benson (2011) p. 5.

knowledge of the parasites' behaviour and a new level of control over them in the laboratory.

As *E. granulosus* allied itself with Schwabe, he responded in kind, relying upon the parasite in his efforts to advance his career. As the sole faculty member of AUB with veterinary training, Schwabe was under especially intense pressure to demonstrate his particular value to his medically trained (and occasionally dubious) colleagues.[28] Working on *E. granulosus* enabled him to elaborate his professional network,[29] building bridges across departments at AUB, actively collaborating, for example, with colleagues in the chemistry department, who had the instruments and techniques he needed to gauge the osmotic balance maintained by his tapeworm subject within the host's body.[30] As with the other animals whose histories are documented in this volume, *E. granulosus* promoted working across disciplinary boundaries as much as species boundaries. It also enabled Schwabe to revitalize AUB as a centre for *E. granulosus* research. In his unpublished autobiography, he writes of the visits of many international researchers, in an expanding network that would continue to be invaluable to him in the coming decades.[31] Indeed, his growing experience with the parasite seems to have been the primary factor that drew many of these researchers and which established him as one of the world's experts on it.[32]

---

[28] In his autobiography, he describes his position as the only veterinarian, writing that his choice of research subject was a consciously strategic decision. By his recollection, he was also the youngest department chair in the history of AUB. He recounts some early challenges to his expertise, including an instance of one of his colleagues bringing him what he (the MD) assumed was a fungal infection but which Schwabe revealed to be a parasite. Schwabe (n.d.) p. 217.

[29] For example, in the Webster and Cameron paper cited above (1961), both Calvin Schwabe and prominent Swiss parasitologist Jean Baer (mentioned above) are thanked for the provision of infective parasitic material and infected hosts. Schwabe sent *E. granulosus* from Lebanon and Baer sent an infected vole from Switzerland. Additionally, researchers from Alaska, Toronto, Chile and other locations contributed material for the research (all thanked on p. 880), thus demonstrating the complex web of professional connection and recognition that was enabled by this parasite.

[30] Farhan et al. (1959).

[31] Schwabe (n.d.) pp. 93, 95.

[32] According to his own recollections in his autobiography, that is, but also—as the following sections will demonstrate—the degree to which the WHO came to rely on him suggests the same.

5.2 *Echinococcus* Leaves the Laboratory: Schwabe's Parasitology at the Population Level

While it was the parasite's dynamic interaction with individual host bodies that first captured Schwabe's attention, leading him to conduct laboratory-based investigations into the bodies of experimental animals, its movement beyond this narrow sphere subsequently pushed him to examine the host–parasite interaction writ large—that is, on the human population of Beirut. For the first time in his career, he began to focus on the *human* animal. Via this new species of host, his parasitic subject led him to develop newly epidemiological pathways of enquiry.

These enquiries began in the hospital operating theatre, where signs of *E. granulosus* infection in humans first typically surfaced in the hydatid cysts made visible through surgical disruptions to bodily integrity. Thanks to a widely ranging and heavily infected dog population, human infection was rampant in Beirut, and for this new component of his research, Schwabe accessed a trove of data. He began with the records of 54 Lebanese hospitals, analysing the detailed records of 918 surgical cases that had addressed or uncovered *E. granulosus* infections between 1949 and 1959. The correlations he found were striking—in pursuing his pet parasite, Schwabe had stumbled onto a powerful set of insights about the importance of human cultural traditions in parasitic infection. Christian patients, he found, numbered twice as many as Muslim.[33] The study, published in 1961, claimed that 'religion was a real epidemiological factor',[34] positing Muslim cultural prohibitions against close contact with dogs as a possible explanation. Later efforts to gather further data suggested that Christian families were more likely to keep dogs as family pets and to encourage children to develop affectionate bonds with them.[35]

---

[33] Schwabe and Daoud (1961) p. 377. They also found that shoemakers experienced the disease disproportionately, surmising that placing shoe tacks and thread in their mouths might make them more susceptible. Later it was recognized that dog faeces was used in the process of tanning leather, which explained infection in shoemakers and other people working with leather in Lebanon.

[34] Ibid. p. 379.

[35] Abou-Daoud and Schwabe (1964).

On the level of the population, then, through a complex of culture-bound interactions between humans and dogs, Schwabe had discovered another way in which *E. granulosus* responded to and shaped its environment. In this case, statistics captured how the parasite infiltrated the cultural ecosystem of Lebanese society. Dogs were ascribed a variety of roles, from companions to stray mongrels, some welcomed into the human sphere and some excluded from it. In either case, canine relationships with humans became a key ecological factor that enabled or obstructed the parasite's passage to humans. In invoking the importance of these domestic social relationships alongside surgical data, Schwabe used ephemeral connections between humans and dogs to follow the parasitic animal as it moved from one host ecosystem to another. The parasitological research tradition had been driven in just this manner, by animals such as *E. granulosus*, which, in responding to their environments, often created new symbiotic relationships that were based on the biological qualities of the host animal—Schwabe expanded on this tradition in his explicit inclusion of their social and cultural behaviours as well.

With his success at AUB, Schwabe's sphere of influence grew and he increasingly took to the global health stage. In Beirut he had pursued *E. granulosus* into the human realm, finding that movement between non-human and human research gave him a fuller sense of the parasite's biology. This work only expanded when the WHO first asked him to travel on their behalf in 1960, contracting him to visit Cyprus and investigate the island's endemic *E. granulosus*. This trip was quickly followed by a series of trips to multiple far-flung centres of *E. granulosus* infection, from New Zealand to Argentina, which would mark the initiation of the WHO's global effort to control the disease.[36] Most critical for his own career at this time, however, was Schwabe's trip to Kenya in January 1961, on a Fulbright Scholarship that would relocate his family to a home outside Nairobi for the entire year.[37]

While Schwabe's explicit goal during his stay in Kenya was to finish writing the manuscript that would become his first edition of *VMHH*, he pursued the *E. granulosus* parasite into this new setting as well. In 1958, a brief 'Note on Human Hydatid Disease in Kenya', published

[36] On his travels see Schwabe (n.d.) p. 260, and p. 8 for a statement that he initiated the programme.

[37] Schwabe (n.d.) pp. 439–41.

in *The East African Medical Journal*, had captured his attention. It suggested an unusually high level of *E. granulosus* infection among the pastoralist tribes of Kenya—the Turkana and the Maasai. In this 'intriguing' note, which Schwabe would still remember decades later,[38] J.R. Wray, a British medical officer in the rural northwest of the country, claimed to have operated on twenty-five human hydatid cysts in three years. Wray also made a series of surprising assertions about the path taken by the *E. granulosus* parasite in this environment, so far from the Lebanese city where Schwabe had first encountered it. Wray suggested that, in Kenya, *E. granulosus* might find its way into the guts of wild carnivores, such as hyenas and jackals, and then infect tribespeople through 'their habit of smearing themselves with earth'. This inference, of the possible involvement of wild carnivores, was based partly on a lack of data on infection in dogs; a 'definitive' host, the role fulfilled by canids, was required for *E. granulosus* to complete its life cycle. However, Wray had an even more intriguing hypothesis about the parasite's movements in store: Because, he wrote, Maasai tribespeople did not inter their dead, but left their bodies where they could be consumed by wild carnivores, *E. granulosus* may even have found a way to cycle directly between humans and carnivores.[39]

The implications of this case for Schwabe—a parasitologist trained in veterinary medicine, just making his first forays into human medicine—would have been extraordinary. The tradition in the parasitological literature of the preceding decades had been to consider the human host a 'dead-end' for *E. granulosus*, an 'accidental host', relative to the sheep, which served as the 'normal', 'natural' or 'usual intermediate host' for the parasite.[40] In fact, graphic depictions of the *E. granulosus* life cycle most often feature a dog and a sheep in the centre; a human host may be excluded entirely from the image,[41] or decentred, visually communicating its 'dead-end' status.[42] After all, the cysts embedded in the sheep's

[38] He recalls the 'intriguing' note in Schwabe (n.d.) p. 444.

[39] Wray (1958).

[40] For example: Bogitsh et al. (2005) p. 288.

[41] For example: ibid. p. 290. The exclusion of a human from the diagram is especially interesting, given that this is a textbook on human parasitology.

[42] For example: 'Parasites—Echinococcosis' (2012).

flesh or organs are far more likely to be eaten by a dog, which then perpetuated the infection. By contrast, owing to culturally contingent burial practices, the human host, while physiologically identical to the sheep from the perspective of *E. granulosus*, is highly unlikely to be consumed by a dog or any other carnivore after death. Thus the infection typically passed from dog to human ends there, and the cysts 'swarming' with larvae die soon after their human host passes away. But the Kenyan case raised a new question: What if an infected human body were actually made available for consumption by canines, upending parasitological expectations with an unusual human cultural practice? In that case, suddenly the assumption that humans were 'accidental' hosts would reveal itself to be a strangely anthropocentric way of dividing human bodies from those of other animals.

Schwabe's interest in how *E. granulosus* might travel through this network of biological and social connections spurred a new investigation into the shared parasites of pastoralist human and wild carnivore populations in Kenya. On arriving in Kenya in 1961, Schwabe quickly teamed up with British parasitologist George Nelson, who worked at the Medical Research Laboratory in Nairobi. Nelson was eager to have Schwabe join him on safari in order to examine the gut contents of hyenas in person. Having killed a zebra as bait, they sought hyenas for hours until eventually Schwabe was rewarded by the clear evidence of *E. granulosus* infection in the guts of three hyenas, which they caught and dissected.[43]

Schwabe also had the opportunity to directly observe the human pastoralist infection that so intrigued him. In March 1961 the medical officer holding Wray's old post, some 200 miles north of Nairobi, contacted Schwabe to invite him to witness—and, ultimately, assist—in the surgical removal of a very large abdominal hydatid cyst. Schwabe combined this powerful surgical experience with an examination of the records of this 'one little bush hospital', after which he estimated that the infection rate of Turkana tribespeople was 'probably higher ... than any other population in the world!'[44] Writing in *VMHH* soon after this

---

[43] Schwabe (n.d.) pp. 445–6

[44] Ibid. p. 448. It is important to note that many of the details found in Schwabe's autobiography, cited here, are corroborated by family correspondence, which he quotes and cites extensively in the text, particularly between his wife, Tippy, and her parents.

experience, he calculated the rate of *E. granulosus* infection in this population to be '40 per 100,000 per year (or approximately three times the highest known national rate, which is that of Cyprus)'.[45]

His description of *E. granulosus* among the Turkana in *VMHH* makes clear, however, that the case represented more than just a startling epidemiological statistic. Bracketed in the text by his account of the parasite's path through Beirut and the mysteriously high rate of infection in human forestry workers in New Zealand, the story of Turkana infection exemplifies Schwabe's mounting interest in the way that intangible social relationships provided opportunities for *E. granulosus* to find new niches and transgress the boundary between non-humans and humans in surprising ways.[46]

The story of *E. granulosus* in Kenyan pastoralists was ultimately revealed to hinge more on the 'intimate contact from a very early age' between Turkana children and the numerous dogs kept by their families (as well as plentiful and *E. granulosus*-laden livestock).[47] Though it did not revolutionize the perception of the human as an 'accidental' host of the parasite, Schwabe's experience in Kenya came at the same time that he was writing the first edition of *VMHH*, when he was just beginning to articulate what would become a lifelong challenge to the validity of the boundary between humans and other animals. First he had followed the parasite through the laboratory, cultivating its health and proliferation as he considered how it moved between different non-human hosts and examining the minuscule biochemical exchanges that made these intimate interactions possible. However, by the time he was completing *VMHH* in 1961, the parasite had drawn him out of the laboratory and across the species boundary between non-humans and humans, where cultural exchanges became just as critical to intimate host–parasite relationships as the biochemical interactions observed in the laboratory.

---

[45] Schwabe (1964) p. 211.

[46] Ibid.

[47] Nelson and Rausch (1963) p. 145.

5.3 Following *Echinococcus* Across the Globe: Schwabe's Persistent Parasitology

The human dimension of Schwabe's research, and particularly his search for the path of the parasite through the cultural practices and social relationships of human hosts, only grew in the next few years. At the same time, the global ubiquity of *E. granulosus* was increasingly acknowledged,[48] which also provided Schwabe, reciprocally, with pathways to new career opportunities. Through the parasite, then, the scope of his work grew, as he took on increasing responsibility and reward with the WHO.[49] It remained at the centre of his work throughout this period, a driving force that is felt only more distinctly after considering the sheer variety of methodological approaches that he took to pursue it between animal bodies, across landscapes and between continents.

As well as a vehicle for Schwabe's professional ambitions, *E. granulosus* also became a medium for the building of bridges across disciplines and between nations. Using his expertise on *E. granulosus* as currency, he gained increasing access to the networking possibilities of the WHO, forging a lasting friendship with Martin Kaplan, head of its Veterinary Public Health (VPH) unit, as he continued to work for the WHO as a contractor. This friendship would prove pivotal for Schwabe when the WHO finally offered him a permanent job in 1964, when he and his family moved to Geneva for two years.[50] Kaplan's work for the WHO is described in detail in Chapter 4, where his efforts to promote human health and nutrition through the prevention of livestock disease are highlighted. Joining the VPH had at first been mentioned to Schwabe.

[48] For example, a Web of Science search for the term 'Echinococcus' between 1940 and 1970 shows a scant 3–6 publications per year through the early 1950s. In the last half of the 1950s there were 7–9 publications per year. Through the 1960s, these numbers grew, reaching 20 in 1966, 20 in 1967, 31 in 1968 and 25 in 1969.

[49] While his research funding had previously been dominated by Pfizer and the US National Institute of Allergy and Infectious Diseases (part of the NIH), his publication record shows that in 1961 he began to receive grants from the WHO. For this shift, see Kilejian et al. (1961).

[50] On the developing friendship and ongoing correspondence between Kaplan and Schwabe, see Schwabe (n.d.) pp. 259–60, 310. Later, after his move to the University of California-Davis, Schwabe attempted to recruit Kaplan to join him. For example: Schwabe (1967).

In the event, however, he became 'second in command' of the Parasitology Disease (PD) unit, which he considered to be the '"nerve centre" of medical parasitology worldwide'. Like VPH, PD took human health to be a goal of primary importance. However, Schwabe's persistently broad interest in the lives of parasites in general, and the fact that *E. granulosus* infection in animals did not immediately threaten human health, made PD a better fit for his work. It offered him the opportunity to keep the parasite at the very centre of enquiry. He helped to track infection rates and run prevention programmes for a number of parasites, from soil-transmitted helminths such as hookworm to fungi that caused animal disease. He combined this pursuit of human health with investigations into a variety of aspects of parasitology, such as taxonomy and evolutionary history, which some medical researchers might have regarded as somewhat esoteric and ancillary to medical concerns. For Schwabe, then, working for PD enabled him, in large part, to follow parasites where they led him.[51]

This was true also in a geographical sense. In 1965 alone, Schwabe visited eight countries during the months of July and August.[52] And while his time at the WHO was a whirlwind of consulting on a range of parasitic infections, coordinating international meetings, and producing technical reports and bulletins, he also continued to focus on *E. granulosus* in these travels and draw conclusions about the array of human social and cultural niches into which the parasite could insert itself. Through Schwabe's efforts to correlate findings in a vast array of different environments and human cultural contexts, *E. granulosus* built increasingly elaborate and transnational connections—for example, bringing Nelson in Kenya into collaboration with a prominent American *E. granulosus* researcher, Robert Rausch, to compare the parasite in the wild hyenas of Kenya with the sylvatic transmission cycles of wolves and moose in Alaska. Enabling such connections inspired Schwabe, and he later recalled that this was 'what I first visualized trying to do for WHO'.[53]

Nevertheless, despite his enthusiasm for some aspects of the job, Schwabe was not long for the WHO, and in his memoir he suggests that

[51] Schwabe (n.d.) pp. 287, 310.

[52] 'Duty Travel' (n.d.).

[53] Schwabe (n.d.) pp. 319, 446.

it was the bureaucracy that ultimately wore him down.[54] In 1966 he was offered a new position at the University of California, Davis, where he could help build connections between the School of Veterinary Medicine and the School of Medicine. After a decade living abroad, he and his family returned to the USA.

For Schwabe, moving to California had one significant scientific drawback: the apparent absence of his 'paradigmatic parasitism'. The search for 'autochthonous' *E. granulosus* infections—those thought to have *originated* in the USA—had turned up only 40 cases by the end of the 1950s, which served as an extreme contrast to Schwabe's previous setting of Beirut.[55] A true symbiont, however, *E. granulosus* had shaped Schwabe's career and his perceptions of successful science so profoundly that he could not entertain the possibility of giving it up, even in a new context that seemed far less promising for the parasite's prospects. Moreover, as he reflected on the importance of the parasite after retirement, Schwabe quoted William Osler, writing that one should '[k]now one disease completely and you will know all of medicine'. For Schwabe, that 'one disease' was echinococcosis and 'that one parasitism' would serve him, in his own words, 'as a sort of paradigm for a modern comprehensive parasitology'.[56] His commitment to this philosophy is vividly expressed here; instead of considering the study of a different parasite, Schwabe began to consider how he might bring *E. granulosus* with him, reflecting on ways to ramp up his previous efforts to develop better laboratory hosts for the parasite.[57]

Fortunately, however, *E. granulosus* had reached California long before Schwabe did, proving again its insidious potential for utilizing

[54] Ibid. p. 324.

[55] For example: Cobgill (1957), Brooks et al. (1959) and Sterman and Brown (1959).

[56] Schwabe (n.d.) p. 333.

[57] This was not a straightforward task, and it was always a challenge to establish secondary infections in rodents and other experimental animals by transferring cysts as he had done at AUB. Schwabe et al. (1964, 1970). He was able to call on his existing network of *Echinococcus* researchers for their help. (See Rausch (1967) on shipping him a vole infected with *Echinococcus*). The patterns of international correspondence, visits and network-building via the study of this parasite, which he had established at AUB, continued at University of California, Davis without interruption.

myriad human movements and connections to colonize new environments. One morning, soon after his arrival in Davis, one of Schwabe's students made an unexpected discovery in a local abattoir. The student was a US Department of Agriculture veterinarian, studying with Schwabe and working in his lab, and he had been sent to collect sheep viscera in order to identify their parasitic fauna. However, he had not expected to uncover his mentor's pet parasite in the process. He returned to Schwabe's laboratory eagerly, impatient to show him the sheep livers he had collected—full, as he believed, of *E. granulosus* cysts. Subsequent examination of local sheep carcasses confirmed that the parasite was present and thriving in California. For example, in a January 1968 examination of a group of 227 sheep sent to a local abattoir (from the farm owned by the family of J.O., in fact), 225 were found to be carrying living *E. granulosus* cysts.[58] Schwabe eagerly reactivated his research programme and undertook to track the worm through its local populations of hosts.

His efforts would overturn assumptions about *E. granulosus* in the USA, showing the parasite to be well established in the state of California. In 1969, Schwabe wrote to a colleague in Tasmania, who was heading up the *E. granulosus* control effort there, telling him:

> You will have to revise your assumption about the absence of hydatid infection in sheep and dogs in North American sheep [*sic*] ... At present we have demonstrated transmission in eight counties of the Central Valley of California, spanning almost the entire length of the state. This included infected coyotes in two counties and several human cases so far. In one recent fatal case, all 13 of the man's dogs were infected!

His Tasmanian colleague replied: 'The paper of course fascinated me, especially after spending a year in California wondering how you had escaped infection.'[59] From the Tasmanian researcher's perspective, the many sheep ranches of the Central Valley of California had presented an obvious conundrum: The conditions suggested an ideal environment for *E. granulosus*, yet the region had ostensibly 'escaped infection'. The

[58] Araujo et al. (1975) pp. 291, 298.

[59] Schwabe (1969).

discovery made by Schwabe's student at the abattoir had revealed, however, that the Central Valley had *not* escaped infection after all. Instead, the parasite had remained concealed, and part of Schwabe's task would be to understand how the parasite had flourished and why it had gone mostly undetected. Previously, Schwabe had laboured to elucidate the network of connections forged by *E. granulosus* in the human and canine populations of Beirut; now he would do the same in the Central Valley of California.[60]

As before, hospital surgical records provided an important starting point for his investigation. Surveying and tabulating data about cysts taken from human patients and from sheep in local abattoirs allowed Schwabe to begin to reconstruct the history of *E. granulosus* in California, following the trail of the parasite back to the initial sites of infection. *Both* sets of traces led to the Basque sheep-farming community from which J.O. and his father, Salvador, hailed. Once Schwabe began to focus on Basque sheep farms, he took multiple tacks: deworming dogs; examining sheep; and interviewing family members and shepherds. Most of the potential human and non-human hosts that he and his team encountered, however, were asymptomatic and healthy, effectively obscuring the real level of infection and requiring immunological testing in order to infer infection. Soon it was clear, from all of these forms of data, both direct and indirect, that humans, sheep and dogs on these farms were all subject to infection by *E. granulosus.*

Following the parasite through the precise points of contact between the hosts, however, required that Schwabe employ the methods he had developed in following the parasite in Beirut, interrogating the social interactions and mores that created the interspecies pathways exploited by *E. granulosus.* In order to understand the relationships between Basque immigrants, sheep, dogs and *E. granulosus*, Schwabe needed a far more intimate look at the workings of these farming operations. In 1972 he sent anthropology graduate student Frank Araujo to live and work on a Central Valley Basque sheep ranch, where—like

[60] He was also able to place this into the context of fairly extensive experience in far-flung locations and diverse cultures (e.g. the Turkana people of Kenya) and control programmes in many different countries (e.g. New Zealand and Iceland). For example, Burridge and Schwabe (1977) consider infection among New Zealand's indigenous Maori population.

the late nineteenth-century British experts whose investigations were described in Chapter 3—he sought to learn about disease directly from sheep farmers. Thanks to his own Basque ethnic heritage, Araujo had a functional knowledge of the language, which allowed him to press family and workers for, in his own words, 'ethno-veterinarian lore' and 'an outline of the decision-making procedures' used on a typical Basque sheep farm.[61]

Though he was trained in anthropology, Araujo examined this community through an ecological lens, seeking the interrelationships that made the system work. In writing up this research, his language demonstrated that each component of the 'ancient transhumant type of man-sheep-dog ecosystem' was invested with agency, including the parasite itself; in addition to the 'close interrelationships between these three [host] species,' he wrote, 'a fourth species, *Echinococcus granulosus*, traditionally derives comfort and prospers too, once it has been introduced'.[62] An ecological perspective is apparent even in Araujo's anthropological observations. In his initial research proposal, he wrote of the exchanges that made the Californian sheep industry function, moving goods like wool and meat from the fairly insulated Basque community to the larger body of consumers, in a manner 'characteristic of a symbiotic relationship'.[63] This mode of description was echoed in his 1975 publication, co-authored with Schwabe and others, where he described the Basque sheepherding economy as the 'successful exploitation' of a 'marginal ecological niche, with a transhumant and complementary utilization [of] … seasonally useless land', which has, as a result, allowed the Californian population of Basques the 'preservation of their ethnicity'.[64]

The system worked by dividing a rancher's ewes into groups of 600–800, and taking them by truck to roam in small bands over leased land in the Sierra Nevada or the Mojave Desert. While one 'camp tender or *kanpero*' would live in a central location in a trailer, providing the sheepherders or *artzainak* with essential supplies, the latter would roam on foot with their bands of sheep, living in a tent along the way. All of these—sheep, humans, dogs and their invisible internal companions—would be taken back to their home ranches in the San Joaquin valley at

[61] Araujo (23 June 1972).

[62] Araujo et al. (1975) pp. 300–1.

[63] Araujo (n.d.) p. 3.

[64] Araujo et al. (1975) p. 295.

critical times.[65] Araujo and Schwabe recorded these transhumant migrations using arrow-laden maps of the state of California, from which they concluded: 'This system of husbandry results in the possibility for large areas of crop and recreational lands in California to be seeded with *E. granulosus* eggs from the feces [*sic*] of infected sheep dogs.'[66]

In addition to mapping out the scale at which *E. granulosus* traversed the state of California, Araujo mapped out the more intimate and detailed passages of the parasite, through a linguistic, figurative understanding of the relationships between the four core species of animals. Most significantly, he observed and participated in farming practices, seeing that sheep were being fed the carcasses of deceased, and often diseased, sheep. Many ranchers denied that this practice continued on their farms. However, evidence pointed to its perpetuation: most transparently, the presence of tapeworms (*E. granulosus* and others) in sheepdogs with little opportunity to be infected elsewhere, which indicated that they had been consuming raw meat. In fact, as Araujo recorded, the practice was common enough: he himself was employed to do it, though he attempted to mitigate the effects by removing suspicious-looking cystic lumps from the eviscerated sheep before letting the dogs loose to feed on them. From the months that he spent living among and communing with the ranch hands and shepherds, Araujo learned that it was generally believed that a good sheepdog *needed* to eat sheep viscera. He also learned that few of the shepherds connected their own hydatid cysts to the 'stones or pebbles' that they saw when they gutted the dead sheep and left them to the dogs.[67] Indeed, he observed, most of the ranchers and sheepherders he had come to know seemed to think nothing of the frequent appearance of abscesses and pathological tissue in the flesh and organs of their dead sheep.[68] In other words, he concluded, 'folk knowledge' had not led the Basque community to make the inferences that they would have needed to arrest the constant cycling of *E. granulosus* between their sheep and dogs.

---

[65] Ibid. pp. 295–6.

[66] Ibid. p. 296.

[67] Araujo (5 July 1972). Writing about his anthropological–epidemiological fieldwork, Araujo said that many of the sheepherders 'don't seem to know (or care!) what causes them', and one proclaimed it to be 'bullshit.' Araujo (14 November 1972).

[68] Araujo (14 November 1972).

Complementing Basque beliefs about sheepdogs' dietary requirements and their lack of knowledge about cysts, the transhumant patterns described above left shepherds, dogs and sheep in joint isolation for long periods of time, on a series of lands located at a distance from the home ranch. In these circumstances, feeding dogs on dead sheep provided a convenient source of sustenance. After all, the profit margins in the industry were small, and wasting the meat of a dead sheep seemed uneconomical. More profoundly, however, Araujo and Schwabe claimed, in this isolating system of ranching, '[r]elationships between shepherds, dogs and sheep are highly mutualistic', with the means of subsistence literally enabled or provided to each other by each member of the tripartite relationship.[69]

Araujo's study also revealed the presence of additional links in this ecosystem. Taking a day to follow a sheep owner and his favourite dog, he carefully recorded the manifold contacts the dog had with people of all ages and stations at the ranch, particularly the children. And in observing the dumping of excess dead sheep, he suggested the possibility that wild canids—coyotes and feral dogs—might also provide new host environments for *E. granulosus.*[70] The entanglement of wild animals in the parasite's movement through domestic and agricultural systems had been verified in multiple contexts, as we have already seen in this chapter. As with the hyenas in Kenya, Schwabe and his collaborators discovered that the parasite had found another cohort of hosts in coyotes and had, in fact, also begun to exploit deer as an intermediate host, in place of sheep.[71]

As American *E. granulosus* continued to draw attention to itself, it soon became apparent that it had found its way to other human communities that practised modes of animal husbandry similar to those of the Basques. Like Californian coyotes and Alaskan moose, these disparate groups of people had been caught up in a series of new, loosely interconnected ecosystems that *E. granulosus*, through its own mode of

---

[69] Araujo et al. (1975) p. 297.

[70] Ibid.

[71] Liu et al. (1970). The story of the parasite's path from the domestic and agricultural settings generated by humans into wild populations of animals is still developing today, particularly as the 'wild' increasingly merges into the borderland around the intensively urban. For example: Catalano et al. (2012). As Chapter 6 describes, the 'wild' is one category of animal that OH advocates attempt to include beneath their umbrella. Animals are primarily regarded in that sphere as disease vectors.

transmission, had created. As Schwabe and his students would report in 1977, the practices of transhumant sheepherding effectively united a motley crew of American subcultures, from the Basque immigrants of California, to Mormon sheepherding communities in Utah, to indigenous Navajo and Zuni in Arizona and New Mexico.[72] Expanding this view to a global scale, farmwives in Iceland, Turkana tribespeople in Kenya and Cypriot islanders were also members of this ecosystem, connected as well to the deer, coyotes, moose, wolves and various other animals in which *E. Granulosus* made its home.

5.4 Conclusion

During the first two decades of his career, Schwabe tracked *E. granulosus* across multiple boundaries. Where the parasite went—from host to host, environment to environment, continent to continent and discipline to discipline—so too did Schwabe, creating professional connections that brought the tapeworm's movements and exchanges into relief. When Schwabe made the leap from studying parasites in the context of non-human bodies and the laboratory to studying parasites in human bodies and human cultural niches, it was not so much a *leap*, in fact, but a transition guided by the parasitic animal itself, and an extension of its biological autonomy. The network of scientists and medical practitioners that collaborated with Schwabe, engaging in the global effort to investigate human and animal health, can also be seen as an extension of the interactive biological networks forged by the parasite. Schwabe's graduate students and collaborators would become vital additions to those organizations that strove to track and prevent the spread of disease, from the Centres for Disease Control to the Pan American Health Organization.[73]

---

[72] Pappanaioanou et al. (1977) pp. 732, 738.

[73] They included: Peter Schantz, who was Schwabe's first PhD student at the University of California, Davis, and the recipient of the first ever PhD in veterinary epidemiology. Schwabe (n.d.) p. 337, Nolen (2013). See Schantz and Schwabe (1969) for an example of their collaboration around *Echinococcus*. Schantz went on to work on *Echinococcus* first at the Pan American Zoonoses Center in Buenos Aires, Argentina, and from 1974 at the Centers for Disease Control (CDC) in Atlanta, Georgia, where he was part of epidemiological research on many parasites that passed between humans and non-humans. Schantz and Colli (1973), Pappaioanou (multiple dates). For his continuing involvement in, and influence on matters concerning *Echinococcus*, see, for example Jones et al. (1980),

Thus, just as the parasite connected far-flung populations of diverse animals and humans, it was also a primary vehicle for the development of careers, and a dispersed, multidisciplinary network of scientists, doctors and veterinarians.

In part, the extended association that Schwabe formed with *E. granulosus* should be seen in terms of the history of the field of parasitology, whose grounding in late nineteenth-century tropical colonial medicine and agriculture gave it a richly contextualized perspective on infectious disease from the beginning.[74] Historians have noted that this field drew from natural history, zoology and medicine, taking ecological environments and evolutionary history seriously, and questioning why particular parasites thrived in some places and not others.[75] This disciplinary background provided Schwabe with an enriched biological conception of interactions between parasites and hosts, which he expressed in writing with Araujo in 1975. Framing *E. granulosus* as the fourth member of the '[hu]man-sheep-dog ecosystem',[76] he placed it on an equal ecological standing with the other animals in the cycle of transmission, and asked how its physiological and ecological needs were met by the body of the host. This was very different from medical and veterinary approaches which tended to identify parasites with disease, and to regard them as threats to humans and animals rather than as interacting organisms in their own right. Schwabe regarded his subject primarily as an animal, and only secondarily in terms of the disease it might cause. This chapter

---

Moro and Schantz (2009). Likewise, Schwabe's graduate student Marguerite Pappaioanou, who also collaborated on the California programme, went on, at his recommendation and with his consultation, to work on Echinococcus on the island of Cyprus. Pappanaioanou et al. (1977), Pappaionanou (April–June 1977). Pappaioanou went on to a long career at the CDC as well, and became an outspoken advocate of OM and OH. For example: Pappanaioanou (2004). These are only two examples out of a plethora of students who still influence the global health community today.

[74] See Chapter 3.

[75] On the origins of parasitology, see Farley (1972, 1992), Worboys (1983), Li (2004). Parasitology became an important basis for the development of disease ecology in the early twentieth century. For example, see Anderson (2004). It also developed a range of complex perspectives on the evolution of pathogens, and the relationship between the evolution of parasites and the evolution of hosts. Méthot (2012), Mason Dentinger (2016).

[76] Araujo et al. (1975) pp. 300–1.

therefore extends the insights gained in Chapters 2 and 3, further exploring how the concurrent study of human and non-human health *enables*, and *is enabled by*, multidisciplinary scientific approaches.

Following the parasite changed the way that Schwabe saw the relationship between humans and non-humans, and between human and veterinary medicine. As he worked to complete *VMHH* in 1961, he was simultaneously exploring the dynamic movement of *E. granulosus* among the hyenas and the humans of Kenya. Here, in the early years of his career, before his shift of focus to epidemiology and advocacy for OM, he developed a critique of the very concept of 'zoonosis', which he described as 'a pre-Copernican notion' that relied on and enforced a '"[hu]man-other animal" dichotomy' that could have no 'real meaning to the student of the natural history of infections'.[77] In other words, thanks to the influence of *E. granulosus*, he was already actively undermining the basic definition of 'zoonoses', given by the WHO as 'diseases and infections which are naturally transmitted between man and animals'.[78] Schwabe challenged the distinction at the core of this definition, insisting that the line between humans and non-humans was not fundamentally biological but, in large part, a product of human cultural variations.[79] He would also ultimately extend this insight into a disciplinary critique of medicine, arguing that human and veterinary medicine were separated only by human traditions and preconceptions and not by essential differences between their subjects. In other words, one of the key innovations in Schwabe's thinking, reiterated throughout the latter half of his life, in multiple writings—that of undermining the very validity of species boundaries in biology and medicine[80]—finds its roots at the

[77] Schwabe (1964) p. 197.

[78] This definition is taken from Joint WHO/FAO (1959).

[79] He would later infuse this sensibility into the next report of the WHO/FAO Expert Committee on Zoonoses, from 1967, when he served on the committee. Though the report suggests that the 1959 definition should be preserved, this recommendation is preceded by a 'Schwabean' disclaimer, stating that while 'the term zoonoses is etymologically inexact and of little biological merit it is generally agreed that it is useful because it creates common ground for the medical veterinary professionals' to work together on disease understanding and prevention. Joint WHO/FAO (1967).

[80] Which then became a central tenet of OM and OH. See Chapter 6 for more information.

beginning, at a time when he was still deeply engrossed in his pursuit of his paradigmatic parasite.

Just as Schwabe tracked *E. granulosus* throughout his career, so too have I in this account. By considering the movements of the parasite and how they have ramified through the careers of Schwabe and his collaborators, I have crisscrossed the historiographical boundaries that typically stand between the history of biology and the history of medicine, and between the history of human medicine and veterinary medicine. Parasitologists have, in their pursuit of parasites, brought natural history, zoology and medicine all to bear on their human and non-human subjects. Likewise, this account has moved between all of these domains, suggesting that while an understanding of disciplinary norms and training is an essential element in our analysis of the history of science and medicine, these must not restrict the ultimate scope of our enquiry. As our subjects, of all species, repeatedly prove their ability to move beyond the many bounds that we have constructed and imagined, so too must historians.

Bibliography

Abou-Daoud, Kamal and Calvin W. Schwabe. "Epidemiology of Echinococcus in the Middle East: III. A Study of Hydatid Disease Patients in the City of Beirut." *American Journal of Tropical Medicine and Hygiene* 13 (1964): 681–5.

Anderson, Warwick. "Natural Histories of Infectious Disease: Ecological Vision in Twentieth-Century Biomedical Science." *Osiris* 19 (2004): 39–61.

Araujo, Frank. "Basque Ecology in the Western United States." n.d. Calvin W. Schwabe Papers, National Library of Medicine, 21:12.

Araujo, Frank. "Correspondence with Calvin Schwabe." 23 June 1972, 5 July 1972, 14 November 1972. Calvin W. Schwabe Papers, National Library of Medicine, 21:12.

Araujo, F.P., C.W. Schwabe, J.C. Sawyer and W.G. Davis. "Hydatid Disease Transmission in California: A Study of the Basque Connection." *American Journal of Epidemiology* 102 (1975): 291–302.

Baer, Jean G. *Animal Parasites.* London: World University Library, 1971.

Barnett, Louis. "Hydatid Disease: Errors in Teaching and Practice." *British Medical Journal* 2 (1939): 593–9.

Beisel, Ulli, Anne H. Kelly and Noémi Tousignant. "Knowing Insects: Hosts, Vectors and Companions of Science." *Science as Culture* 22 (2013): 1–15.

Benson, Etienne, "Animal Writes: Historiography, Disciplinarity, and the Animal Trace." In *Making Animal Meaning*, edited by L. Kalof and G.M. Montgomery, 3–16. East Lansing, MI: Michigan State University Press, 2011.

Bogitsh, Burton, Thomas Oeltmann and Clint Carter (eds). *Human Parasitology, Third edition.* Burlington, MA: Academic Press, 2005.

Brooks, T.J., W.R. Webb and K.M. Heard. "Hydatid Disease: A Summary of Human Cases in Mississippi." *American Medical Association Archives of Internal Medicine* 104 (1959): 562–7.

Burridge, M.J. and C.W. Schwabe. 'Hydatid Disease in New Zealand: An Epidemiological Study of Transmission among Maoris'. *American Journal of Tropical Medicine and Hygiene* 26 (1977): 258–65.

Bynum, William. *The Western Medical Tradition: 1800–2000*. New York, NY: Cambridge University Press, 2006.

Cameron, Thomas W.M. "The Helminth Parasites of Animals and Human Disease." *Proceedings of the Royal Society of Medicine, Section of Comparative Medicine* 20 (1927): 547–56.

Catalano, Stefano et al. "*Echinococcus multilocularis* in Urban Coyotes, Alberta, Canada." *Emerging Infectious Diseases* 18 (2012): 1625–8.

Cobgill, Charles L. "Echinococcus Cyst." *American Medical Association Archives of Surgery* 75 (1957): 267–71.

Craig, Charles F. and Ernest Carroll Faust. *Craig and Faust's Clinical Parasitology*. Philadelphia: Lea & Febiger, 1964.

"Curriculum Vitae." n.d. Calvin W. Schwabe Papers, National Library of Medicine, 1:1.

Dew, Harold. "Some Complications of Hydatid Disease." *British Journal of Surgery* 18 (1930): 275–93.

Dew, Harold. "Morphological Variation in Hydatid Disease." *The British Journal of Surgery* 45 (1958): 447–53.

"Duty Travel Report." n.d. Calvin W. Schwabe Papers, National Library of Medicine, 28:2.

Farhan, Ishak, Calvin W. Schwabe and C. Richard Zobel. "Host-Parasite Relationships in Echinococcosis: III. Relation of Environmental Oxygen Tension to the Metabolism of Hydatid Scolices." *American Journal of Tropical Medicine and Hygiene* 8 (1959): 473–8.

Farley, John. "The Spontaneous Generation Controversy (1700–1860): The Origin of Parasitic Worms." *Journal of the History of Biology* 5 (1972): 95–125.

Farley, John. "Parasites and the Germ Theory of Disease." In *Framing Disease: Studies in Cultural History*, edited by Charles Rosenberg and Janet Golden, 33–49. New Brunswick, NJ: Rutgers University Press, 1992.

Farley, John. *Bilharzia: A History of Imperial Tropical Medicine*. Cambridge: Cambridge University Press, 2003.

Joint WHO/FAO Expert Committee on Zoonoses. "Second Report." *World Health Organization Technical Report Series* 169 (1959): 1–83.

Joint WHO/FAO Expert Committee on Zoonoses. "Third Report." *World Health Organization Technical Report Series* 378 (1967): 1–127.

Jones, Wesley E., Peter M. Schantz, Kate Foreman, Linda Kay Smith, Ernest J. Witte, David E. Schooley and Dennis D. Juranek. "Human Toxocariasis in a Rural Community." *American Journal of the Diseases of Children* 134 (1980): 967–9.

Jones, Susan. *Death in a Small Package: A Short History of Anthrax.* Baltimore: John Hopkins University Press, 2010.

Kilejian, Araxie, Lewis A. Schinazi and Calvin W. Schwabe. "Host-Parasite Relationships in *Echinococcus*: V. Histochemical Observations on Echinococcus Granulosus." *American Journal of Tropical Medicine and Hygiene* 47 (1961): 181–8.

Huxley, Thomas Henry. *The Scientific Memoirs of Thomas Henry Huxley.* London: Macmillan and Co., 1898.

Li, Shang-Jen. "The Nurse of Parasites: Gender Concepts in Patrick Manson's Parasitological Research." *Journal of the History of Biology* 37 (2004): 103–30.

Liu, Irwin K. M., Calvin W. Schwabe, Peter M. Schantz and Malcolm N. Allison. "The Occurrence of Echinococcus Granulosus in Coyotes (*Canis latrans*) in the Central Valley of California." *Journal of Parasitology* 56 (1970): 1135–7.

Mason Dentinger, Rachel. "Patterns of Infection and Patterns of Evolution: How a Malaria Parasite Brought 'Monkeys and Man' Closer Together in the 1960s." *Journal of the History of Biology* 49 (2016): 359–95.

Méthot, Pierre-Olivier. "Why do Parasites Harm Their Host? On the Origin and Legacy of Theobald Smith's 'Law of Declining Virulence' – 1900–1980." *History and Philosophy of the Life Sciences* 34 (2012): 561–601.

Mitchell, T. "Can the Mosquito Speak?" In *Rule of Experts: Egypt, Technopolitics, Modernity*, by T. Mitchell, 19–53. London: University of California Press, 2002.

Moro, Pedro and Peter M. Schantz. "*Echinococcus*: A Review." *International Journal of Infectious Diseases* 13 (2009): 125–33.

Nelson, George S. and Robert L. Rausch. "*Echinococcus* Infections in Man and Animals in Kenya." *Annals of Tropical Medicine and Parasitology* 57 (1963): 136–49.

Noble, Elmer R. and Glenn A. Noble. *Parasitology: The Biology of Animal Parasites.* Philadelphia: Lea & Febiger, 1964.

Nolen, R. Scott. "LEGENDS: The Accidental Epidemiologist." *Journal of the American Veterinary Medical Association News*, 1 July 2013. Accessed April 2, 2017. https://www.avma.org/News/JAVMANews/Pages/130701m.aspx.

Packard, Randall. *The Making of a Tropical Disease: A Short History of Malaria.* Baltimore: Johns Hopkins University Press, 2011.

Pappanaioanou, Marguerite. "Correspondence with Calvin Schwabe." April–Jul 1977 and multiple other dates. Calvin W. Schwabe Papers, National Library of Medicine, 21:21, 21:23.

Pappanaioanou, Marguerite, Calvin W. Schwabe and Diana M. Sard. "An Evolving Pattern of Human Hydatid Disease Transmission in the United States." *The American Journal of Tropical Medicine and Hygiene* 26 (1977): 732–42.

Pappanaioanou, Marguerite. "Veterinary Medicine Protecting and Promoting the Public's Health and Well-Being." *Preventive Veterinary Medicine* 62 (2004): 153–63.

"Parasites – Echinococcosis." Centers for Disease Control, 2012. Accessed April 2, 2017. https://www.cdc.gov/parasites/echinococcosis/biology.html.

Patterson, James T. "Disease in the History of Medicine and Public Health." In *Major Problems in the History of American Medicine and Public Health: Documents and Essays,* edited by John Harley Warner and Janet Tighe, 17–23. Boston: Houghton Mifflin, 2001.

Rausch, Robert. "Correspondence with Calvin W. Schwabe." 9 January 1967. Calvin W. Schwabe Papers, National Library of Medicine, 11:10.

Rausch, Robert L. "Hydatid Disease in Boreal Regions." *Arctic: Journal of the Arctic Institute of North America* 5 (1952): 157–74.

Sapp, Jan. *Evolution by Association: A History of Symbiosis.* New York: Oxford University Press, 1994.

Schantz, Peter M. and Calvin W. Schwabe. "Worldwide Status of Hydatid Disease Control." *Journal of the American Veterinary Medical Association* 155 (1969): 2104–21.

Schantz, Peter M. and Cristina Colli. "*Echinococcus oligarthrus* (Diesing, 1863) from Geoffroy's Cat (*Felis Geoffroyi* D'Orbigny y Gervais) in Temperate South America." *The Journal of Parasitology* 59 (1973): 1138–40.

Schwabe, Calvin W. "Hoofprints of Cheiron." n.d. Calvin W. Schwabe Papers, National Library of Medicine, vol. 12.

Schwabe, Calvin W. "Correspondence with Martin Kaplan." 3 April 1967. Calvin W. Schwabe Papers, National Library of Medicine, 9:3.

Schwabe, Calvin W. "Correspondence with Trevor Beard." 14 July 1969, 26 Jul 1969. Calvin W. Schwabe Papers, National Library of Medicine, 5:4.

Schwabe, Calvin W. "Studies on *Oxyspirura mansoni*, the Tropical Eyeworm of Poultry. II. Life History." *Pacific Science* 5 (1951): 18–35.

Schwabe, Calvin W. "Observations on the Respiration of Free-Living and Parasitic *Nippostrongylus muris* Larvae." *American Journal of Hygiene* 65 (1957): 325–37.

Schwabe, Calvin W. "Effects of Normal and Immune Rat Sera upon the Respiration of Free-Living and Parasitic *Nippostrongylus muris* Larvae." *American Journal of Hygiene* 65 (1957): 338–43.

Schwabe, Calvin W. "Host-Parasite Relationships in *Echinococcus*: I. Observations on the Permeability of the Hydatid Cyst Wall." *American Journal of Tropical Medicine and Hygiene* 8 (1959): 20–8.

Schwabe, Calvin W. *Veterinary Medicine and Human Health.* Baltimore: Williams & Wilkins Co., 1964.

Schwabe, Calvin W., 'Curriculum Vitae', *Preventive Veterinary Medicine* 62 (2004): 207–216.

Schwabe, Calvin W. and Kamal Abou Daoud. "Epidemiology of *Echinococcus* in the Middle East I. Human Infection in Lebanon, 1949–1959." *American Journal of Tropical Medicine and Hygiene* 9 (1961): 374–81.

Schwabe, Calvin W., Lewis A. Schinazi and Araxie Kilejian. "Host-Parasite Relationships in *Echinococcus*: II. Age Resistance to Secondary Echinococcus in the White Mouse." *The American Journal of Tropical Medicine and Hygiene* 8 (1959): 29–36.

Schwabe, Calvin W., G.W. Luttermoser, M. Koussa and S.R. Ali. "Serial Passage of Fertile Hydatid Cysts of *Echinococcus granulosus* in Absence of the Definitive Host." *Journal of Parasitology* 50 (1964): 260.

Schwabe, Calvin W., Araxie Kilejian and Gerasimos Lainas. "The Propagation of Secondary Cysts of *Echinococcus granulosus* in the Mongolian Jird, *Meriones unguiculatus*." *The Journal of Parasitology* 56 (1970): 80–3.

Sterman, Max M. and Harold W. Brown. "*Echinococcus* in Man and Dog in the Same Household in New York City." *Journal of the American Medical Association* 169 (1959): 938–40.

Tenenbaum, Joseph. "*Echinococcus* Cyst of Kidney." *Journal of the American Medical Association* 108 (1937): 1704–5.

Turner, E.L., D.A. Berberian and E.W. Dennis. "The Production of Artificial Immunity in Dogs against *Echinococcus granulosus*." *The Journal of Parasitology* 22 (1936): 14–28.

Webster, Gloria and T.W.M. Cameron. 'Observations of Experimental Infections with *Echinococcus* in Rodents'. *Canadian Journal of Zoology* 39 (1961): 877–91.

Worboys, Michael. "The Emergence and Early Development of Parasitology." In *Parasitology: A Global Perspective*, edited by Kenneth S. Warren and John Z. Bowers, 1–18. New York: Springer-Verlag, 1983.

Wray, J.R. "Human Hydatid Disease in Kenya." *East African Medical Journal* 35 (1958): 37–9.

CHAPTER 6

Humans, Other Animals and 'One Health' in the Early Twenty-First Century

Angela Cassidy

In 2002 the US-based Association for Veterinary Epidemiology and Preventive Medicine (AVEPM) co-organized a symposium in St. Louis, Missouri, to honour the lifetime achievements of Calvin W. Schwabe, who had served as professor of epidemiology in both the medical and veterinary schools of the University of California, Davis until his retirement in 1991.[1] At the symposium, Schwabe gave a keynote address summarizing his ideas about how veterinary medicine should relate to other disciplines—particularly human medicine—and the wider world. Arguing against the compartmentalization of medicine by species, into human and veterinary strands, he used the opportunity to restate his longstanding arguments for a philosophy of One Medicine (OM), which sees veterinary medicine as a close collaborative partner with human medicine, working together towards the broader endeavours of healthcare and furthering knowledge in the life sciences.[2] He claimed that this positioning reflected and recognized the contributions that veterinary medicine made to a range of other fields, including comparative zoology, parasitology, epidemiology, human public health, agriculture

[1] At the time the group was known as the Association of Teachers of Veterinary Public Health and Preventive Medicine. The symposium became an annual event, at which a senior member of the field is presented with the Calvin W. Schwabe Award. For details of the original meeting, see AVEPM (2002) p. 3.

[2] Schwabe (2004).

A. Woods et al., *Animals and the Shaping of Modern Medicine*, Medicine and Biomedical Sciences in Modern History,
https://doi.org/10.1007/978-3-319-64337-3_6

and conservation.[3] Schwabe's philosophy of OM was inspired by and expressed in his own career trajectory, which cut across many of these disciplines, as exemplified by his work on the tapeworm *Echinococcus granulosus*, described in Chapter 5. He had first written about bringing 'Veterinary Medicine and Human Health' together during the early 1960s, while working at the (AUB) University of Beirut and consulting on parasitology for the World Health Organization (WHO). However, he elaborated his ideas and first described them using the term OM during the 1980s, following his return to the USA.[4]

The other contributors to the 2002 symposium, who included some of Schwabe's many students and collaborators (now senior academics and policy-makers in their own right), discussed the relevance of OM to their own work in areas such as disease surveillance, veterinary public health and epidemiology.[5] The event was particularly timely because Schwabe was becoming a figurehead for a wide network of scientists and health professionals working across human, animal and environmental health. While many of these individuals had been grappling with scientific and policy problems lying at the intersection of these fields for some time, Schwabe's ideas helped them articulate why it was necessary to think in this integrative way. His ideas about OM also provided a key foundation for the later emergence of One Health (OH), a broader reconfiguration of research, policy and clinical practice across human and animal health, which also brought in environmental concerns.

The term OH first appeared in 2003, when it was adopted by several groups working across human and animal health, and subsequently by policy-makers, clinicians and researchers.[6] Its initial impetus came from renewed fears about the emergence and spread of zoonotic diseases passing between humans and other animals.[7] In November 2002, as the veterinary epidemiologists celebrated Schwabe's career, a previously unidentified coronavirus that originated in an as yet unidentified animal was causing a global outbreak of severe acute respiratory syndrome (SARS),

---

[3] Schwabe (1984) pp. 1–2.

[4] Compare Schwabe (1964, 1969) with Schwabe (1984).

[5] See all papers in *Preventive Veterinary Medicine* 62 (2004).

[6] Osofsky et al. (2003) p. 63, Zinsstag et al. (2005).

[7] Anderson (2004). The WHO defines 'zoonosis' as 'diseases and infections which are naturally transmitted between man and animals'. World Health Organisation (1959) p. 6.

which took six months to contain and killed more than 700 people. This was the first of a series of crises and near-crises related to zoonoses, including the emergence of new strains of highly pathogenic avian influenza (HPAI) in the mid-2000s. Such events refocused scientific and policy attention on the transmission of infectious diseases from animal to human populations.[8] They also brought wider recognition of the problems posed by the traditional separation of human and animal health in science, policy and the professions, particularly when (as in the case of HPAI) they created 'silos' that limited the ability to share knowledge or coordinate policy across international health organizations.[9] This situation resulted in calls for more effective and integrated working across these domains.

Since 2010, OH ideas have spread across the world, with research and advocacy groups forming in, for example, South Korea, Japan, Sweden and Australia. Postgraduate courses in OH have been launched in several countries, while in the USA, universities are experimenting with joint teaching across medical and veterinary schools. Alongside this institutionalization, the scientific literature has matured, with journal citation rates shooting up, two textbooks being published in 2014[10] and new journals being launched in 2011 and 2015.[11] Within this literature, Schwabe is widely referenced as a key source of its ideas, a visionary who coined the term OM,[12] and whose career established him as the 'father of veterinary epidemiology'.[13]

This chapter turns the spotlight on the recent history of OH as a self-conscious movement in the twenty-first century, analysing its emergence and the roles that Calvin Schwabe played in it. While it is a more human-centred chapter than the others in this volume, it follows them in demonstrating the zoological foundations of medicine by examining

---

[8] King (2004).

[9] Jerolmack (2013).

[10] Atlas and Maloy (2014), Zinsstag et al. (2015).

[11] *Infection Ecology & Epidemiology—The One Health Journal* (Co-Action Publishing, Sweden) was launched in 2011, while *One Health: The Official Journal of the OH Platform* (Elsevier) and *International Journal of One Health* (Veterinary World, Gujurat, India) were launched in 2015.

[12] Kaplan and Scott (2011).

[13] Nolan (2013).

the human–animal health relations that underpin the OH movement. The first half identifies Schwabe as a key source of ideas and inspiration, as well as the latest in a series of historical progenitors for OH today. It documents how the idea of OH was developed by different academics, clinicians and policy-makers working in specific institutional contexts to produce not one but many OHs, which awarded different roles to animals, offered different portrayals of their health relationships with humans, presented multiple interpretations of the term 'zoonosis' and held different visions of how disciplinary relationships needed to change in order to achieve the desired integration of human and animal health.[14] It argues that, like the earlier intersections of human and animal health and medicine explored in the other chapters, OH is a response mounted by specific researchers (and policymakers) to problems manifesting at particular times and in particular places. In contrast to advocates' claims, it is not a self-evidently beneficial phenomenon, nor the result of inevitable progress, but a contingent and context-bound activity that is actively and continually created through persuasive rhetoric and alliance-building.[15]

The second half of the chapter focuses on the animal subjects of OH. It asks what sorts of animal feature in the images and scientific literatures associated with OH, and in what types of roles and relationships with humans. Where in the world do they come from? How are they perceived in relation to each other and to humans, and what can this tell us about the relative prioritization of human and animal health within the OH agenda?[16] As in earlier chapters, this analysis involves the scrutiny of traces left by animals on the medical historical record.[17] The photographs, infographics and logos used by advocates as they make their case for OH offer a particularly distinctive type of animal trace that—like other cultural material, such as films, photographs, artistic portrayals, fictions, illustrations, advertising and even clipart—provide a rich source of information about the roles that animals play in medicine

[14]These differences persist. For example, see Gates Foundation (2013), BBSRC (2014), Barrett and Boulay (2015).

[15]Craddock and Hinchliffe (2015), Cassidy (2016).

[16]Degeling et al. (2015).

[17]Benson (2011).

and society.[18] Such sources have been used previously to investigate human–animal relationships, and to illuminate how human recipients of care are represented and understood, particularly in health and international development contexts.[19] While the symbolic representations of animals that they contain constitute less direct animal traces than those in the scientific and other sources analysed elsewhere in this volume, they are traces nonetheless that are left on and remade by the human imagination. They might differ wildly from animals themselves, up to and including completely imaginary animals, but it is unlikely that humans could create these images without encountering animals in the first place. Therefore their analysis can offer meaningful insights into human–animal relationships. In the case of OH, they are all the more important because they are created and used with the intention of shaping how humans interact with animals in the future.

Drawing on these analyses of animal images, and the imagery used in campaigns for public health, global health and international development, the second half of the chapter identifies the contradictions inherent in the OH portrayal of animals, the implications for the trajectories of OH research and practice, and for the health of the humans and animals on which they are projected to impact. Distinguishing between the portrayal of 'animals' as a generic category and as specific living beings, it will argue that animals feature in OH primarily in roles that either threaten or promise to advance human health, such as transmitters of infectious disease, sources of nutrition and companionship, and experimental models for the advancement of medical science and technology. In contrast to the case studies presented in some of the earlier chapters, which similarly examined the intertwining of human and animal health, knowledge about and concern for animals in their own right does not appear to be a major topic of interest in OH. Despite the stated aim—to bring human and animal health closer together—this substantive focus on ultimately advancing human health may create a paradoxical situation where OH advocacy ends up reinforcing the very anthropocentrism that it seeks to change.

[18] Nicholls (2011), Molloy (2011).

[19] Cassidy (2012), Calain (2013), Wilkinson (2013), Lupton (2015).

6.1 One Health or Many?

> The One Health concept is a worldwide strategy for expanding interdisciplinary collaborations and communications in all aspects of health care for humans, animals and the environment.[20]

This definition of OH was developed by the OH Initiative, a US-based advocacy group: an unfunded group of public health physicians and veterinarians in favour of human–animal health collaboration.[21] While useful for advocates, this definition has not gone uncontested, and the broad and flexible nature of the OH concept has been widely debated. While some believe that this breadth risks losing all meaning and has been detrimental to implementing ideas in practice,[22] others have argued that OH acts as a usefully flexible 'boundary object' or 'umbrella' under which a range of topics, disciplines and forms of collaboration can shelter, facilitating interdisciplinary cooperation up to and including the social sciences and humanities.[23] The metaphor of OH as an umbrella (originally formulated by policy analyst Aline Leboeuf) has proved to be popular among OH advocates. Fig. 6.1 shows a graphic created by One Health Sweden, depicting fields dealing with zoonosis sheltering on one side, and those involved in clinical research and practice on the other.[24] While this metaphor evidently helps OH advocates to articulate both the breadth and the limits of their endeavour, it abstracts the idea away from the personal, practical and institutional contexts where it originated and is now being adopted worldwide. While OH presents itself as bridging human and animal health, the majority of advocates and actors taking on the idea can be located in the veterinary sciences. The veterinary origins of the agenda has provoked criticism from some doctors, who perceive OH to be a threat to their professional boundaries: this may account for the limited uptake of OH in mainstream medicine. At the same time, some veterinarians have expressed concern that OH will lead to a loss of the specific status and interest in animal health for

[20] Kahn et al. (2012) p.1.

[21] Kahn et al. (2015).

[22] Lee and Brumme (2012) pp. 1–8.

[23] Leboeuf (2011), Wood et al. (2012), Chien (2013).

[24] Gibbs (2014), One Health Sweden (2014).

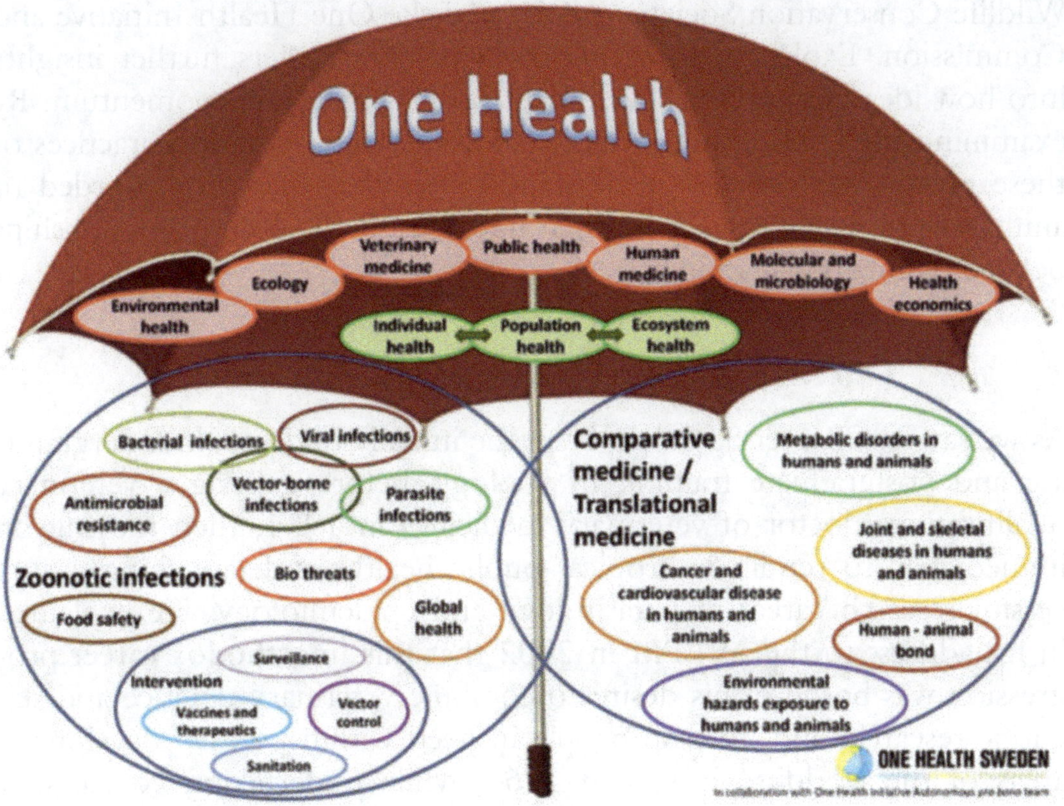

Fig. 6.1 The One Health umbrella. *Source* OH Sweden, 2014

its own sake.[25] This defensiveness over disciplinary boundaries, alongside competitiveness over professional status between veterinarians and their more dominant, better-resourced neighbours, would have been familiar to Schwabe and has repeatedly surfaced in veterinary–medical interactions since the nineteenth century.[26]

To gain a more nuanced understanding of how the ideas associated with OH came about and came together, the specific contexts where the agenda was first developed bear more detailed examination. To this end, I will now explore the longstanding interests and activities of four interlinked advocacy and research networks that were central to the formation of the OH movement: that of Calvin Schwabe, his students and collaborators; the Swiss Tropical and Public Health Institute (STPH); the

[25] Cassidy (2016).

[26] For Schwabe's experiences, see Chapter 5, p. 172. For other examples of veterinary-medical tensions, see Chapters 2 and 3. Also see Bresalier et al. (2015).

Wildlife Conservation Society (WCS); and the One Health Initiative and Commission. Exploring these networks in detail offers further insights into how ideas about OH have moved around and built momentum. By examining the publications, activities, locations and working practices of these groups, we can also understand better the roles they awarded to animals within OH, and how they understood the health relationships between humans and animals.

6.1.1 *Calvin Schwabe and One Medicine*

As we saw in Chapter 5, Calvin Schwabe initially undertook undergraduate and postgraduate training in zoology, before gaining a veterinary qualification (doctor of veterinary medicine) in 1954, then moving on immediately to retrain in tropical public health, and launching a successful research career in parasitology and epidemiology. He explained in his address to the AVEPM in 2002 that this unorthodox career progression was borne of his desire to combine veterinary practice and scientific research, and 'to help people in need within poorly "developed" areas of the world'.[27] It was in 1964, while undertaking consultancy work for the WHO Communicable Diseases Programme and researching the parasitic tapeworm *E. granulosus* at the AUB, that he published the first edition of his most famous work, *Veterinary Medicine and Human Health* (*VMHH*). A combination of textbook and magnum opus, *VMHH* was a product of an age in which (as described in Chapter 4) interactions between veterinarians and public health experts were increasing. It was intended to advance Schwabe's view that 'the veterinarian possesses unique qualifications which can not only be increasingly directed to the investigation of human diseases, but also to their management'.[28] Written with the support of a Fulbright fellowship and grant from the WHO, the book did not use the term OM. However, its structuring around the well-established domains of public health, epidemiology and comparative medicine, with additional sections on food hygiene and research methods, foregrounded those areas of medicine where animals frequently brought vets and doctors together. The book

---

[27] Schwabe (2004) pp. 194–5.

[28] Schwabe (1964) p. vii.

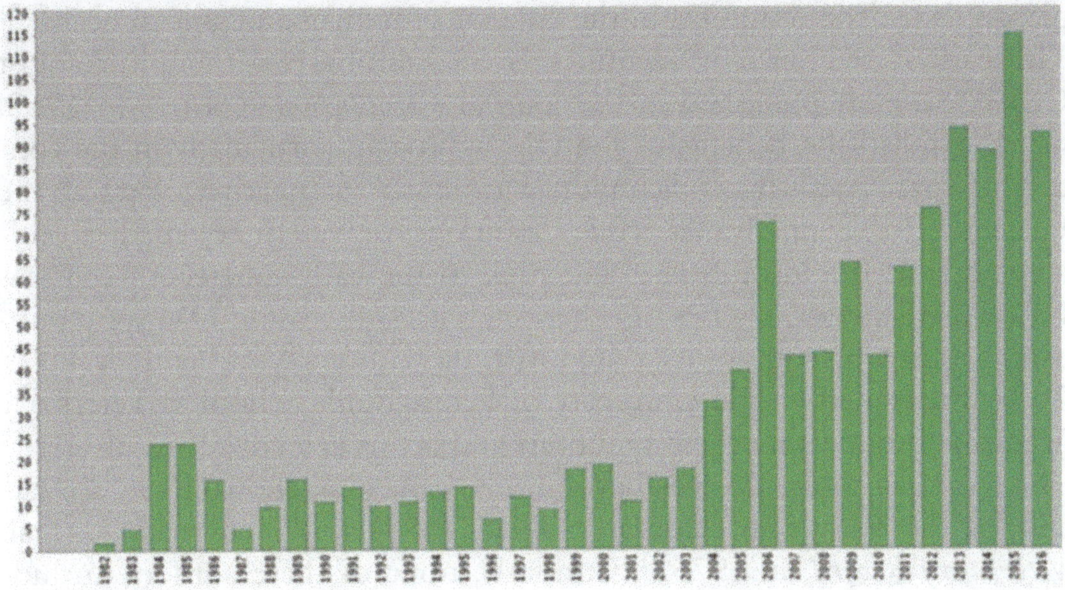

Fig. 6.2 Citations to Schwabe's *VMHH*, 1964, 1969, 1984. *Source* Web of Science, searched January 2017

was reviewed widely in veterinary and medical journals on both sides of the Atlantic (including at least three times by Schwabe's friend and collaborator James Steele), and it was republished in a second edition in 1969. Later in his career, with the support of a Rockefeller Foundation writing retreat,[29] Schwabe revised, updated and extended *VMHH* into a third edition, published in 1984. It was here that OM first featured—as a central organizing framework for the volume, in several chapter headings, and throughout the text.

As shown in Fig. 6.2, a citation search for *VMHH* suggests that its impact at the time of publication was relatively limited, at least on research publications, and it was not until the mid-2000s that the book was widely cited. The third (1984) edition accounts for about half of the post-2000 citations of *VMHH* and is often referred to in support of the idea that Schwabe devised the concept of OM.[30] However, searching bibliographic databases reveals that in fact Schwabe was not the first

[29]The Bellagio Centre Residency Program is still active. See Rockefeller Foundation (2017).

[30]Monath et al. (2010), Kaplan and Scott (2011).

person to use the term OM in the context of human and animal health.[31] The earliest reference it identifies is an editorial by the physiologist Carl F. Schmidt published in the journal *Circulation Research* in 1962, which extolled the benefits of the OM approach, particularly in the context of space medicine.[32] Schmidt, a professor of pharmacology at the University of Pennsylvania, cited traditions of veterinary–medical collaboration at the institution going back to the early nineteenth century. Following Schmidt, a series of other references discussing OM were published, mostly by authors associated with the University of Pennsylvania.[33] Today the leaders of the University of Pennsylvania School of Veterinary Medicine proudly cite these traditions and act as key advocates of OH.[34] The term had some currency beyond this context, as shown by its appearance as the title of an editorial in the UK's premier veterinary journal, *Veterinary Record*, in 1975.[35] Curiously, none of these authors (including Schwabe in the 1984 edition of *VMHH*) provided a definition of OM, instead treating it as a self-evident term which would already be familiar to the reader. This colloquial usage suggests that OM may have arisen organically, perhaps in veterinary-medical teaching or clinical collaborations taking place in and around Pennsylvania, and that rather than inventing it—as claimed by some OH advocates[36]—Schwabe adopted the term and greatly elaborated the idea when working on the third edition of his book.[37] Further support for this idea comes from following the career of Lord Lawson Soulsby, a recently deceased British veterinarian who served as president of both the Royal College of Veterinary Surgeons and

[31] The bibliographic databases Web of Science and PubMed (which index the contents of medical, natural science and humanities research journals) were searched for the phrase 'one medicine' in journal publications from 1900 to the present. Seven citations were found using the term 'OM' prior to Schwabe (1984).

[32] Schmidt (1962). On animals in American space medicine at this time, see Bimm (2013).

[33] Ravdin (1965), Allam (1966), Lechner (1968), Parish and Schwartzmann (1971), Cass (1973).

[34] Hendricks et al. (2009).

[35] Editorial (1975) p. 535.

[36] Kaplan and Scott (2011).

[37] While Schwabe never held a position at the University of Pennsylvania, after his retirement he moved from California to nearby Haverford, Pennsylvania, suggesting personal or professional connections to the area. Schwabe (2003), Nolan (2013).

the Royal Society of Medicine. Soulsby, now also claimed posthumously as a 'One Health pioneer' and like Schwabe a parasitologist specializing in helminths, held a position as professor of parasitology and chair of the Department of Pathobiology in the University of Pennsylvania School of Veterinary Medicine between 1964 and 1978. He then returned to Britain to head the University of Cambridge Veterinary School. Soulsby was a lifelong practitioner and advocate of integrating human and animal health. It therefore seems plausible that he also picked up the term at Pennsylvania, and influenced the *Veterinary Record*'s consistent support of OM prior to the rise of OH.[38]

As well as treating OM as a self-evident concept, many of these early authors attributed its origins to their own historical forebears—medical men such as Rudolf Virchow, William Osler and Benjamin Rush, alongside veterinarians such as John McFadyean—whose work transcended the human–animal divide and brought benefits to both. Schwabe went a step further by tracing the origins of OM back to medical and agricultural practices in classical and even prehistoric societies. Twenty-first-century OH advocates have continued this pattern of grounding and legitimizing their work by citing that of leading historical figures, often citing Schwabe's own historical research as a supporting reference.[39] Such processes of retrospective citation and celebration of historical individuals and publications are well understood as an important aspect of discipline-building.[40] However, for scholarly historians, the teleological, progressive historical narratives that they generate are deeply problematic. In attributing the pursuit of a twenty-first-century agenda to intelligent, successful and forward-looking nineteenth- and twentieth-century scientists, advocates for OM and OH have failed to engage with what, in the language of the time, these individuals thought they were doing and why. They have also neglected to consider the specific historical circumstances that encouraged the coming together of human and animal medicine in different times and places, as we describe in this volume and elsewhere.[41]

---

[38] Editorial (1975), Editorial (2005), Obituary (2017).

[39] Examples include: King et al. (2008), Monath et al. (2010).

[40] Examples include: the construction of Charles Darwin as a scientific icon for contemporary evolutionary biology (Rees 2009), and the epidemiologist John Snow as a historical hero of public health (Vandenbroucke et al. 1991).

[41] Bresalier et al. (2015).

Despite the widespread recent citation of *VMHH*, the book has been out of print for many years, even if it is widely retained in the libraries of veterinary schools. Its increasing citation rate correlates closely with the increasing usage of the term OH in academic journal articles.[42] This suggests that it may have taken on some of the features of a 'citation classic'—a piece written in the past which is widely referenced by contemporary scholars for symbolic or strategic purposes—in this case OH advocacy.[43] Beyond the book, the figure of Schwabe appears to have been co-opted into this process, playing the role of the latest in a long series of visionary 'founding fathers' who each played their part in the foundation of today's OH agenda. This symbolic role obscures the historical specificities of Schwabe's own life and work, which, as shown in Chapter 5, ranged widely across parasitology, epidemiology, anthropology, and human and veterinary medicine. His integrated thinking around health and medicine persisted in his retirement, when he continued his studies on the religious symbolism of cattle in Ancient Egypt, and animal medicine in prehistory.[44] From his writings on veterinary epidemiology through to the cookbook on utilizing unusual sources of animal protein (*Unmentionable Cuisine*), most of Schwabe's work supported his continually restated argument that veterinary medicine was important for human public health, and that there should be a legitimate space for veterinarians to contribute to that goal.[45]

During his lifetime, Schwabe influenced wider thinking on health and medicine, primarily via his immediate, largely veterinary, network of collaborators and students, and in turn their collaborators and students. As exemplified by the contributors to the 2002 Schwabe symposium, over time, members of this network moved into positions of power and influence both within US health policy and across international health. Two years after the symposium, the contributing papers were published in a special issue of the journal *Preventative Veterinary Medicine*.[46] While we do not have access to the attendee list, the stories presented below suggest that this event may have had a catalysing influence on

---

[42] See Cassidy (2016) p. 221.

[43] Weisz and Olszynko-Gryn (2010).

[44] Majok and Schwabe (1996), Gordon and Schwabe (2004).

[45] Schwabe (1979). For a full bibliography, see Schwabe (2004).

[46] See all papers in *Preventive Veterinary Medicine* 62 (2004).

the subsequent construction and promotion of the OH agenda in several institutions.

6.1.2 *The Wildlife Conservation Society*

The Wildlife Conservation Society (WCS) constitutes a very different working context from that experienced by Schwabe, yet one in which his ideas about human and animal health helped to provide a foundation from which new interconnections across these domains developed. The WCS is a USA-based non-governmental organization. Today it describes its core vision as 'a world where wildlife thrives in healthy lands and seas, valued by societies that embrace and benefit from the diversity and integrity of life on earth'.[47] It can be regarded as a US equivalent to the Zoological Society of London, and it runs several zoos and wildlife parks in the USA, including the Bronx Zoo. In addition the WCS runs an international programme of field research and conservation projects; fundraising, policy-making and campaigning; and it has pioneered veterinary wildlife research and practice in its zoos and in the field.

From the late 1990s, a small group of veterinarians working at the WCS (including William Karesh and Steven Osofsky) started building collaborative links between themselves, scientists studying emerging infectious diseases, and veterinary scientists and clinicians involved with global livestock health.[48] In 2003 they co-organized a workshop in Durban, South Africa, with the Veterinary Specialist Group of the International Union for the Conservation of Nature (IUCN). The purpose of the meeting was to further this collaborative agenda, bringing in practitioners working in government, international health and conservation non-governmental organizations to launch a new international network for health, environment and development, entitled AHEAD. In the workshop briefing, the organizers laid out an agenda for developing better collaborative relationships across these fields, which they described as "One Health".[49] The following year the WCS group organized an

[47] Wildlife Conservation Society (2015, 2016).

[48] Wolfe et al. (1998), Karesh, et al. (2002), Wildlife Conservation Society (2016).

[49] AHEAD stands for Animal and Human Health for the Environment and Development. This global network is still active. For the earliest usage of OH, see Osofsky et al. (2003) p. 63.

international conference on the theme of One World, One Health (OWOH), which was sponsored by the Rockefeller Foundation and held at the foundation's university campus in New York. Over the next few years it built links with the international Food and Agriculture Organisation (FAO) and the World Organisation for Animal Health (OIE), contributed to international responses to HPAI, and continued to publish its ideas about OH in academic and policy journals.[50] The proceedings of the AHEAD workshop outlined the WCS group's ideas about OH in more detail. Starting with the WHO's widely accepted definition of 'health' as a state of positive wellbeing (rather than the absence of disease), advocates of 'ecosystem health' argue by analogy that ecosystems can also be regarded as patients and evaluated as healthy or otherwise. The WCS veterinarians built on this idea, bringing it together with Schwabe's 'visionary attempts … to construct a bridge between medicine and agriculture' to argue for a broader collaborative approach to improving the health of humans, animals and environments, which they described as OH.[51]

These wildlife veterinarians developed the idea of OH primarily to advance their conservation agenda, but it was particularly grounded in thinking about problems of infectious disease, especially zoonoses. Their thinking around zoonotic diseases was, and is, unusually broad. While the WHO defines 'zoonosis' as disease transmission between animals and humans, most actors in global public health today use the term to denote the transmission of infections *from* animals *to* humans. By contrast the WCS group and their collaborators discuss the movement of infectious diseases between multiple species, back and forth across wildlife and livestock, humans and animals, much as Schwabe did when challenging the human–animal distinction at the core of 'zoonosis'.[52] If anything, the WCS group took this even further, highlighting the particular risks of transmitting common human infectious diseases *to* endangered species of wildlife. This understanding—that humans form part of an interconnected network of organisms including wildlife, domestic animals and microorganisms—was underlined by the logo the group used for OWOH, which depicted a 'parade' of silhouetted wild and domestic

[50] For example: Cook et al. (2004), Karesh and Cook (2009) pp. 259–60.

[51] Osofsky (2005) p. 83. For further details on ecosystem health, see for example Rapport et al. (1998).

[52] See Chapter 5, p. 188.

animal species alongside a human adult and child.[53] In the WCS group's writing on OH, animals commonly appear as specific species rooted in specific places, such as buffalo suffering from rinderpest in Uganda; or gorillas, bushmeat and Ebola in the Congo. While authors award animals key roles as transmitters of infectious diseases, they also present them as charismatic wildlife that need to be protected from disease; or, in the case of livestock animals, as potential food for humans whose productivity (like that of the cows discussed in Chapter 4) must be safeguarded and promoted. While the WCS veterinarians' ultimate priority was (in line with their institutional orientation) the protection and preservation of wildlife, the version of OH that they fashioned argues that this is best pursued through means that jointly protect human, animal and ecological health, for the benefit of all species. While drawing heavily on older ideas about OM, by broadening the scope from medicine to health, and bringing in the idea of care for ecosystems and wildlife alongside livestock and humans, it decentred humans significantly.

6.1.3 The Swiss Tropical and Public Health Institute

Drawing on these developments, in 2005, Professor Jakob Zinsstag and a group of his colleagues at the Swiss Tropical Public Health Institute (STPH) published an article in the international medical journal *The Lancet* arguing for the OH approach.[54] Bringing OH to a much bigger audience, including medical doctors and public health professionals, Zinsstag et al. started their article with a discussion of Schwabe and OM (citing *VMHH*) before proceeding to discuss the importance of ecosystem health (citing the WCS). They argued that OH needed to extend beyond the specifics of human and veterinary medicine and include broader ideas about health as wellbeing. They, in turn, added their own perspectives, to place a greater emphasis on research into tropical medicine and livestock health. They also introduced the public health concept of 'health systems', defined by the WHO as 'all organizations, people and actions whose primary intent is to promote, restore or maintain health. This includes efforts to influence determinants of health as well as more direct health-improving activities'.[55] This further broadened

[53] For examples of the OWOH logo, see Cook et al. (2004).

[54] Zinsstag et al. (2005).

[55] Tanner (2005) pp. 403–404, World Health Organisation (2007) p. 2.

OH by highlighting the social and administrative aspects of healthcare. Zinsstag and his colleagues applied this idea to human and animal health by arguing that, for example, vaccinating animals against diseases such as brucellosis or rabies can simultaneously protect human populations.[56]

The STPH is a partly state-funded research institute, devoted to research and clinical practice in tropical diseases and global public health. It was founded in 1943 by the zoologist Rudolf Geigy, who directed the institute until 1975.[57] The original aim of the then Swiss Tropical Institute was twofold: to perform research into tropical diseases—a field that straddled human medicine, biology and agriculture from its very foundation, as explained in Chapter 5[58]—and to train scientists, administrators and others preparing to live and work in French and British colonies.[59] Geigy himself worked across multiple disciplines, including zoology, physiology and embryology, and the institute was organized along these lines. From early in its history, the STPH worked with an affiliated research institute in Cote D'Ivoire, the Centre Suisse de Recherches Scientifiques (CSRS), to enable longstanding collaborative partnerships between Swiss and Ivoirian scientists investigating tropical medicine.[60] Today it is a large and thriving organization, with divisions focused on epidemiology, parasitology, international health, diagnostics, drug development and education.

Working in this tradition, Jakob Zinsstag joined the STPH during the 1990s to perform postdoctoral research on trypanosomiasis in the Gambia. After spending four years directing the CSRS in Cote D'Ivoire, he then returned to Switzerland to head up the STPH's animal health research group. For many years this group has worked on topics in and around global livestock health and international development, including the epidemiology of zoonotic and parasitic diseases, and also public health interventions such as vaccination, as described above. As

[56] Zinsstag et al. (2005).

[57] Rudolf was a member of the Geigy family, of the pharmaceutical and chemical company J.R. Geigy, inventors of dichlorodiphenyltrichloroethane (DDT), and now part of the contemporary Swiss pharmaceutical firm Novartis AG (Meier 2017).

[58] See Chapter 5, also Worboys (1996).

[59] Meier (2014, 2015).

[60] The CSRS was administered by the Swiss Academy of Sciences until 2001, after which it was gradually handed over to Ivoirian scientists and national government.

suggested by the STPH's institutional orientation towards tropical medicine, the group's work is mostly conducted in the global South, with a particular focus on working with pastoralist communities. It is clear from the STPH group's publications that—like the WCS veterinarians—they were working across human and animal health long before it started using the term OH in the mid-2000s.[61]

Alongside their emphasis on health systems, the STPH group also advocate a 'transdisciplinary' approach to OH research and practice, which involves working in participatory partnerships with local communities.[62] In contrast to the WCS group, who work across science and policy from within a non-governmental organization, the engagement of Zinsstag and his colleagues with OH has involved primarily academic activities, such as organizing professional societies, attending conferences, and writing and editing research articles. When they write about OH, the STPH group move rapidly beyond generic discussions of humans and animals towards the specific: it works with particular kinds of people and animals (e.g. mothers, herders, cattle, dogs) on particular diseases (e.g. rabies, brucellosis, Q fever) and in specific places (e.g. Chad, Cote d'Ivoire, Morocco). Highlighting how animals and humans live together in communities or as part of ecosystems, they consider it essential to care for the health of all. While the WCS group sometimes refer to wild animals, usually as disease vectors, the core of their work is with domestic animals, which are awarded roles as food sources, working animals, companions and community members.[63] As STPH's overall focus on human public health implies, this group's version of human–animal health is, like Schwabe's, anthropocentric, albeit with an intense interest in the shared lives and wellbeing of humans and animals, the transmission of infections between the two and the ambition to protect both.

6.1.4 *The One Health Initiative and Commission*

In 2006, the year after the STPH group's *Lancet* article, the incoming president of the American Veterinary Medical Association (AVMA), Dr Roger Mahr, addressed the association's annual conference. He argued

[61] For an overview of the group's work, see Zinsstag (2017).

[62] For example: Allen-Scott et al. (2015).

[63] Zinsstag et al. (2012).

that twenty-first-century challenges of global food security and zoonotic diseases meant that 'the continuing convergence of animal health, human health, and ecosystem health is the new reality', which must be responded to with a 'One World, One Health, One Medicine' approach. Mahr argued that veterinarians should adopt OH. Through building partnerships with public and environmental health professionals, they should assume leading roles in meeting these challenges—and growing the profession along the way.[64] Over the following year, he gained the support of his counterpart at the American Medical Association (AMA), public health physician Ronald M. Davis, who had pre-existing concerns about the risks that zoonotic diseases pose to humans. While this alliance resulted in OH being endorsed by the AMA in 2007, Davis died of cancer the following year and the resolution was subsequently dropped, indicating that the US medical profession more widely did not share his enthusiasm for OH.[65]

Mahr was more successful in persuading his colleagues in the AVMA, who passed their own resolution supporting OH. They also established a One Health Commission to investigate ways of improving veterinary-medical collaborations and moving the agenda forward, chaired by Lonnie King, one of the 2002 Schwabe symposium contributors. In parallel, Laura Kahn, Thomas Monath and Bruce Kaplan formed the One Health Initiative, an unfunded advocacy group dedicated to making the case for OH. Kahn is a physician based at Princeton University who by 2006 was already working on biosecurity and the risks of pandemic disease.[66] Kaplan had worked on food-borne illnesses for the Centres for Disease Control and Prevention (CDC) before his retirement, and Monath is a physician and consultant working in the pharmaceutical industry.[67] The OH Initiative quickly launched a website and organized a series of meetings and publications on OH/OM, including a piece entitled 'Confronting Zoonoses' co-authored by Kahn and Kaplan with veterinary public health pioneer James H. Steele (whose role in the 1948 establishment of the WHO's Veterinary Public Health

[64] Mahr (2006), Enserink (2007).

[65] Kahn and Davis (2008).

[66] Kahn (2006).

[67] Monath et al. (2010).

unit is described in Chapter 4.)[68] When the OH Commission published its report in 2008, it acknowledged the central influence of Schwabe's *VMHH*, cited Zinsstag et al.'s *Lancet* paper, the literature on emerging infectious diseases and the OH Initiative's publications. However, it did not cite the WCS veterinarians, instead tracing their influences directly back to Schwabe and OM—a move which emphasized veterinary medicine and de-emphasized environments and wildlife.[69]

The differences between the OH Initiative and WCS versions of OH are reflected in the imagery used by each group: unlike the WCS's 'parade' of humans and other animals, the OH Initiative's logo depicts the twinned icons of human and veterinary medicine in front of planet Earth.[70] This signals that for the Initiative—as for the Commission—OH is a project for changing professional relationships that is grounded in and legitimized by human–animal health relationships. Its assumption that closer veterinary–medical partnerships are universally relevant and beneficial perhaps explains the somewhat generic status of many of the animals that feature in their writings. The categories of animals, animal health, animal disease and animal science feature much more frequently than specific instances, and diseases (e.g. bovine spongiform encephalopathy—BSE) are named as or more often than the animals involved (e.g. cows). The key roles awarded to animals are those of patients; transmitters of zoonotic infections *from* animals *to* humans; victims of environmental pollution; and models and subjects of biomedical research.[71] The animal whose health has been of central concern to these groups has tended to be the human animal, with a particular focus on the USA. Like the immediate network around Calvin Schwabe, the OH Initiative and OH Commission maintain close connections with US health policy organizations such as the CDC and the Food and Drug Administration.[72]

In October 2008 a group of international agencies, including the WHO, FAO, OIE and World Bank, published a 'Strategic Framework for

[68] Kahn et al. (2007), Kaplan et al. (2009), Kahn et al. (2015).

[69] King et al. (2008).

[70] See, for example, the banner image used by Kahn et al. (2012).

[71] King et al. (2008), Day (2010).

[72] For further discussions of pandemic science and policy, and its tendency to orient towards publics in the developed world, see, for example, Caduff (2013).

Reducing Risks of Infectious Diseases at the Animal–Human–Ecosystems Interface.' This 70-page document drew upon the OH Commission report alongside the work of the WCS group to reflect on problems encountered during the avian influenza outbreak, when the division of health between animal- and human-focused organizations prevented effective communication and the ability to quickly coordinate responses to this 'hybrid' disease.[73] The agencies put forward proposals to improve the situation, using OH as an organizing framework and as shorthand to signal their collaborative intent.[74] In 2010 they followed up with a shorter policy briefing that reinforced their commitment to OH.[75] These publications brought the ideas and terminology of OH to the attention of a wider range of audiences than ever before. After 2010, OH became much more coherent and continued to grow, with increases in academic citations, the establishment of academic journals, textbook publications, the adoption of the term in health policy in several countries, and its uptake by major funders of global health agencies, including the Gates Foundation.

This pattern—of slow emergence, usefully flexible terms, intense negotiation followed by broad consensus, and then widespread adoption—was first described as a 'scientific bandwagon' in studies of the emergence and spread of molecular biology into cancer research during the 1980s.[76] However, while OH broadly fits this description, there are some key differences. In particular, it works across multiple disciplines and beyond science into the policy sphere; it is aimed at large institutional as well as individual actors; and it employs 'buzzwords' which are not only usefully flexible but also help advocates gather rhetorical support and financial resources from supporters. OH can therefore be viewed as an example of a newer form of scientific agenda-building, the 'interdisciplinary bandwagon', which works in concert with other agendas such as food security and translational medicine.[77]

[73] Jerolmack (2013).

[74] FAO, WHO, OIE et al. (2008).

[75] FAO, OIE and WHO (2010).

[76] Fujimura (1996, 1998).

[77] Maye and Kirwan (2013), Bensaude Vincent (2014), Cassidy (2016).

While the networks associated with Schwabe, the WCS, the STPH and the OH Initiative have by no means been the only groups involved in building OH, they can be understood as core to the early negotiation and development of its agenda. By looking at their writing and activities, we can identify the range of different influences, institutions and intentions that have given rise to not one but many OHs. We can also see that while the widespread belief that Schwabe founded OH/OM is inaccurate, his ideas, as propagated by his collaborators, students and readers, did exert a profound influence on the early formation of OH. In this sense, Schwabe was indeed crucial to the development of OH. However, the rise of OH also drove the popularity and fame of Schwabe, particularly after his death in 2006. It is also important to note that, in the majority of cases, the OH advocates discussed here were *already working and thinking across human and animal health* before OH rose to prominence. For them, Schwabe and the OH concept provided a concise and compelling way of articulating the advantages of working in this way—to themselves, to colleagues, to researchers beyond their immediate fields, and to wider audiences including policy-makers and funding bodies. In turn, each of these groups has been successful in persuading and enrolling each other, alongside an increasingly wide circle of individuals and organizations, into their common cause.

Despite these successes, it would appear that the consensus around what OH is, and, perhaps more importantly, what it should be, is still quite fragile. As we have seen, while the various groups described above have been able to develop and adapt each other's ideas, recrafting OH to fit their own contexts while also working together, multiple versions of OH remain in play. In particular, the two sides of the OH umbrella (Fig. 6.1) align not only with different fields of interest but also with different versions of human–animal relations. OWOH, the slogan originally used by the WCS group, can be broadly characterized as the left-hand side of the umbrella, involving veterinarians but also conservation, global health and development specialists. As we have seen with both the WCS and the STPH groups, OWOH sees humans, animals and environments as part of an interconnected network which requires care, decentring humans partially or completely. In contrast, the twenty-first-century version of OH/OM broadly but not completely aligns with the right-hand side of the umbrella: in something of a departure from Schwabe's original ideas it mobilizes zoonoses as a concern primarily because of the risk posed to humans. It then interconnects into clinical practice and human medicine via translational medicine, where it highlights the benefits of veterinary–medical collaboration for developing new drugs, gaining financial and symbolic support from pharmaceutical companies.[78] The emphasis on human health risks alongside veterinary–medical professional relationships creates a version of OH which appears to be significantly more anthropocentric than that seen in OWOH.

While there is no direct evidence of active tensions between OWOH and OM, the OH consensus does appear to be fracturing somewhat. For example, the WCS group have reoriented themselves towards 'ecohealth'—a restatement of the ideas of ecosystem health, with key personnel such as William Karesh taking on leadership roles in a new Ecohealth Alliance.[79] Jakob Zinsstag and his colleagues have also taken on core roles in the international academic association for EcoHealth. Other researchers working across human and animal health are adopting newer buzzwords alongside or instead of OH. A good example of this is 'the nexus',[80] an idea that originated in environmental governance during the late 2000s and that describes the need for interlinked thinking in response to environmental challenges that cut across multiple domains. Unlike OH, it has avoided defining what these domains are, and this increased flexibility may be helping 'the nexus' to avoid becoming as entangled in disciplinary politics.[81]

6.2 The Animal Subjects of One Health

While the above stories bring depth to our account of the rise of OH in the early twenty-first century, so far this chapter has told a mostly human story, albeit one involving several groups of people professionally involved with animals. In keeping with the overall aims of this book, I shall now analyse the place of animals within OH, both in their own right and in their relationships with humans. Looking at how animals are conceptualized, represented and acted on by those who research, practice and advocate OH offers important insights into the roles awarded to these animals and their relative valuation in society, health and medicine. In revealing how humans perceive and have elected to respond to the health threats and opportunities presented by animal bodies, it also

[78] Twine (2013), Hobson-West and Timmons (2016).

[79] Gunelius (2010), Ecohealth Alliance (2017).

[80] For example: Davies et al. (2016), Mwangi et al. (2016).

[81] Cairns and Krzywoszynska (2016).

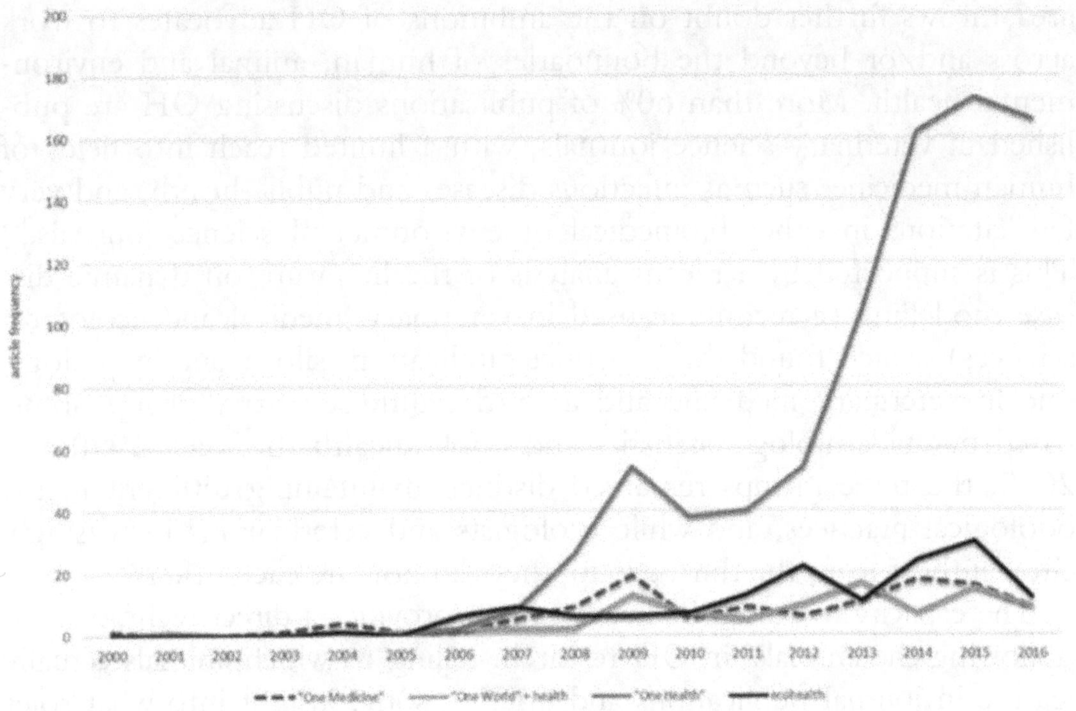

Fig. 6.3 Growth of the One Health bandwagon. *Source* Web of Science, searched March 2017

illuminates the ways in which animals have inadvertently shaped OH, and how OH aspires to shape them. These insights derive from analysis of the literal and symbolic traces that animals have left on the scientific journal articles, websites, policy documents and media outputs created by human participants in OH.

6.2.1 *Animals in One Health Research Texts*

While OH encompasses research, policy and clinical practice, the preceding stories show that scientists and their research lie at its core. Consequently, scientific citation databases can reveal its entry into, and expression in, research agendas, as shown in the earlier analysis of Schwabe's *VMHH*. The development of the OH bandwagon can be traced in the same way: usage of the term in journal articles spiked after the WHO-FAO-OIE joint statement, and increased sharply between 2012 and 2016 (Fig. 6.3).[82] Analysis of these references by subject

[82] Source: Web of Science (Science, Social Science and Humanities Indices), excluding conference proceedings and incidental usage such as 'one health authority'.

area throws further doubt on the ambitions of OH advocates to work across and/or beyond the boundaries of human, animal and environmental health. More than 60% of publications discussing OH are published in veterinary science journals, with a limited reach into fields of human medicine, such as infectious diseases and public health, and very few citations in other biomedical or environmental science journals.[83] This is supported by a recent analysis of the literature on dynamic disease modelling (a technique used in veterinary, medical and ecological sciences), which found three distinct publication 'silos': one in ecology, one in veterinary medicine and a third multidisciplinary group dominated by epidemiology, statistics and public health. Between 1990 and 2015, the three groups remained distinct, maintaining different methodological practices, and while ecologists and veterinarians increasingly cited authors from the third group, they did not cite each other.[84]

The capacity to search by keyword also provides a direct technique for 'following the animals' in OH research, telling us which animals actually feature in journal publications and offering some insight into what roles they are awarded by researchers. The Web of Science database was therefore searched for 'one health', alongside a series of animal names and roles. The relative frequency of these terms and the scientific content of the articles in which they feature were recorded. The results of this process are shown in Tables 6.1 and 6.2. Perhaps the most striking finding is that the most frequently mentioned animal in the scientific literature on

Table 6.1 One Health and animal categories

Search term	*Article hits*
'One Health'	1737
OH AND human	1178
OH AND animal OR animals	727
OH AND model	293
OH AND food	170
OH AND wildlife OR 'wild animal'	125
OH AND livestock	115
OH AND pet OR companion	85

Source Web of Science, 2004–2015, searched January 2017

[83] Galaz et al. (2015), Cassidy (2016). See also Friese and Nuyts (2017).

[84] Manlove et al. (2016).

Table 6.2 One Health and animal species

Search term	*Article hits*	*Research topics*
OH AND canine OR dogs	121	zoonosis (46), rabies (38), vector (31), bite (22)
OH AND avian OR poultry OR birds	94	influenza (66), zoonosis (42), food (28)
OH AND bovine OR cows OR cattle	80	zoonosis (34), TB (25), food/milk (24), brucellosis (11),
OH AND swine OR pig	57	zoonosis (27), influenza (16), model (15), food (15)
OH AND feline OR cat	39	zoonosis (15), parasite (10),
OH AND horse OR equine	25	zoonosis (11), hendra (6)
OH AND rat OR mouse OR rodents	18	model (11), zoonosis (6), leptospirosis (3)
OH AND sheep OR goat	18	zoonosis (6), rift valley fever (3); brucellosis (2)
OH AND bat	17	rabies (7), zoonosis (6), hendra (5)
OH AND deer	12	TB (5), zoonosis (2)
OH AND gorilla OR chimpanzee OR ape OR monkeys	10	conservation (5), zoonosis (4)

Source Web of Science, 2004–2015

OH is actually the *human* animal, while non-human animals are referred to mostly in generic terms. The roles that animals were awarded in scientific research are indicated via the use of categories such as 'models' (model organisms employed as experimental material in human biomedical research), 'food' (as a source of human infection, rather than nutrition, as discussed in Chapter 4), 'wildlife' (hosts and transmitters of zoonotic infections), 'livestock' (intermediate hosts and transmitters of parasites, as described in Chapter 5, and as zoonotic disease transmitters), and 'pets/companion animals' (again as zoonotic disease transmitters). Many of the journal articles using these terms demonstrate a lack of specificity about what aspects of health or disease are actually of concern.

Far fewer OH articles mention specific types of animal, and when they do, a few species dominate (Table 6.2). This makes it possible to examine the articles more closely and analyse the specific animal contributions to human health that researchers are interested in. Dogs feature most commonly, primarily as vectors of zoonotic disease, particularly rabies, and as direct threats to human health via bites (which also carry risks of disease transmission); then birds, primarily as vectors of influenza, but domestic poultry specifically feature as a major source of gastrointestinal infections, such as *Salmonella*. Cows are the third most common animal type, featuring usually in relation to zoonotic infections carried in milk and meat, such as bovine tuberculosis and brucellosis.[85] A second key animal role that emerges is that of the experimental model for human disease, and it is usually assigned to rodents or pigs, reflecting the intersection between OH and translational medicine.[86] Despite the prominence of the category 'wildlife', specific species are rarely named. When they are it is in relation to certain infections, such as rats and leptospirosis, or bats and viral infections such as rabies or Hendra.[87]

From these figures it appears that much of the research literature using the term OH tends to discuss animals in terms of generic categories (e.g. animal-livestock-wildlife). When specific types of animal are named, they tend to be domestic species which pose certain risks (as disease vectors, e.g. dogs-rabies, birds-influenza, cows-tuberculosis) or offer benefits (as experimental models, e.g. rodents) to humans. This strong focus on the animal roles of disease vector and experimental model represents the continuation of existing interests in their relationships to human health that date back to the nineteenth century.[88] It supports the idea that OH can be understood in part as a rebranding of existing fields of enquiry. While OH advocates may claim to pursue an expansive vision of health at the interface of humans, animals and environment, in practice OH is primarily shaped by pre-existing, longstanding human–animal health relationships. This analysis suggests that the majority of researchers adhere to an anthropocentric perspective in which animals matter only insofar as their bodies threaten human health or offer opportunities for its advancement.[89] Animals are thereby sidelined

[85] Bovine tuberculosis, caused by the bacterium M. bovis, is a zoonotic form of tuberculosis which can infect all mammal species, caused by the bacterium *M. bovis*. Brucellosis is a bacterial infection which causes abortion in cattle and fever and wasting in humans. Both infections are passed from animals to humans via contaminated meat and milk.

[86] Davies (2012), Cassidy (2016).

[87] Leptospirosis is a zoonotic bacterial infection carried primarily by rodents which can be fatal in severe cases. Rift Valley Fever and Hendra are both zoonotic viruses carried by livestock animals with a wildlife reservoir in bat populations.

[88] Clarke and Fujimura (1992), Waddington (2006), Pemberton and Worboys (2007). See also Appendix: Annotated Bibliography of Animals in the History of Medicine.

[89] Woods (2017).

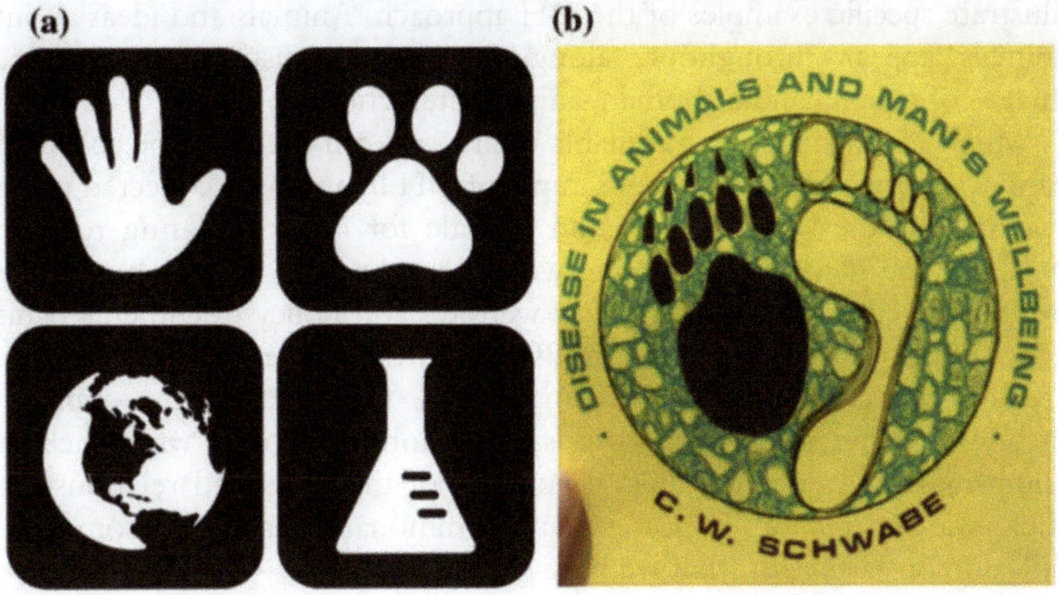

Fig. 6.4 Human–animal partnerships. *Sources* a) Cornell One Health workshop, 2015; b) Calvin Schwabe, *Disease in Animals and Man's Wellbeing* (1970)

as prospective beneficiaries of OH. Despite this, it is worth noting that searches of Web of Science for these animal types alongside terms such as 'zoonosis' reveals an abundance of scientific research primarily concerned with animal health and its relationships with humans and/or environments. However, for reasons which merit further investigation, the individuals who conduct this research do not appear to find OH a useful term for advancing their ideas.

6.2.2 *Animals in One Health Imagery*

Animal images are central to the visual strategies employed by OH advocates as they seek to persuade colleagues, funders and policy-makers of OH's merits. These images appear occasionally in journal articles, but more prominently in the 'grey' literature of policy reports, the websites of conference and advocacy groups, and mass media coverage of OH. This material can offer further insights, beyond the more constrained form of scientific publishing, into the place of animals in OH. Its imagery consists of logos, infographics, diagrams and photographs, which are used in a variety of ways: most obviously to envisage ideal relationships between human, animal and environmental health; as logos highlighting the 'brand' of particular organizations and events; and to illustrate specific examples of the OH approach. Animals and ideas about animals appear throughout, alongside more 'realistic' photographic images of people, and of human–animal interactions.

Much of this material is available online and can therefore be collected easily via keyword searching. A sample of OH images was collected using two main routes: by searching on Google for images relating to 'one health', 'one medicine' and 'one world, one health'; and by harvesting images directly from OH advocacy websites and policy documents. This activity was performed initially in 2013 and then repeated in late 2015, creating a total sample of 217 image files. Of these images, approximately 60% were drawn illustrations, infographics or logos, while the rest comprised photographic images. Analysis of the roles and relationships they award to animals indicates some commonalities and also some significant contrasts with what we have seen so far.

Given that the core idea of OH involves intersecting domains, the vast majority of these images provide visual interpretations of this concept, depicting the human–animal dyad of OM, a triad of humans, animals and the environment and so on. The images used to convey these broad, abstract categories have been, on the whole, correspondingly broad and abstract. Indeed, the most abstract of these dispense with any form of direct representation, opting instead for interconnected spirals or swirls.[90] The logo of the OH Initiative (as described above) depicts the paired icons of human and veterinary medicine. A minority of images in the sample use this same idea. An alternate approach depicts the subjects of OH rather than the professions concerned with it. Several versions of this strategy can be seen in the sample. The simplest and most popular version uses the iconography of a human hand or foot alongside animal feet, most commonly a paw (Fig. 6.4).

While the 'human' in these images is universal, the 'animal', while deeply abstracted, is not. The animals with paws indicated in Fig. 6.3 tend to be carnivores: in veterinary contexts, paws often indicate pet dogs and cats. This inference is backed up by the photographic images in the sample, which includes eight pictures of dogs, all depicted as companion animals and sometimes as veterinary patients (one cat features,

---

[90] See, for example, the banner logo of the OH Commission and that designed for the annual OH Day, initiated in 2016 (One Health Commission 2017) or that of the OH Platform and journal (One Health Platform 2017).

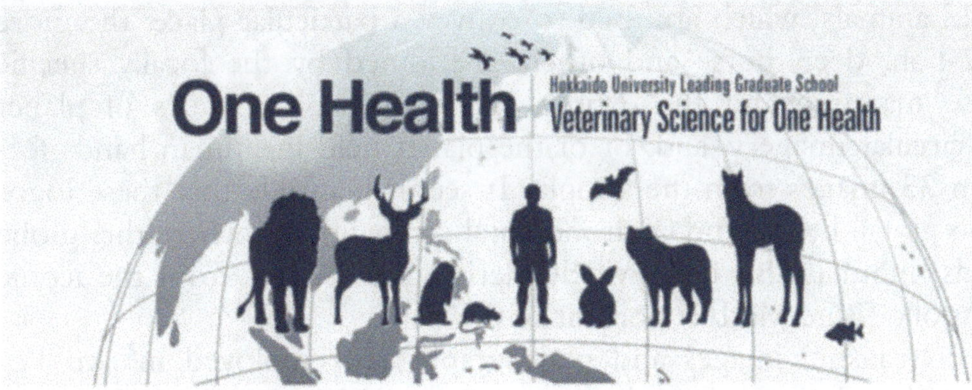

Fig. 6.5 OH contextualised. *Source* One Health Graduate School, Hokkaido University, Japan

accompanied by a dog). By contrast, in the scientific articles analysed above, these roles rarely feature. There, dogs appear primarily as risks to humans either via bites or as a source of rabies infection.

The transition from OM to OH involved a shift from a clinical, medical focus to broader concepts of health and wellbeing. It also extended beyond human–animal health relationships to include the idea of health across the natural environment. This shift is reflected in the usage of tripartite imagery depicting humans, animals and environments, which was first employed by the WCS vets in their 2003 AHEAD workshop.[91] In these logos, the hands and paws are joined by leaves, trees or sheaves of wheat. Alternatively, humans, animals and plants are depicted as silhouettes, and this strategy introduces a little more variety into the imagery. Humans are joined by smaller figures evoking families, and, while paws still feature, livestock animals such as cows or pigs also appear.[92] Human and animal silhouettes are also used in an alternative strategy to depict humans–animals–environment, bringing together the 'parade' used by the 2004 OWOH meeting with the planetary imagery of the OH Initiative. A good example of this type can be seen in the logo designed by Hokkaido University (Fig. 6.5). Humans and animals are depicted together, in or on the planet Earth. While most of these images remain universal and generic, others like this one display a diversity of domestic

[91] Osovsky et al. (2003).

[92] See, for example, the logo of the EU Veterinary Week 2010 conference. EU Vet Week (2010).

and wild animals, which are used to convey a particular place: the more generic lion, deer, horse and others are joined by the locally specific Japanese macaque and the extinct Hokkaido wolf. Images of planet Earth, circular imagery, and/or of the planet held in human hands featured in 35 images from the sample. It seems plausible that these logos draw on global health and environmental campaigning, where the 'globe in hands' motif is also used widely, deriving as it does from the iconic 1972 Apollo 'Blue Marble' portrait of the Earth.[93]

More 'realistic' images and photographs are employed in two key ways: as a less design-oriented version of the OH 'tripartite' of humans-animals-environment, or to illustrate examples of problems or research issues which OH can address (e.g. influenza illustrated by chickens). The animals portrayed in these realistic tripartites are usually domesticated—both agricultural animals and pets, although more frequently the former—while images of plants (representing the environment) tend to suggest food crops.[94] Photographic images are also employed to illustrate examples of problems that can be addressed through the OH approach. Conveying 'success stories' in this way is so important that one OH advocacy site hosts an online archive of images specifically for promotional usage.[95] Almost all of these types of image include animals, but they are dominated by very particular types of animal, playing particular roles in particular places. For example, of the 11 photographs of cows in our sample, 7 are of zebu-type cattle, often depicted with African pastoralist farmers. As we have seen in Chapter 4, the zebu was a core animal of concern for veterinarians involved in international health and nutrition in the mid-twentieth century, whose work Schwabe was closely associated with. Their visual presence suggests that pastoralist contexts remain a key site for OH in the present day. Chickens and pigs also feature. Their presence reflects OH's entanglement with contemporary concerns about pandemic influenza, and resonates with the content of the scientific journal literature, as analysed above. These species are shown with humans in small-scale, global South farming contexts; being transported or contained for sale in 'wet markets' in East Asia; or (in the case of chickens)

93 For further analysis and commentary on the Blue Marble image, see Gurevitch (2014), Höhler (2015).

94 See the covers of Osofsky et al. (2003) and King et al. (2008).

95 One Health Global Network (2017).

with humans in medical protective clothing. Here, animals and humans are portrayed in close proximity, in open air and/or muddy, messy situations, implying that the source of zoonotic disease risks are not solely the animals but the intimacy of human–animal relationships in these parts of the world.

Wild animals appear in some of these photographs, usually large charismatic species, including ostriches, giraffes, seals, elephants, lions and great apes. They are depicted alone, or in about a third of the images with humans, usually as recipients of veterinary care, but occasionally as 'hands and paws', evoking the imagery seen in Fig. 6.5, and the famous *National Geographic* image of Jane Goodall and a chimpanzee hand in hand. These images seem to be drawing on conservation and animal welfare campaigning to advance ideas of human care for, and custodianship of, animals.[96] While occasionally wild animals appear in relation to zoonotic disease transmission, these are usually less sympathetic animals such as bats, at times manipulated to look more threatening.[97] The prominence of wildlife in these images contrasts heavily with the published literature on OH, where beyond the generic category of 'wild animals', individual species barely feature.

Eight photographs in the sample show animals as patients, with human clinicians working directly with them in one way or another. They are split evenly between images of dogs being cared for in clinical settings (by implication in the global North), and wild or agricultural species being cared for in the field (by implication in the global South). Finally, 18 images of humans without animals feature. About half of these are pictures taken at conferences and other scientific or policy meetings, while most of the rest depict people working in laboratories. With the exception of a still from the 2011 film *Contagion*, no images of human patients were found. Indeed, the plot of *Contagion*, which plays out the imagined scenario of an emerging infectious disease pandemic, can be seen as part of a broader cultural case for OH. The film

---

[96] For a fuller analysis of this kind of human-paw imagery, see Haraway (1999) pp. 134–9.

[97] Examples include the first edition cover of David Quammen's popular science book *Spillover* (2013), depicting a baboon baring its fangs; and the process of creation of a 'scarier looking' computer-generated imagery (CGI) bat for the 2011 film *Contagion* (Failes 2011).

starts with an American businesswoman who becomes sick after a trip to Hong Kong, passing on the disease to several others before dying and setting off a civilization-threatening pandemic. While much of the film focuses on victims, survivors and scientists' efforts to understand, trace the source of and treat the outbreak, the end of the film provides a critical 'reveal'. A series of brief shots shows the destruction of rainforest, disrupted bats taking refuge in a pig house, a pig sold at a wet market being prepared in a restaurant, an Asian chef with unwashed hands, and an American businesswoman, who then becomes ill, taking the viewer back to the start of the story. This narrative brings together many of the themes found across OH advocacy images. Indeed, Professor Ian Lipkin of Columbia University (an expert in emerging infectious diseases and OH ally) was a key scientific adviser for the film.[98]

Taken together, what can these images tell us about the sorts of animal bodies and disease that have shaped OH, and which are, in turn, shaped by it? Generic animals, humans and plants play a central role—with outlined images of human figures, common animals such as cows, hand-foot-paw prints, and leaves often appearing in OH logos. Reinforcing the verbal messages of OH advocates, they convey an idea of OH as a generic, universal approach that addresses all types of health problem arising at the intersections of humans, animals and environment—even though, as shown above, the work performed by researchers adopts a more selective approach to those problems. Once we move beyond the generic animal, more differences begin to open up between their portrayal in OH images, advocacy arguments and OH research. For example, while cows feature in a small number of OH research papers which are largely devoted to bovine tuberculosis and brucellosis, they are extremely common in the visual sample. While dogs appear in both, in visual images they feature as family members and veterinary patients, not—as in scientific articles—as carriers of rabies. Images of charismatic wildlife such as great apes and giraffes are prominent in OH advocacy but extremely rare in OH research. By contrast, animals as experimental models are rarely depicted despite their presence in the research literature. These are obvious promotional choices, making the most of publicly appealing imagery while avoiding drawing attention

[98] Hernendez (2017).

to more controversial animal roles. However, this once again highlights contrasts between OH promotion and practice.

These images can also tell us how OH advocates understand relationships between humans, animals and environments—as they are and how OH believes they should be. Humans appear regularly, talking to each other, caring for animals, working in laboratories, or as human hands. OH depicts itself as a form of care of animals, environments and the planet. Implicitly or explicitly, this imagery shares the assumption that humans must care via forms of custodianship where only human agency is made visible. In first world contexts we see familial or clinical scenes, most often with pets; in images of the global South and East we see small-scale, direct agricultural care and veterinary care of wildlife. In this way, OH indicates its globalizing ambition alongside its awareness of key differences in human–animal relationships in different parts of the world. Care and risk are held in balance, particularly in the context of zoonotic diseases, which by implication come from less appealing wildlife species and from modes of human–animal interactions that occur in traditional food and farming systems. This narrative casts animals and certain kinds of human as 'guilty victims', geographically far away from the global North, or socially excluded, who must be kept out at all costs.[99] It is also at odds with emerging OH research which suggests that pandemic disease risks may be accentuated not by traditional but by modern intensive farming systems and the global distribution of their products.[100] Finally, it is worth observing that as time goes on, the imagery of OH has become more and more abstracted: following John Berger, the animals are literally disappearing from a movement primarily led by people concerned with animal health.[101]

6.3 Conclusion

This chapter has examined attempts in the early twenty-first century to develop integrated OH approaches to problems lying at the intersection of human health, animal health and the environment. It has explored in

---

[99] Washer (2010), Cassidy (2012).

[100] See, for example, Ducrotoy et al. (2015), Hinchliffe et al. (2016).

[101] Berger (1980).

detail the early formation and negotiation of OH, teasing out the diverse institutional contexts in which it emerged and the different versions of OH they gave rise to. The roles played by Calvin Schwabe in the development of these many versions of 'One Health' have been investigated: while he was not in fact the originator of OH or OM, he has provided a common point of connection and inspiration across the key scientific networks involved in building what has, in very recent years, become an 'interdisciplinary bandwagon'. Alongside a series of august forebears, Schwabe is now cited as a key precedent, informant and source of authority for OH today. However, as this chapter has demonstrated, the OH agenda developed this role for Schwabe, just as much as he—through his ideas, publications and personal connections—developed the modern movement for OH.

In keeping with the overall aims of this book, this chapter has also indicated the sorts of animal and animal health concern that have attracted attention from across human medicine, veterinary medicine and the life sciences, and contributed to the development of new relationships between individuals working in these fields under the banner of OH. Both scientific journal articles and images in OH advocacy documents deal overwhelmingly with animals in the abstract: as broad categories such as 'animal' or 'wildlife', and as literal abstractions in the form of silhouettes and logos. This abstraction matches the generic claims made for OH by its advocates, as a universally applicable and beneficial approach to health that has demonstrated its value repeatedly through history. It also recalls to mind how often and how persistently animals continue to be viewed as 'mere blank pages onto which humans wrote meaning'.[102] At the same time, when tracing the origins and practical applications of OH, very specific types of animal, context and problem are shown to be involved.

Zoonotic diseases (as transmitted by agricultural animals, dogs and wildlife) feature prominently in both the research and policy/advocacy literatures analysed here, while animals as 'models' in laboratory research appear much more commonly in the scientific literature. As our annotated bibliography indicates, both are extremely longstanding animal roles. When considered alongside the institutional origins of OH, their prominence suggests that much of what goes by the name of OH today is in fact a rebranding of existing health agendas.

[102] Fudge (2006).

They also indicate an anthropocentric character to OH, its greater concern for the human than the animal health benefits that may arise from an integrated approach to their health. While OH imagery demonstrates an additional objective of care for valued animals (livestock, pets and aesthetically pleasing charismatic wildlife), which it portrays in the roles of patients and subjects of human custodianship, this has yet to be realized substantially in scientific work that claims to pursue a OH approach. This situation indicates the peculiar contradictions at the heart of OH: a movement trying to bring together human and animal health does so by arguing—and working to ensure—that attending to animal health will benefit humans.

These anthropocentric contradictions may be related to ongoing anxieties about the ability of OH to move 'from rhetoric to reality'.[103] As both advocates and observers have noted, OH has tended to flip from very broad generalities to specific 'success stories', but with little discussion of how researchers, policy-makers and clinicians might move from one to the other.[104] The analysis presented here suggests that these problems persist at the level of research practice. Yet OH continues to be mobilized in international health. Over the past two years the WHO has published strategies for action on antimicrobial resistance and rabies elimination, which both prominently reference OH as a conceptual support for coordinating across organizations in human and animal health.[105] Time will tell what impact such activities have on the roles that animals perform in OH, on how OH is practised, and on how it presents itself to the wider world.

Bibliography

Allen-Scott, Lisa K., Bonnie Buntain, Jennifer M. Hatfield, Andrea Meisser and Christopher James Thomas. "Academic Institutions and One Health: Building Capacity for Transdisciplinary Research Approaches to Address Complex Health Issues at the Animal-Human-Ecosystem Interface." *Academic Medicine* 90 (2015): 866–71.

[103] Marks (2014), Okello et al. (2011), Cork et al. (2016).

[104] Stephen and Karesh (2014), Galaz et al. (2015).

[105] World Health Organisation (2015, 2016).

Allam, M.W. "The M.D. and the V.M.D." *Pennsylvania Medicine* 69 (1966): 57–60.

Anderson, Warwick. "Natural Histories of Infectious Disease: Ecological Vision in Twentieth-Century Biomedical Science." *Osiris* 19 (2004): 39–61.

Atlas, R.M. and S. Maloy (eds). *One Health: People, Animals, and the Environment.* ASM Press, 2014.

AVEPM *Newsletter, Spring/Summer 2002.* Accessed March 29, 2017. http://www.avepm.org/files/AVEPMnewsletterspring02.pdf?attredirects=0.

Barrett, Meredith A. and Timothy A. Bouley. "Need for Enhanced Environmental Representation in the Implementation of One Health." *EcoHealth* 12 (June 2015): 212–9.

Bimm, J. "Primate Lives in Early American Space Science." *Quest: History of Spaceflight Quarterly* 20(4) (2013): 29–40.

BBSRC. *Strategic Plan: 2010-2015.* Swindon: UK Biology and Biotechnology Research Council. Published online 2014. Accessed March 29, 2017. http://www.bbsrc.ac.uk/documents/strategic-plan-pdf/.

Bensaude Vincent, Bernadette. "The Politics of Buzzwords at the Interface of Technoscience, Market and Society: The Case of 'Public Engagement in Science.'" *Public Understanding of Science* 23 (2014): 238–53.

Benson, Etienne. "Animal Writes: Historiography, Disciplinarity, and the Animal Trace." In *Making Animal Meaning*, edited by Linda Kalof and Georgina M. Montgomery, 3–16. East Lansing: Michigan State University Press, 2011.

Berger, John. "Why look at animals?" In *About Looking*, edited by J. Berger, 1–26. London: Writers and Readers, 1980.

Bresalier, M., A. Cassidy and A. Woods. "One Health in History." In *One Health: The Theory and Practice of Integrated Health Approaches*, edited by J. Zinsstag, E. Schelling, D. Waltner-Toews, M. Whittaker and M. Tanner, 1–15. Wallingford: CABI, 2015.

Caduff, Carlo. "Whose World? Which Health? What Security? The Facts and Fictions of Global Health Security." *BioSocieties* 8(1) (2013): 94–6.

Cairns, Rose and Anna Krzywoszynska. "Anatomy of a Buzzword: The Emergence of 'the Water-Energy-Food Nexus' in UK Natural Resource Debates." *Environmental Science & Policy* 64 (2016): 164–70.

Calain, Philippe. "Ethics and Images of Suffering Bodies in Humanitarian Medicine." *Social Science & Medicine* 98 (2013): 278–85.

Cass, J. "One Medicine – Human and Veterinary." *Perspectives in Biology and Medicine* 16 (1973): 418–26.

Cassidy, A. "Vermin, Victims and Disease: UK Framings of Badgers In and Beyond the Bovine TB Controversy." *Sociologia Ruralis* 52(2) (2012): 192–204.

Cassidy, A. "One Medicine? Advocating (Inter)disciplinarity at the Interfaces of Animal Health, Human Health and the Environment." In *Investigating*

Interdisciplinary Collaboration: Theory and Practice across Disciplines, edited by S. Frickel, M. Albert and B. Prainsack, chapter 10. Rutgers University Press, 2016. Accessed March 29 2017. https://www.ncbi.nlm.nih.gov/books/NBK395883/.

Chien, Yu-Ju. "How Did International Agencies Perceive the Avian Influenza Problem? The Adoption and Manufacture of the 'One World, One Health' Framework." *Sociology of Health & Illness* 35(2) (2013): 213–26.

Clarke, A.E. and J.H. Fujimura (eds). *The Right Tools for the Job: At Work in the Twentieth Century Life Sciences.* Princeton: Princeton University Press, 1992.

Cook, R.A., W.B. Karesh and S.A Osofsky. "One World, One Health: Building Interdisciplinary Bridges." Published online, 2004; Accessed March 29, 2017. https://web.archive.org/web/20170211045743/http://www.oneworldonehealth.org/.

Cork, Susan C., David Hall and Karen A. Liljebjelke. *One Health Case Studies: Addressing Complex Problems in a Changing World.* Sheffield: 5M Publishing, 2016.

Craddock, Susan and Steve Hinchliffe. "One World, One Health? Social Science Engagements with the One Health Agenda." *Social Science & Medicine* 129 (2015): 1–4.

Davies, G. "What is a Humanized Mouse? Remaking the Species and Spaces of Translational Medicine." *Body & Society*, 18(3–4) (2012): 126–55.

Davies, Gail, Beth Greenhough, Pru Hobson-West, Robert Kirk, Ken Applebee, Laura Bellingan and others. "Developing a Collaborative Agenda for Humanities and Social Scientific Research on Laboratory Animal Science and Welfare." *PLoS ONE*, 11(7): e0158791 (2016). Accessed March 29, 2017. doi:10.1371/journal.pone.0158791.

Day, M.J. "One Health: The Small Animal Dimension." *Veterinary Record* 167 (2010): 847–9.

Degeling, C., Jane Johnson, Ian Kerridge, Andrew Wilson, Michael Ward, Cameron Stewart and Gwendolyn Gilbert. "Implementing a One Health Approach to Emerging Infectious Disease: Reflections on the Socio-Political, Ethical and Legal Dimensions." *BMC Public Health* 15 (2015): 1307. Accessed March 29, 2017. doi: 10.1186/s12889-015-2617-1.

Ducrotoy, M.J., Khaoula Ammary, Hicham Ait Lbacha, Zaid Zouagui, Virginie Mick, Laura Prevost et al. "Narrative Overview of Animal and Human Brucellosis in Morocco: Intensification of Livestock Production as a Driver for Emergence?" *Infectious Diseases of Poverty*, 4(57) (2015): 1–21.

EcoHealth Alliance, "Scientists - Dr. William Karesh - Executive Vice President for Health and Policy." EcoHealth Alliance, accessed March 29, 2017. http://www.ecohealthalliance.org/personnel/dr-william-karesh.

Editorial. "Two Disciplines, One Medicine." *Veterinary Record* 96 (1975): 535.

Editorial. "One Medicine?" *Veterinary Record* 157 (2005): 669.

Enserink, M. "Medicine: Initiative Aims to Merge Animal and Human Health Science to Benefit Both." *Science* 316 (2007): 1553.

'EU Vet Week to Focus on Food Traceability.' *Vet Times*, June 14, 2010. Accessed November 8, 2017. https://www.vettimes.co.uk/news/eu-vet-week-to-focus-on-food-traceability/.

Failes, Ian. "Incredible, Invisible Effects." Fxguide, 30 September 2011. https://www.fxguide.com/featured/incredible-invisible-effects/.

FAO, OIE and WHO. *The FAO-OIE-WHO Collaboration: Tripartite Concept Note.* World Health Organisation, 2010. Accessed March 29, 2017. http://www.who.int/influenza/resources/documents/tripartite_concept_note_hanoi/en/.

FAO, WHO, OIE et al. *Contributing to One World, One Health A Strategic Framework for Reducing Risks of Infectious Diseases at the Animal – Human – Ecosystems Interface.* Food and Agriculture Organisation, 2008. Accessed March 29, 2017. http://www.fao.org/docrep/011/aj137e/aj137e00.htm.

Friese, Carrie and Nathalie Nuyts. "Posthumanist Critique and Human Health: How Nonhumans (Could) Figure in Public Health Research." *Critical Public Health*, 27(3) (2017): 303–13.

Fudge, Erica. "Ruminations 1: The History of Animals." (2006). Accessed February 19, 2017. https://networks.h-net.org/node/16560/pages/32226/history-animals-erica-fudge.

Fujimura, Joan. *Crafting Science: A Sociohistory of the Quest for the Genetics of Cancer.* London: Harvard University Press, 1996.

Fujimura, Joan. "The Molecular Biological Bandwagon in Cancer Research: Where Social Worlds Meet." *Social Problems* 35(3) (1998): 261–83.

Galaz, Victor, Melissa Leach, Ian Scoones and Christian Stein. "*The Political Economy of One Health Research and Policy.*" STEPS Working Paper 81, 2015. Accessed April 2, 2017. http://steps-centre.org/wp-content/uploads/One-Health-wp3.pdf.

Gates Foundation. "The 'One Health' Concept: Bringing Together Human and Animal Health for New Solutions: Grand Challenges Explorations 11." 2013. Accessed March 29 2017. http://gcgh.grandchallenges.org/challenge/one-health-concept-bringing-together-human-and-animal-health-new-solutions-round-11.

Gibbs, E.P.J. "The Evolution of One Health: A Decade of Progress and Challenges for the Future." *Veterinary Record* 174 (2014): 85–91.

Gordon, A.H and C.W. Schwabe. *The Quick And The Dead: Biomedical Theory In Ancient Egypt.* Leiden: Brill, 2004.

Gunelius, S. "Wildlife Trust Rebrands as Ecohealth Alliance." *Corporate Eye*, September 21, 2010. Accessed 2 April, 2017. http://www.corporate-eye.com/main/wildlife-trust-rebrands-as-ecOHealth-alliance/.

Gurevitch, L. "Google Warming: Google Earth as Eco-Machinima." *Convergence* 20(1) (2014): 85–107.

Haraway, D. *Primate Visions: Gender, Race, and Nature in the World of Modern Science.* London: Verso, 1999.

Hendricks, J., C.D. Newton and A. Rubenstein. "'One Medicine – One Health' at the School of Veterinary Medicine of the University of Pennsylvania – The First 125 years." *Veterinaria Italiana* 45 (2009): 183–94.

Hernendez, D. "Responding to Emerging Threats: An Article for the One Health Newsletter." Accessed March 29 2017. https://www.mailman.columbia.edu/research/center-infection-and-immunity/cii-%E2%80%94-responding-emerging-threats-article-one-health.

Hinchliffe, Steve, Nick Bingham, John Allen and Simon Carter. *Pathological Lives: Disease, Space and Biopolitics.* Chichester, West Sussex: Wiley Blackwell, 2016.

Hobson-West, Pru and Stephen Timmons. "Animals and Anomalies: An Analysis of the UK Veterinary Profession and the Relative Lack of State Reform." *The Sociological Review* 64(1) (2016): 47–63.

Höhler, S. *Spaceship Earth in the Environmental Age, 1960–1990.* London: Routledge, 2015.

Jerolmack, Colin. "Who's Worried about Turkeys? How 'Organisational Silos' Impede Zoonotic Disease Surveillance." *Sociology of Health & Illness* 35 (2013): 200–12.

Joint WHO/FAO Expert Committee on Zoonoses. "Second Report." *World Health Organization Technical Report Series* 169 (1959): 1–83.

Kahn, L.H. "Confronting Zoonoses, Linking Human and Veterinary Medicine." *Emerging Infectious Diseases*, 12 (2006): 556–61.

Kahn, L.H. and R.M. Davis. "One Medicine – One Health. Interview with Ronald M. Davis, MD, President of the American Medical Association, 14 May 2008." *Veterinaria Italiana* 45 (2009): 19–21.

Kahn L.H., B. Kaplan and T.P. Monath. "About the One Health Initiative." One Health Initiative Website, 2012. Accessed May 11, 2015. http://www.onehealthinitiative.com/about.php.

Kahn, L.H., B. Kaplan, T. Monath, J. Woodhall and L.A. Conti. "History of the One Health Initiative team." One Health Initiative Website, 2015. Accessed March 29, 2017. http://www.onehealthinitiative.com/publications/Draft%205%20NEWS%20OHI%20ONE%20HEALTH.pdf.

Kahn, L.H., B. Kaplan and J.H. Steele. "Confronting Zoonoses Through Closer Collaboration Between Medicine and Veterinary Medicine (as 'One Medicine')." *Veterinaria Italiana* 43 (2007): 5–19.

Kaplan, B., L.H. Kahn and T. Monath (eds). "Special Issue: One Health - One Medicine: Linking Human, Animal and Environmental Health." *Veterinaria Italiana* 45 (2009): 1–211.

Kaplan, B. and C. Scott. "One Health History Question: Who Coined the Term 'One Medicine'?" One Health Initiative Website, 2011. Accessed February 24, 2017. http://www.onehealthinitiative.com/publications/Who%20coined%20

the%20term%20One%20Medicine%20by%20B%20%20Kaplan%20and%20C%20%20Scott%20May19%202011-CS.pdf.

Karesh, W.B., S. Osofsky, T.E. Rocke and P.L. Barrows. "Joining Forces to Improve Our World." *Conservation Biology* 16(5) (2002): 1432–4.

Karesh, W.B. and R.A. Cook. "One World – One Health." *Clinical Medicine, Journal of the Royal College of Physicians of London* 9(3) (2009): 259–60.

King, Lonnie et al. *One Health: A New Professional Imperative. One Health Initiative Task Force: Final Report.* American Veterinary Medical Association, 2008. Accessed March 29, 2017. https://www.avma.org/KB/Resources/Reports/Documents/onehealth_final.pdf.

King, Nicholas. "The Scale Politics of Emerging Diseases." *Osiris*, 19 (2004): 62–76.

Kirk, Robert G. "'Life in a Germ-Free World': Isolating Life from the Laboratory Animal to the Bubble Boy." *Bulletin of the History of Medicine* 86(2) (2012): 237–75.

Leboeuf, Aline. "Making Sense of One Health Cooperating at the Human-Animal-Ecosystem Health Interface." *IFRI Health and Environment Reports* 7, April 2011. Institut Français des Relations Internationales (IFRI), Paris. Accessed April 2, 2017. http://www.ifri.org/en/publications/enotes/notes-de-lifri/making-sense-one-health.

Lechner, C.B. "One Medicine." *Pennsylvania Medicine* 71 (1968): 50–1.

Lee, K. and Z.L. Brumme. "Operationalizing the One Health Approach: The Global Governance Challenges." *Health Policy and Planning* 28(7) (2012): 1–8.

Lupton, Deborah. "The Pedagogy of Disgust: The Ethical, Moral and Political Implications of Using Disgust in Public Health Campaigns." *Critical Public Health* 25(1) (2015): 4–14.

Majok, A.A. and C.W. Schwabe. *Development among Africa's Migratory Pastoralists.* London: Bergin & Garvey, 1996.

Mahr, R.K. "AVMA President-Elect Address to the House of Delegates." American Veterinary Association, July 14, 2006. Accessed March 29, 2017. https://www.avma.org/News/PressRoom/Pages/Speeches-onehealth-mahr-060714.aspx.

Manlove, Kezia, Josephine Walker, Meggan Craft, Kathryn Huyvaert, Maxwell Joseph, Ryan Miller, Pauline Nol et al. "'One Health' or Three? Publication Silos Among the One Health Disciplines." *PLoS Biology* 14(4) (2016): e1002448. Accessed March 29, 2017. doi:10.1371/journal.pbio.1002448.

Marks, N. "The Politics of Delivering One Health." *STEPS Centre Briefing*. November 17, 2014. Accessed April 2, 2017. http://steps-centre.org/publication/politics-delivering-one-health/.

Maye, Damian and James Kirwan. "Food Security: A Fractured Consensus." *Journal of Rural Studies* 39 (2013): 1–6.

Meier, L. *Swiss Science, African Decolonization, and the Rise of Global Health, 1940–2010.* Basel: Schwabe Verlag, 2014.

Meier, L. "The Other's Colony: Switzerland and the Discovery of Cote D'Ivoire." In *Colonial Switzerland: Rethinking Colonialism From the Margins*, edited by P. Purtschert and H. Fischer-Tiné, 73–87. Basingstoke: Palgrave Macmillan, 2015.

Meier, L. "Rudolf Geigy." R.Geigy Foundation website. Accessed February 24, 2017. http://www.geigystiftung.ch/en/rudolf-geigy.html.

Molloy, C. *Popular Media and Animals*. Basingstoke: Palgrave Macmillan, 2011.

Monath, T.P., L.H. Kahn and B. Kaplan. "Introduction: One Health Perspective." *ILAR Journal* 51 (2010): 193–8.

Mwangi, W., P. de Figueiredo and M.F. Criscitiello. "One Health: Addressing Global Challenges at the Nexus of Human, Animal, and Environmental Health." *PLoS Pathogens* 12(9) (2016): p.e1005731. Accessed March 29, 2017. doi:10.1371/journal.ppat.1005731.

Nicholls, Henry. "The Art of Conservation." *Nature* 472 (21 April 2011): 287–9.

Nolan, R.S. "LEGENDS: The Accidental Epidemiologist." *Journal of the American Veterinary Medical Association: News*. July 1, 2013. Accessed April 2, 2017. https://www.avma.org/News/JAVMANews/Pages/130701m.aspx.

Obituary. "Lord Soulsby of Swaffham Prior." *Veterinary Record* 180 (2017): 504.

Okello A.L. et al. "One Health and the Neglected Zoonoses: Turning Rhetoric into Reality." *Veterinary Record* 169 (2011): 281–5.

One Health Commission. "One Health Day." One Health Commission Website, accessed March 29, 2017. http://www.onehealthcommission.org/en/eventscalendar/one_health_day/.

One Health Global Network. "Photo Archive" One Health Global Network website, accessed March 29, 2017. http://www.onehealthglobal.net/resources/photo-archive/.

One Health Platform. "Creating a Healthy Future for Humans, Animals and Environments." One Health Platform Website, accessed March 29, 2017. http://www.onehealthplatform.com/.

One Health Sweden. "One Health Sweden Steering Committee Visit to Florida, December 2013." *One Health Sweden*, 2014. Accessed March 29, 2017. http://www.onehealth.se/ohs/node/176.

Osofsky, S., W. Karesh, R. Kock and M. Kock. "AHEAD Invitees Briefing Packet." Wildlife Conservation Society, 2003. Accessed March 29, 2017. http://www.wcs-ahead.org/wpcongress.html.

Osofsky, Steven A. (ed.) "Conservation and Development Interventions at the Wildlife / Livestock Interface: Implications for Wildlife, Livestock and Human Health." *Occasional Paper of the IUCN Species Survival Commission* 30 (2005). Accessed March 29, 2017. http://www.wcs-ahead.org/documents/aheadbriefingbooklet.pdf.

Parish L.C. and R.M. Schwartzman. "There is but One Medicine." *Pennsylvania Medicine* 74 (1971): 65–6.

Pemberton, Neil and Michael Worboys. *Mad Dogs and Englishmen: Rabies in Britain 1830–2000*. Basingstoke: Palgrave Macmillan, 2007.

Quamman, D. *Spillover: Animal Infections and the Next Human Pandemic*. New York: W.W. Norton, 2012.

Rapport D., R. Costanza, P.R. Epstein, C. Gaudet and R. Levins (eds). *Ecosystem Health*. Oxford: Oxford University Press, 1998.

Ravdin, I.S. "One Medicine – Human, Dental, Animal." *Pennsylvania Medicine*, 68(11) (1965): 48–50.

Rees, A. "The Undead Darwin: Iconic Narrative, Scientific Controversy and the History of Science." *History of Science*, 47(4) (2009): 445–447.

Rockefeller Foundation. "The Bellagio Centre Residency Programme" Accessed March 29 2017. https://www.rockefellerfoundation.org/our-work/bellagio-center/residency-program/.

Schmidt, C.F. "Editorial: One Medicine for More than One World." *Circulation Research* 11 (1962): 901–3.

Schwabe, C.W. *Veterinary Medicine and Human Health*. 1st ed. Baltimore: Williams and Wilkins Co., 1964; 2nd ed. Baltimore: Williams and Wilkins Co., 1969; 3rd ed. Baltimore: Williams and Wilkins Co., 1984.

Schwabe, C.W. *Unmentionable Cuisine*. Charlottesville: University of Virginia Press, 1979.

Schwabe, C.W. "A Spiritual Haven for Scientists" *Friends Journal*, January 1, 2003. Accessed June 13 2017. https://www.friendsjournal.org/2003006/.

Schwabe, C.W. "Keynote Address: The Calculus of Disease – Importance of an Integrating Mindset." *Preventive Veterinary Medicine* 62(3) (2004): 193–205.

Stephen, C. and W.B. Karesh. "Introduction: Is One Health Delivering Results?" *Revue scientifique et technique (International Office of Epizootics)* 33(2) (2014): 375–9.

Tanner, Marcel. "Strengthening District Health Systems." *Bulletin of the World Health Organisation* 83 (2005): 403–4.

Twine, Richard. "Animals on Drugs: Understanding the Role of Pharmaceutical Companies in the Animal-Industrial Complex." *Journal of Bioethical Inquiry* 10(4) (2013): 505–14.

Vandenbroucke, J.P., H.M. Eelkman Rooda and H. Beukers. "Who Made John Snow a Hero?" *American Journal of Epidemiology* 133 (1991): 967–73.

Waddington, Keir. *The Bovine Scourge: Meat, Tuberculosis and Public Health, 1850-1914*. Woodbridge: Boydell & Brewer, 2006.

Washer, P. *Emerging Infectious Diseases and Society*. Basingstoke: Palgrave Macmillan, 2010.

Wildlife Conservation Society. "2020 Strategy." Wildlife Conservation Society website, published online 2015. Accessed March 29, 2017. https://www.wcs.org/our-work/2020-strategy.

Wildlife Conservation Society. "120 Years: A Conservation Legacy." Wildlife Conservation Society website, published online 2016. Accessed March 29, 2017. http://fscdn.wcs.org/2016/03/01/9kmyv16g9x_WCS_historical_timeline_February_2016.pdf.

World Health Organisation. Everybody's Business. Strengthening Health Systems to Improve Health Outcomes: WHO's Framework for Action. Published online 2007. Accessed March 29, 2017. http://www.who.int/healthsystems/strategy/everybodys_business.pdf.

World Health Organisation. Global Action Plan on Antimicrobial Resistance. Published online 2015. Accessed March 29, 2017. http://www.who.int/antimicrobial-resistance/global-action-plan/en/.

World Health Organisation. Global Framework to Eliminate Human Rabies Transmitted by Dogs by 2030. Published online 2016. Accessed March 29, 2017. http://www.who.int/neglected_diseases/news/Global_framework_eliminate_human_rabies_transmitted_dogs_2030/en/.

Weisz, G. and J. Olszynko-Gryn. "The Theory of Epidemiologic Transition: The Origins of a Citation Classic." *Journal of the History of Medicine and Allied Sciences* 65(3) (2010): 287–326.

Wolfe, N.D., A. Escalante, W.B. Karesh, A. Kilbourn, A. Spielman and A. Lal. "Wild Primate Populations in Emerging Infectious Disease Research: The Missing Link?" *Emerging Infectious Diseases* 4 (1998): 149–58.

Wood, James, Melissa Leach et al. "A Framework for the Study of Zoonotic Disease Emergence and Its Drivers: Spillover of Bat Pathogens as a Case Study." *Philosophical Transactions of the Royal Society of London. Series B, Biological Sciences* 367(1604) (2012): 2881–92.

Woods, Abigail. "Animals in the History of Human and Veterinary Medicine." In *Routledge Companion to Animal-Human History*, edited by H. Kean and P. Howell. Basingstoke: Palgrave, 2017, forthcoming.

Worboys, M. "Germs, Malaria and the Invention of Mansonian Tropical Medicine: From 'Diseases in the Tropics' to 'Tropical Diseases.'" *Clio Medica* 35 (1996): 181–207.

Wilkinson, I. "The Provocation of the Humanitarian Social Imaginary." *Visual Communication* 12(3) (2013): 261–76.

Zinsstag, J. "Unit: Human and Animal Health" Swiss Tropical Public Health Institute website. Accessed March 29, 2017. https://www.swisstph.ch/en/about/eph/human-and-animal-health/.

Zinsstag, Jakob, Esther Schelling, Kaspar Wyss and Mahamat Bechir Mahamat. "Potential of Cooperation between Human and Animal Health to Strengthen Health Systems." *Lancet* 366 (2005): 2142–5.

Zinsstag, Jakob, Andrea Meisser, Esther Schelling, Bassirou Bonfoh and Marcel Tanner. "From 'Two Medicines' to 'One Health' and Beyond." *Onderstepoort Journal of Veterinary Research* 79 (2012): 1–5.

Zinsstag, J., E. Schelling, D. Waltner-Toews, M. Whittaker and M. Tanner (eds). *One Health: The Theory and Practice of Integrated Health Approaches*. Wallingford: CABI, 2015.

CHAPTER 7

Conclusion

The volume has aimed to break new ground in developing an animal history of medicine and a medical history of animals. Despite burgeoning interest in animal history in recent years, its scholars have seldom followed their subjects into the realms of health and medicine, while in medical history, the animal presence is largely implicit. Reduced to their diseases, bodily processes and products, animals typically provide the stage on which human history is enacted. This volume has argued instead for studying them in their own right, as subjects and shapers of medicine. As documented in our annotated bibliography (Appendix), the few scholars who have previously adopted this approach have tended to focus on the fashioning of animals into experimental subjects in laboratories. However, this volume has demonstrated that laboratory medicine was just one node in a multi-centred network of enquiry into animals and their diseases, which stretched into, and helped to fashion and connect up, domains situated at the borderlands of medicine: comparative anatomy and pathology, natural history, zoology, veterinary medicine, agriculture, nutritional science, veterinary public health, parasitology and epidemiology. In studying these networks, we have revealed what humans did to animals in their efforts to advance health and medicine, and what difference animals made to medicine through shaping its knowledge-practices, institutional settings and the lives of its investigators. The result is a richly contextualized series of case studies which not only add to our understandings of animals in medicine, but also change

A. Woods et al., *Animals and the Shaping of Modern Medicine*, Medicine and Biomedical Sciences in Modern History, https://doi.org/10.1007/978-3-319-64337-3_7

our conceptions of what constituted medicine in particular times and places.

The relationships that animals forged within medicine are central to these studies. It was through such relationships that they influenced medicine and were, in turn, shaped by it. One important observation that arises in our studies is that these relationships involved *multiple species.* Generally, in medicine today, in historical writing on the subject (as summarised in our annotated bibliography), and in research outputs employing the banner of One Health (OH) (Chapter 6), interspecies relationships are portrayed in dualistic terms: a particular type of animal spreads infection to humans, or is manipulated in the laboratory to shed light on human disease. Such animals tend to be farmed livestock or laboratory rodents, and are of interest to medicine and its history because of the threats and benefits they present to human health.

Our studies have shown that this is a reductionist and anthropocentric view of medicine which fails to recognize the rich multiplicity of interspecies relationships that were forged through medical practices—not simply for the purpose of advancing human health but also to learn about relationships between species, to study the disease processes they had in common, and to advance animal health for its own sake (although here, too, humans have been the ultimate beneficiaries because healthier animals could better perform their human-designated roles). Chapters 2 and 3 have described medical interventions pursued in zoos and on Scottish hill farms for the benefit of animal, not human health, while Chapter 4 has shown how, under the post-war campaign against world hunger, such interventions were intended to benefit human and animal health simultaneously. The comparative pathology described in Chapter 2 sought similarities and differences between the diseases affecting human beings and the zoos' various vertebrates. Some investigators interpreted their findings in evolutionary terms, suggesting that disease drove, and was a product of, evolutionary differences between species. Chapter 3 described how sheep became enmeshed in relationships with ticks, bacteria, experimental animals belonging to the same and different species, and the human and animal victims of analogous diseases. Chapter 5 extended this ecological network to include tapeworms, dogs, wild carnivores and multiple types of human communities, and showed that for Calvin Schwabe, the elucidation of this network was as important a research objective as the prevention of human disease. Chapter 6 examined the somewhat uneven portrayal of these multispecies networks in the texts and images used to illustrate and advertise OH today.

Collectively, these findings serve to expand historical understandings of the numbers and types of animal that participated in medicine. They show that the foundations—and indeed the objectives—of medicine have been more broadly zoological than historians have previously acknowledged. Furthermore, analysis of the roles that these animals have performed within medicine shows that they shaped it in previously unrecognized ways. While prevailing anthropocentric perspectives on medical history have generated insights into animals as experimental models of disease and transmitters of zoonotic infections to humans, in shifting to a more animal-centred perspective, our chapters bring to the fore a host of other animal roles: as disease victims, patients, pathological specimens, points of comparison with other species, products and shapers of their environments, suppliers of human nutrition, subjects of international health policy and commercially lucrative products of medicine (such as more productive livestock, more appealing visitor attractions in zoological gardens, dead specimens for museum display, and post-experimental sheep sold for knackers' meat).

Performed simultaneously or sequentially through animal lives and afterlives, these roles were awarded by humans and legitimated by human relationships with, and valuations of animals. They also have their own histories which merit further elucidation. As the chapters have shown, these roles opened up certain opportunities for animals to shape health and medicine. For example, as patients, pathological specimens and points of comparison, monkeys in the zoo illuminated the cause of rickets (Chapter 2); as victims of their environments and as experimental subjects, sheep influenced the geography and timing of scientific enquiry and its practices (Chapter 3); as suppliers of human nutrition, cows pushed forward the campaign against world hunger (Chapter 4); while as shapers of their environments, *E. granulosus* informed laboratory investigations into its biology and wider epidemiological movements within communities (Chapter 5). In performing their roles, animals did not only impact on the knowledge-practices of medicine but also on its social and organisational aspects. As pathological specimens, animals brought doctors into the zoo. They also advanced the career of John Bland Sutton (Chapter 2), just as the tapeworm's shaping of its environment advanced Calvin Schwabe's (Chapter 5). As victims of their environments, sheep forged diverse research networks, while as hosts and transmitters of infection, they enabled ambitious vets to make a bid for professional recognition (Chapter 3). As sources of human health and nutrition, dairy cows brought departments of the Food and Agriculture Organization and World Health Organization into existence, and forged interdisciplinary connections that granted vets the authority to make international health policy (Chapter 4). Tracing the sequential and overlapping roles that animals held also links institutions, disclosing, for instance, that Schwabe's laboratory-based studies of *E. granulosus* fed into, but did not dominate, parallel fieldwork and epidemiological investigations, indicating not only more complex multispecies relationships but also more intricately interlaced sites and disciplinary worlds than usually feature in histories of medicine and biology.

Roles also had implications for the animals that performed them, because they affected how humans treated them. We have seen how, as patients or potential victims of disease, zoo animals, sheep and dairy cows were closely monitored and subjected to interventions such as dosing, dipping, dressings, surgical operations, special feeding or pasturing, and new housing. Pathological specimens were created through natural or deliberate deaths, post-mortem examination and sometimes the preservation of animal remains. Experimental animals had their bodily integrity disrupted, while environmental shapers had their surroundings studied and manipulated. Through the practice of medicine, therefore, animal identities, bodies, habits, environments, relationships and lived experiences were profoundly and continually altered. By attending to these processes and circumstances, we can begin to understand how animals have been changed by medicine, and how they made a difference to it, thereby elucidating their deeply intertwined histories.

Studying this process of co-constitution prompts us to rethink not only the subjects and objectives of medicine, but also how, where and by whom it was practised. In following animals through medicine, our chapters have revealed a host of spaces in which medical enquiries have took place—not just in laboratories, but on farmland and ranches, in zoos and homes, and in the wild. The incorporation of these spaces expands the known geographies of medicine as well as the species that have participated in it. We have also highlighted the involvement of various humans who rarely feature in existing medical histories: zoological society doctors, zoo vets, keepers and superintendents in Chapter 2; the farmers, labourers, landowners, natural historians and medical experts of Chapter 3; the vets in Chapter 4 who worked to enrol animals in the post-war international campaign against world hunger; and in Chapter 5, the dog-owning communities of Beirut, the pastoralists, ranchers and sheepherding communities of Kenya and North America, and the experts in anthropology and parasitology who studied them.

These findings show firstly, that the keepers and carers of animals were important contributors to the development of knowledge about their diseases and should therefore be incorporated into histories of animals and medicine. Secondly, that the health of animals attracted the attention of diverse scientific experts, whose engagement with them forged intersections between human medicine, veterinary medicine and biology. Chapters 2 and 3 revealed how human doctors applied medical ideas and practices to the health of zoo and agricultural animals; Chapters 4, 5 and 6 demonstrated the application of veterinary ideas and approaches to human health agendas; Chapters 2, 3 and 5 showed how the biological perspectives of comparative anatomy, zoology, botany, entomology and parasitology were brought to bear on human health, animal health and the relationships between them. While the nature of these intersections was context specific, they highlight the shared capacity of animal subjects of medicine to cut across and forge connections across disciplines. The medicine that was produced through them was not bounded by species. Indeed, some of its practitioners were outspoken in their rejection of species and disciplinary boundaries: Chapter 4's veterinary public health experts proclaimed their work as a contribution to human health and wellbeing, while for Calvin Schwabe the line between humans and non-humans was not fundamentally biological but cultural in character.

The backgrounds and positions occupied by many of the medical experts whose activities we have documented do not give an obvious indication of their interest in animal health. Similarly, the medical associations of the work performed by our experts in veterinary medicine and the natural world are not always apparent. This may explain why their activities at the borderlands of these disciplines have evaded historical detection. However, historians' traditionally anthropocentric conceptions of what constituted modern medicine are also to blame. The standard assumptions that, except in its direct bearings on human health, the health of animals was a veterinary matter and the life of animals a subject for biologists have served to obscure the actual historical relationships between veterinary medicine, biology and medicine. In showing that diseased animals featured within all three of them, we have demonstrated the need for historians to generate more empirically grounded, historically sensitive understandings of their characteristics and boundaries. One meaningful approach to this issue is through the history of animals because, as we have shown, in attracting the attention of different types of expert, animals have helped to fashion the activities of and relationships between different fields of science and medicine.

The case studies presented here have also offered novel and important historical precedents to the current way of working known as One Health (OH), which seeks to develop integrated perspectives from across human medicine, veterinary medicine and the life sciences. Chapters have illuminated circumstances in which such integrated perspectives were developed in the past, and shown how this way of working was shaped, advanced and at times challenged by the human and animal participants, and the wider political, economic, institutional and scientific contexts. We have seen how, drawing on a longer tradition of medical involvement in animal health, the doctors who attended Britain's nineteenth-century zoos were quick to import human medical methods and concepts. However, animals did not always comply with their efforts to construct them as subjects of public health, bedside medicine and hospital medicine. Sick sheep were similarly recalcitrant pathological and experimental subjects. In studying them, the ambitious veterinarians of Chapter 3 sought to distance investigators in medicine and zoology from what had previously been a cross-cutting field of endeavour. Aided by institutional shifts in research funding and ideas of disease causation, these vets contributed to the compartmentalization of the disciplines. As a consequence, during the interwar period, the pursuit of healthy humans and healthy animals occurred largely along parallel tracks. However, as Chapter 4 revealed, the outbreak of war, and the post-war discovery of hunger and protein malnutrition, helped to break down the disciplinary compartments, and to forge new connections between healthy animals, healthy humans and their experts. This provided a fertile context for the work of parasitologist Calvin Schwabe, who crossed multiple disciplinary domains in his pursuit of the tapeworm *E. granulosus*. These findings offer a preliminary trajectory for the practice of OH from the mid-nineteenth to the late twentieth century.

It is notable that the 'OH' practices documented here do not feature in scholarly medical histories, or in the history that OH advocates have constructed for themselves. The former is primarily concerned with the uses of experimental animals in medicine, not the multispecies, multicentred activities that we have described. The latter relies on a highly selective narrative of famous 'OH' practitioners. By contrast, with the exception of Schwabe, whose life and work merits further scrutiny, we have elected to study, and embed within their historical contexts, the work of individuals who were more representative of their age. OH advocates also posit a mid-twentieth-century low point for OH that they attribute to reductionist tendencies that abolished earlier holistic thinking about health. The trajectory we have sketched out challenges this claim by showing how, in the context of international health, OH was actually reinvigorated in this period.

Our findings therefore suggest that in modern medicine the practice of OH is both more frequent and more significant than either historians or OH advocates have realized. This finding strengthens the case for why medical historians need to move beyond the human, to incorporate animals into their frame of reference. It also boosts the claims made by OH advocates about the historical importance of OH ways of working. At the same time, however, in revealing the historical specificity of OH, our findings challenge their conviction that it constitutes a universally applicable and self-evidently beneficial approach. We have shown that the health problem under investigation, the animals affected, the humans involved, the institutional setting, the funding regime, the intended outcomes, and the wider social, political and economic contexts may all have a bearing on whether the practice of 'OH' proved feasible, desirable, and capable of achieving its desired objectives. There is no universal scientific logic of OH. History shows that its merits can only be determined on a case-by-case basis, with due regard to social, political and economic circumstances.

In addition to providing precedents for the practice of OH today, the later chapters in this volume have also elucidated its historical roots as a self-conscious scientific and policy agenda. As described in Chapter 6, this movement emerged in the early twenty-first century. Partly in response to a series of emerging zoonotic disease threats, a number of research groups began to call for a reconfiguration of research, policy and clinical practice, which would break down the professional, scientific and policy silos of human health, veterinary medicine and environmental health. Such groups were often already working in this way, but with distinctively different approaches, resulting in not one OH but many. We have traced a direct connection between OH today and the post-war context of international health. As shown in Chapter 4, the realisation within this context that the health and nutrition of humans depended on the health and nutrition of animals produced new institutional settings in which new relationships were formed across human and animal medicine. Chapter 5 shows that this context both resonated with and granted further opportunities for parasitologist Calvin Schwabe to pursue his discipline-crossing research on *E. granulosus.* This work proved crucial to his formulation of an integrated philosophy of 'One Medicine', which both drove and was enhanced by the twenty-first-century OH movement. Such findings reinforce the observation made above that OH—like OM before it—is not a universal good but a product of very specific historical circumstances, which this volume has gone some way to elucidate.

While the discrete case studies presented here function synergistically to shed important light on how animals and modern medicine have shaped each other, they have only begun to scratch the surface of this long neglected historical problem. In this volume we have deliberately sought the commonalities between our case studies in efforts to generate overarching insights into the integrated practice of human and animal health and its development over time and place. However, much more work remains to be done in drawing out some of the specificities: in the capacity of particular animals performing particular roles to influence the course of medicine, as practised by specific individuals working in specific institutions, countries and contexts. Further investigations will elucidate how the lives of different animals were affected by health and medicine. They will enable our preliminary trajectory of OH approaches in modern medicine to be tested and expanded, and will help to clarify the circumstances that facilitated its pursuit in certain times and places.

This is a fertile ground for enquiry, for there are many other contexts beyond those addressed here in which animals have made a difference to, and were changed by medicine. While the experimental laboratory, with its dogs and rodents, represents an obvious focus of enquiry, our case studies have revealed that it was just one of many contexts in which histories of animals and medicine were intertwined. Beyond its bounds lies a richer animal history of medicine, comprising a greater diversity of spaces, species, specialisms, modes of enquiry and human participants. We urge historians to seek out animals within the comparative fields of medicine (such as psychology, neurology, therapeutics, physiology and pathology), at the intersections of human and veterinary medicine (notably epidemiology and veterinary public health), and at the borderlands of medicine and biology (such as agriculture, nutrition science, parasitology and biomedicine). As this volume has demonstrated, such investigations can do more than simply add animals to existing medical historical narratives. They also have the potential to reconfigure understandings of what medicine was, and therefore what medical history might become.

Appendix: Annotated Bibliography of Animals in the History of Medicine

This bibliography aims to orient readers in the literature addressing animals within modern medical history, from c.1800 to the present day. It is confined to works published in the English language, virtually all of which focus on Western and colonial contexts, and in which agricultural and experimental animals—particularly cattle and laboratory rodents—are heavily represented. The discussion is structured according to the roles that humans awarded to animals in medical science, practice and policy. As the chapters in this volume make clear, these roles were extremely diverse and they had their own particular histories. Their awarding was informed partly by human–animal relationships and how they were disrupted by animal disease. Prevailing scientific understandings of animal disease, and the tools available to conceptualize, investigate and manage it, also exerted important influences. These roles had important implications for how animals were perceived and treated by humans in life and afterlife. Through performing them, animals shaped the ideas, practices and social configurations of medicine, with ramifications for the health of humans and animals. Their analysis therefore offers important insights into the human–animal relationships that developed in medicine and society, and allows the reconstruction of the processes through which animals and medicine were co-constituted.

Often animals performed multiple roles—simultaneously or sequentially—in the course of their lives and afterlives. Consequently, it

A. Woods et al., *Animals and the Shaping of Modern Medicine*, Medicine and Biomedical Sciences in Modern History,
https://doi.org/10.1007/978-3-319-64337-3

may seem a little artificial to separate them here. We do this to draw out their individual histories and to highlight the extent to which existing literature privileges certain roles (most notably the experimental animal) over others. It must be acknowledged, however, that because historians tend to regard animals as part of the backdrop of human history rather than as historical subjects in their own right, most accounts offer only an implicit acknowledgement of the roles they performed. More interested in the diseases than their animal subjects, authors rarely historicize or interrogate how animals acted in medical science, practice and policy. This bibliography is intended to make their roles explicit, thereby providing a jumping-off point for future studies that adopt a less anthropocentric approach to medical history.

Animal Patients

Surprisingly little is known about the history of animal patients. This is partly because many animal victims of disease were not awarded this role: they were killed or left to suffer and die rather than being cared for clinically by owners and healers. It is also because historians have not tended to study the sorts of animals and diseases that resulted in the treatment of animals as patients. In focusing on the interests of humans rather than animals, their accounts privilege the effects of infectious animal diseases on the health of humans, animal populations and the agricultural economy. They rarely consider the implications of disease for individual and small groups of highly valued animals that were more likely to be subjected to clinical interventions: Abigail Woods. "Animals and Disease." In *Routledge History of Disease*, edited by Mark Jackson, 147–64. London: Routledge, 2016.

The few authors who have addressed the history of animals as patients show how, as the valuation of animals changed, for example with the rise and decline of horse-drawn society, the increased demand for livestock food in wartime, or the growth of affective bonds with pets, so, too, did their construction as patients: Susan Jones. "Framing Animal Disease: Housecats with Feline Urological Syndrome, Their Owners, and Their Doctors." *Journal of the History of Medicine and Allied Sciences* 52 (1997): 202–35; Susan Jones. *Valuing Animals: Veterinarians and their Patients in Modern America*. Baltimore: John Hopkins University Press, 2003; Chris Degeling. "Picturing the Pain of Animal Others:

Rationalising Form, Function and Suffering in Veterinary Orthopaedics." *History and Philosophy of the Life Sciences* 31 (2009): 377–403; Abigail Woods. "Animals in Surgery." In *Handbook of the History of Surgery*, edited by Thomas Schlich. Basingstoke: Palgrave, 2017.

Particularly high-status animal patients sometimes benefited from similar levels of care and clinical intervention as human patients. In fact their experiences sometimes informed the treatment of human patients, revealing the historically connected nature of human and veterinary surgery: C. Degeling. "Negotiating Value: Comparing Human and Animal Fracture Care in Industrial Societies." *Science, Technology, & Human Values* 34 (2009): 77–101; Andrew Gardiner. "The Animal as Surgical Patient: A Historical Perspective in the Twentieth Century." *History and Philosophy of the Life Sciences* 31 (2009): 355–76; M. Schlünder and T. Schlich. "The Emergence of 'Implant-Pets' and 'Bone-Sheep': Animals as New Biomedical Objects in Orthopedic Surgery (1960s–2010)." *History and Philosophy of the Life Sciences* 31 (2009): 433–66.

Authors have explored how the social and scientific status of veterinary surgeons, their gender and perceived expertise, and their personal and professional interests impacted on the selection and treatment of animals as veterinary patients: Abigail Woods. "The Farm as Clinic: Veterinary Expertise and the Transformation of Dairy Farming, 1930–50." *Studies in History and Philosophy of Biological and Biomedical Sciences* 38 (2007): 462–87; Abigail Woods and Stephen Matthews. "'Little, If At All, Removed from the Illiterate Farrier or Cow-Leech': The English Veterinary Surgeon, c.1860–85, and the Campaign for Veterinary Reform." *Medical History* 54 (2010): 29–54; Andrew Gardiner, "Small Animal Practice in British Veterinary Medicine" (Ph.D. dissertation, University of Manchester, 2010); Julie Hipperson, "Veterinary Training and Veterinary Work: A Female Perspective, 1919–2000" (Ph.D. dissertation, King's College London, 2015); Kenneth Woodger and Elizabeth Stone. "Equine Surgery at the Ontario Veterinary College in the Early Twentieth Century." *Canadian Bulletin of Medical History* 32 (2015): 181–202. By comparison, virtually nothing has been written about how other types of healers, including owners and doctors, fashioned animals into patients, except for W. Beinart and K. Brown. *African Local Knowledge and Livestock Health.* Woodbridge: Boydell and Brewer, 2013.

Animals as Pathological Specimens

The role of pathological specimen was performed after death by many of the animals that feature in this volume. Its frequency reveals how important animal bodies were to the building of pathological knowledge—about diseases that afflicted particular animals, the distribution of diseases across the species, and the disease relationships between species. We have seen how animals were transformed into pathological specimens through post-mortem examination. Their organs, tissues and bodily fluids could be observed directly, removed for exhibition to interested parties, preserved for deposition and inspection within museums, or prepared for microscopic examination within laboratories.

In existing historical literature, these processes and practices are generally sidelined by, or conflated with, the animal's role as experimental material. The key exception is in accounts of the state control of certain late nineteenth-century animal diseases. Woods shows that in Britain, policies for the eradication of contagious bovine pleuropneumonia and swine fever were predicated on the belief that they could be diagnosed accurately during post-mortem examination. Experience demonstrated that this was not, in fact, the case: Abigail Woods. "From Practical Men to Scientific Experts: British Veterinary Surgeons and the Development of Government Scientific Expertise, c.1878–1919." *History of Science* li (2013): 457–80. Other authors have explored the diagnosis, in animal pathological specimens, of diseases that spread to humans via meat consumption. Here the animals performed simultaneously as food, a role that is discussed further below. Starting in Germany, and spreading subsequently to other European countries and the USA, specimens of pig muscle were subjected to microscopic inspection to see if they contained the parasitic disease trichinosis, which could cause death to human consumers: J. Gignilliat. "Pigs, Politics and Protection: The European Boycott of American Pork, 1879–1891." *Agricultural History* 35 (1961): 3–12; J. Cassedy. "Applied Microscopy and American Pork Diplomacy: Charles Wardell Stiles in Germany 1898–1899." *Isis* 62 (1971): 4–20; Dorothee Brantz. "Animal Bodies, Human Health, and the Reform of Slaughterhouses in Nineteenth Century Berlin." In *Meat, Modernity and the Rise of the Slaughterhouse*, edited by P.Y. Lee, 71–85. London: University of New Hampshire, 2008.

The fear that tuberculosis could spread in this way stimulated the post-mortem inspection of bovine bodies. In identifying them as diseased, vets claimed authority over the measures required for their control, often in the face of medical opposition: Susan Jones. *Valuing Animals: Veterinarians and Their Patients in Modern America*, 74–90. Baltimore: Johns Hopkins University Press, 2003; Keir Waddington. *The Bovine Scourge: Meat, Tuberculosis and Public Health, 1850–1914.* Woodbridge: Boydell Press, 2006; Alan Olmstead and Paul Rhodes. *Arresting Contagion: Science, Policy, and Conflicts over Animal Disease Control.* Cambridge: Harvard University Press, 2015; Tatsuya Mitsuda. "Entangled Histories: German Veterinary Medicine, 1770–1900." *Medical History* 61 (2017): 25–47. During the twentieth century, vets working as meat inspectors in slaughterhouses continued their search for pathologies in the bodies of dead livestock: Peter Koolmees. "Veterinary Inspection and Food Hygiene in the Twentieth Century." In *Food, Science, Policy and Regulation in the Twentieth Century*, edited by D. Smith and J. Phillips, 53–68. London: Routledge, 2000; Anne Hardy. "Professional Advantage and Public Health: British Veterinarians and State Veterinary Services, 1865–1939." *Twentieth Century British History* 14 (2003): 1–23.

The transformation of animals into pathological specimens was also important in working out the pathologies of anthrax and tuberculosis, and the relationships between these diseases in humans and animals: Michael Worboys. *Spreading Germs*, 193–233. Cambridge: Cambridge University Press, 2000; Keir Waddington. "The Science of Cows: Tuberculosis, Research and the State in the United Kingdom, 1890–1914." *History of Science* 34 (2001): 355–81; Susan Jones. *Death in a Small Package: A Short History of Anthrax.* Baltimore: John Hopkins University Press, 2010.

Experimental Animals

The experimental animal is the animal role studied most extensively by historians of modern medicine, to the extent that many fail to look beyond it when considering animal contributions to medicine. Although the practice of experimenting on animals stretches back to antiquity, authors recognize that the nineteenth-century development of the laboratory-based sciences of experimental physiology and bacteriology brought new kinds of experiment and experimental animal into existence: William F. Bynum. "'C'est une Malade!' Animal Models and

Concepts of Human Diseases." *Journal of the History of Medicine and Allied Sciences* 45 (1990): 397–413. Their adoption, standardization and use expanded with the emergence of pharmacology, endocrinology, nutritional science and immunology in the decades around 1900, and with the post-Second World War growth of biomedicine. It was underpinned by the belief that it was morally justifiable to experiment on animals in order to advance the ideas and practices of human medicine, and that animal and human bodies were sufficiently similar in health and disease to permit extrapolation from one to the other.

There are a number of historical overviews of animal experimentation: Lise Wilkinson. *Animals and Disease: An Introduction to the History of Comparative Medicine*. Cambridge: Cambridge University Press, 1992; Anita Guerrini. *Experimenting with Humans and Animals: From Galen to Animal Rights*. Baltimore: John Hopkins University Press, 2003; Ilana Lowy. "The Experimental Body." In *Companion Encyclopedia of Medicine in the Twentieth Century*, edited by Roger Cooter and John Pickstone, 435–49. London: Routledge, 2003; Karen Rader. "Scientific Animals: The Laboratory and Its Human-Animal Relations, from Dba to Dolly." In *A Cultural History of Animals, Volume 6: The Modern Age (1920–2000)*, edited by Linda Kalof and Brigitte Resl, 119–37, London: Bloomsbury, 2007; Thomas Schlich, Eric Mykhalovskiy and Melanie Rock. "Animals in Surgery—Surgery in Animals: Nature and Culture in Animal-Human Relations and Modern Surgery." *History and Philosophy of the Life Sciences* 31 (2009): 321–54; Nuno Henrique Franco. "Animal Experiments in Biomedical Research: A Historical Perspective." Animals 3 (2013): 238–73; Abigail Woods. "Between Human and Veterinary Medicine: The History of Animals and Surgery." In *Palgrave Handbook of the History of Surgery*, edited by Thomas Schlich. Basingstoke: Palgrave Macmillan, 2017. These accounts focus predominantly on Western Europe and North America. For colonial perspectives, see Pratik Chakrabarti. "Beasts of Burden: Animals and Laboratory Research in Colonial India." *History of Science* 48 (2010): 125–52; Peter Hobbins. *Venomous Encounters: Snakes, Vivisection and Scientific Medicine in Colonial Australia*. Manchester: Manchester University Press, 2017.

This literature is generally more concerned with the growth of scientific knowledge deriving from experimental animals than with the processes involved in their creation and use. These processes receive more dedicated treatment in studies of how animals were selected and fashioned into the 'right tools for the job' of biomedical research. Authors show that while the animal's biology was important, so, too, was its cost, ease of acquisition, temperament, the experimenters' skills and the baseline information already gathered about its behaviour under experimental conditions. Once established, experimental animals could be turned into more reliable, 'standard' tools through selective breeding, acquisition and maintenance: A.E. Clarke and J.H. Fujimura (eds). *The Right Tools for the Job: At Work in the Twentieth Century Life Sciences.* Princeton: Princeton University Press, 1992; Bonnie Clause. "The Wistar Rat as a Right Choice: Establishing Mammalian Standards and the Ideal of a Standardized Mammal." *Journal of the History of Biology* 26 (1993): 329–49; Frederick Holmes. "The Old Martyr of Science: The Frog in Experimental Physiology." *Journal of the History of Biology* 26 (1993): 311–28; Robert Kohler. "Drosophila: A Life in the Laboratory." *Journal of the History of Biology* 26 (1993): 218–310; Soraya de Chadarevian. "Of Worms and Programmes: Caenorhabditis Elegans and the Study of Development." *Studies in History and Philosophy of Biological and Biomedical Sciences* 29 (1998): 81–105; I. Löwy and J.-P. Gaudillière. "Disciplining Cancer: Mice and the Practice of Genetic Purity." In *The Invisible Industrialist: Manufactures and the Production of Scientific Knowledge*, edited by J.-P. Gaudillière and I. Löwy, 209–49. Basingstoke: Macmillan, 1998; Nick Hopwood and John Gurdon. "The Introduction of Xenopus Laevis into Developmental Biology: Of Empire, Pregnancy Testing and Ribosomal Genes." *International Journal of Developmental Biology* 44 (2000): 43–5; Karen Rader. *Making Mice: Standardizing Animals for American Biomedical Research, 1900–55.* Woodstock: Princeton University Press, 2004; Robert G.W. Kirk. "'Wanted—Standard Guinea Pigs': Standardisation and the Experimental Animal Market in Britain Ca. 1919–1947." *Studies in History and Philosophy of Biological and Biomedical Sciences* 39 (2008): 280–91. While this literature is primarily concerned with how animals were fashioned into quasi-human 'models' of disease, Slater offers an interesting counterexample of avian models of human malaria that were valued in spite of their lack of congruence with humans: Leo Slater. "Malarial Birds: Modeling Infectious Human Disease in Animals." *Bulletin of the History of Medicine* 79 (2005): 261–94.

Moving beyond the selection and breeding of experimental animals, Lynch's classic ethnographic study describes how they were actually used in, and constituted through, experimental practices: Michael Lynch. "Sacrifice and the Transformation of the Animal Body into a Scientific

Object: Laboratory Culture and Ritual Practice in the Neurosciences." *Social Studies of Science* 18 (1988): 265–89. Historically, such procedures can be difficult to reconstruct, although scientists' notebooks offer important clues: Daniel Todes. "Pavlov's Physiology Factory." *Isis* 88, 1997: 205–46; Christoph Gradmann. *Laboratory Disease: Robert Koch's Medical Bacteriology*. Baltimore: Johns Hopkins University Press, 2009. Insights also arise obliquely from studies of the controversies that surrounded animal experimentation. Through documenting antivivisectionists' efforts to expose the treatment of experimental animals, and scientists' attempts to conceal or defend their actions, authors offer glimpses of experimental practices: Richard French. *Antivivisection and Medical Science in Victorian Society*. London: Princeton University Press, 1975, 112–58; Nicolaas Rupke (ed.). *Vivisection in Historical Perspective*. London: Routledge, 1990; Susan Lederer. "Political Animals: The Shaping of Biomedical Research Literature in Twentieth-Century America." *Isis* 83 (1992): 61–79; Hilda Kean. "The 'Smooth Cool Men of Science': The Feminist and Socialist Response to Vivisection." *History Workshop Journal* 40 (1995): 16–38.

Some authors have begun to look beyond the rhetoric that surrounded animal experimentation to interrogate how scientists related to their animal subjects. They show that contrary to the criticisms directed at them, scientists often felt affection, emotion and a sense of moral obligation towards animals, which shaped the experiments they performed and the experiences of their animal subjects. This line of analysis has been developed most productively by Robert Kirk. For example: R.G.W. Kirk. "The Invention of the 'Stressed Animal' and the Development of a Science of Animal Welfare, 1947–86." In *Stress, Shock, and Adaptation in the Twentieth Century*, edited by D. Cantor and E. Ramsden, 241–63. Rochester: University of Rochester Press, 2014; R.G.W. Kirk. "Care in the Cage: Materializing Moral Economies of Animal Care in the Biomedical Sciences, c.1945–." In *Animal Housing and Human–Animal Relations: Politics, Practices and Infrastructures*, edited by K. Bjørkdahl and T. Druglitrø, 167–85. London: Routledge, 2016. See also Daniel Todes. "Pavlov's Physiology Factory." *Isis* 88 (1997): 205–46; O.E. Dror. "The Affect of Experiment. The Turn to Emotions in Anglo-American Physiology, 1900–1940." *Isis* 90 (1999): 205–37; Rob Boddice. "Vivisecting Major: A Victorian Gentleman Scientist Defends Animal Experimentation, 1876–1885." *Isis* 102 (2011): 215–37.

Several authors have drawn attention to the experimental animal's capacity to advance animal as well as human health, and to forge connections between human and animal medicine, for example by illuminating animal diseases that had a bearing on human health and vice versa, or by testing therapeutic interventions intended for application in both human and animal patients. Their findings challenge the anthropocentric assumption that humans were the intended beneficiaries of animal experiments: Chris Degeling. "Negotiating Value: Comparing Human and Animal Fracture Care in Industrial Societies." *Science, Technology and Human Values* 34 (2009): 77–101; Thomas Schlich and Martina Schlünder. "The Emergence of 'Implant-Pets' and 'Bone-Sheep': Animals as New Biomedical Objects in Orthopedic Surgery (1960s–2010)." *History and Philosophy of the Life Sciences* 31 (2009): 433–66; Michael Bresalier and Michael Worboys. "'Saving the Lives of Our Dogs': The Development of Canine Distemper Vaccine in Interwar Britain." *The British Journal for the History of Science* 47 (2014): 305–34.

In their accounts of experimental medicine, authors often conflate the role of the experimental animal with that of the 'animal model' of human disease. In fact the term 'animal model' was rarely used before the 1940s and its genealogy awaits investigation. Like the 'experimental animal', it was an umbrella term that encompassed a cluster of different roles whose significance waxed and waned over time and space. Logan begins to dissect these in her study of late nineteenth-century German experimental physiology. She differentiates between general physiological approaches, in which diverse species were studied in order to work out the similarities between them, and increasingly dominant, biomedically orientated efforts to create new knowledge from animals whose resemblance to humans was assumed. The former method involved comparison between species, therefore experimental animals performed roles also as 'points of comparison' (see below). In the latter they were regarded as homologous: Cheryl Logan. "Before there Were Standards: The Role of Test Animals in the Production of Empirical Generality in Physiology." *Journal of the History of Biology* 35 (2002): 329–63.

Social scientific analyses of the life sciences go further in differentiating between experimental animals that did not necessarily represent species other than themselves, and those which performed as 'models'—by generating fundamental knowledge of a larger group, or by acting as surrogates for species that were difficult to study experimentally. They show that the epistemological status of the animal influenced its fashioning and use, the social organization of studies that employed it, and the nature and perceived validity of the resulting knowledge. These processes merit further historical elucidation: Jessica Bolker. "Exemplary and Surrogate Models: Two Modes of Representation in Biology." *Perspectives in Biology and Medicine* 52 (2009): 485–99; Niall Shanks, Ray Greek and Jean Greek. "Are Animal Models Predictive for Humans?" *Philosophy, Ethics, and Humanities in Medicine* 4(2) (2009); Bruno Strasser and Soraya de Chadarevian. "The Comparative and the Exemplary: Revisiting the Early History of Molecular Biology." *History of Science* 49 (2011): 317–36; Sabina Leonelli and Rachel Ankeny. "What Makes a Model Organism?" *Endeavour* 37 (2013): 209–12; J. Lewis et al. "Representation and Practical Accomplishment in the Laboratory: When Is an Animal Model Good-Enough?" *Sociology* 47 (2013): 776–92; Pierre-Luc Germain. "From Replica to Instruments: Animal Models in Biomedical Research." *History and Philosophy of the Life Sciences* 36 (2014): 114–28.

Experimental animals did not only produce knowledge. Another role, which emerged with the development of smallpox vaccination and grew more significant in the late nineteenth and twentieth centuries, was that of supplier and standardizer of biological products for use in humans. There are several accounts of how animal bodies were used to culture vaccines and sera: Bruno Latour. *The Pasteurization of France*, translated by Alan Sheridan and John Law. London: Harvard University Press, 1988; J. Simon. "Monitoring the Stable at the Pasteur Institute." *Science in Context* 21 (2008): 181–200; S.L. Kotar and J.E. Gessler. *Smallpox: A History*. Jefferson: McFarland & Company, 2013. Animals also supplied hormones and organs: Nelly Oudshoorn. "On the Making of Sex Hormones: Research Materials and the Production of Knowledge." *Social Studies of Science* 20 (1990): 5–33; Chandak Sengoopta. "'Dr Steinach Coming to Make Old Young!': Sex Glands, Vasectomy and the Quest for Rejuvenation in the Roaring Twenties." *Endeavour* 27 (2003): 122–26; Catherine Rémy. "The Animal Issue in Xenotransplantation: Controversies in France and the United States." *History and Philosophy of the Life Sciences* 31 (2009): 407–32. In addition, they helped to test the safety and efficacy of biological products: E.M. Tansey. "The Wellcome Physiological Research Laboratories 1894–1904: The Home Office, Pharmaceutical Firms, and Animal Experiments." *Medical History* 33 (1989): 1–41.

Animal Hosts and Transmitters of Infection

As hosts and transmitters of infection, animals feature frequently in medical historical literature. However, it is the diseases they spread rather than the animals themselves that form the focus of historical enquiry. Medical historians are primarily interested in diseases known as zoonoses that spread from animals to humans. Infectious diseases that did not affect humans are usually relegated to veterinary history. For an overview, see Abigail Woods. "Animals and Disease." In *Routledge History of Disease*, edited by Mark Jackson, 147–64. London: Routledge, 2016. However, medical historians have noted cases in which the animal-to-animal transmission of disease was studied by doctors, with implications for general understandings of disease: Christoph Gradmann. "Robert Koch and the Invention of the Carrier State: Tropical Medicine, Veterinary Infections and Epidemiology around 1900." *Studies in History and Philosophy of Biological and Biomedical Sciences* 41 (2010): 232–40. In this regard, medical investigations into the British cattle plague epidemic of 1865–1867 have recieved particular attention: Michael Worboys. "Germ Theories of Disease and British Veterinary Medicine, 1860–1890." *Medical History* 35 (1991): 308–27; John Fisher. "British Physicians, Medical Science and the Cattle Plague, 1865–6." *Bulletin of the History of Medicine* 67 (1993): 651–99; T. Romano. "The Cattle Plague of 1865 and the Reception of the Germ Theory." *Journal of the History of Medicine* 52 (1997): 51–80.

In the late nineteenth century, the development of empire, international trade, railways and steamships generated new opportunities for animals to perform as hosts and transmitters of infection to humans. Concurrently, the pathways through which these diseases were transmitted were elucidated by newly developed epidemiological and bacteriological methods: Lise Wilkinson. *Animals and Disease: An Introduction to the History of Comparative Medicine*. Cambridge: Cambridge University Press, 1992; Anne Hardy. "Animals, Disease, and Man: Making Connections." *Perspectives in Biology and Medicine* 46 (2003): 200–15; Mark Harrison. *Contagion: How Commerce has Spread Disease*, 211–46. New Haven: Yale University Press, 2012.

Some animals transmitted diseases to humans via their meat and milk. They are discussed further in the sections on 'animals as food' and as 'pathological specimens'. Others transmitted diseases directly or via the environment, as in the transmission of influenza. Investigations into its spread involved fashioning certain animals into experimental models: Michael Bresalier. "Neutralizing Flu: 'Immunological Devices' and the Making of a Virus Disease." In *Crafting Immunity: Working Histories of Clinical Immunology*, edited by Kenton Kroker, Jennifer Keelan and Pauline Mazumdar, 107–44. Aldershot & Burlington: Ashgate, 2008. The effects of influenza on horses is explored by Floor Haalboom. "'Spanish' Flu and Army Horses: What Historians and Biologists Can Learn from a History of Animals with Flu during the 1918–1919 Influenza Pandemic." *Studium: Tijdschrift Voor Wetenschaps-En Universiteits-Geschiedenis | Revue d'Histoire Des Sciences et Des Universités* 7 (2014): 124–39.

The resurgence of influenza in the twenty-first-century-inspired studies of how animals became the focus of human fears about disease pandemics, with consequences for the animals themselves: Charles Mather and Amy Marshall. "Living with Disease? Biosecurity and Avian Influenza in Ostriches." *Agriculture and Human Values* 28 (2010): 153–65; Steve Hinchliffe et al. *Pathological Lives: Disease, Space and Biopolitics.* Chichester: Wiley Blackwell, 2016. Authors highlight the organizational barriers that separated responses to influenza in humans and animals, and helped to drive today's One Health agenda: Yu-Ju Chien. "How Did International Agencies Perceive the Avian Influenza Problem? The Adoption and Manufacture of the 'One World, One Health' Framework." *Sociology of Health & Illness* 35 (2013): 213–26; Colin Jerolmack. "Who's Worried about Turkeys? How 'Organisational Silos' Impede Zoonotic Disease Surveillance." *Sociology of Health & Illness* 35 (2013): 200–12. A final theme is how claims and concerns over zoonotic disease risk are constructed and contested, and with what consequences for human–animal relationships: Brigitte Nerlich, Brian Brown and Paul Crawford. "Health, Hygiene and Biosecurity: Tribal Knowledge Claims in the UK Poultry Industry." *Health, Risk & Society* 11 (2009): 561–77; David Gerber, Claudine Burton-Jeangros and Annik Dubied. "Animals in the Media: New Boundaries of Risk?" *Health, Risk & Society* 13 (2011): 17–30.

Another zoonosis that has received significant historical attention is rabies. Its transmission by 'man's best friend' and the horrific symptoms it caused often provoked disproportionate fear and panic, leading to measures such as mass slaughter, vaccination, muzzling and quarantine of dogs. These have been explored in late nineteenth-century South Africa: Lance Van Sittert. "Class and Canicide in Little Bess:

The 1893 Port Elizabeth Rabies Epidemic." *South African Historical Journal* 48 (2003): 207–34; the USA: Philip M. Teigen. "Legislating Fear and the Public Health in Gilded Age Massachusetts." *Journal of the History of Medicine and Allied Sciences* 62 (2007): 141–70; colonial Madagascar: Eric T. Jennings. "Confronting Rabies and Its Treatments in Colonial Madagascar, 1899–1910." *Social History of Medicine* 22 (2009): 263–82; France: Kathleen Kete. "La Rage and the Bourgeoisie." *Representations* 22 (1988): 89–107; and most extensively, Britain: Neil Pemberton and Michael Worboys. *Mad Dogs and Englishmen: Rabies in Britain 1830–2000*. Basingstoke: Palgrave Macmillan, 2007; Philip Howell, *At Home and Astray: The Domestic Dog in Victorian Britain*, London: University of Virginia Press, 2015, 150–74. The distinctive manifestations of rabies in Southern Africa, where it circulated and spread through meerkats, jackals and other animals, have also been explored: Karen Brown, *Mad Dogs and Meerkats: A History of Resurgent Rabies in Southern Africa*. Athens: Ohio University Press, 2011.

Other key late nineteenth-century zoonoses were glanders, a respiratory disease of horses that proved fatal in humans: Lise Wilkinson. "Glanders: Medicine and Veterinary Medicine in Common Pursuit of a Contagious Disease." *Medical History* 25 (1981): 363–84; J. Brian Derbyshire. "The Eradication of Glanders from Canada." *Canadian Veterinary Journal* 43 (2002): 722–26; and anthrax, a sporadic but potentially devastating disease of horses, sheep and cattle, which spread via sheep fleeces to cause 'woolsorters disease' and 'malignant pustule' in late nineteenth-century wool workers: Daniel Gilfoyle. "Anthrax in South Africa: Economics, Experiment, and the Mass Vaccination of Animals, c.1910–45." *Medical History* 50 (2006): 465–90; Maurice Cassier, "Producing, Controlling and Stabilising Pasteur's Anthrax Vaccine: Creating a New Industry and a Health Market", *Science in Context* 21 (2008): 253–78; Susan Jones. *Death in a Small Package: A Short History of Anthrax*. Baltimore: Johns Hopkins University Press, 2010; James Stark. *The Making of Modern Anthrax, 1875–1920*. London: Pickering & Chatto, 2013.

New zoonotic disease threats were identified in the twentieth century. Rats and other rodents were identified as vectors of bubonic plague: Christos Lynteris. *Ethnographic Plague—Configuring Disease on the Chinese-Russian Frontier*. London: Palgrave Macmillan, 2016. Species of malaria thought to be specific to monkeys were found to transmit to humans: Rachel Mason Dentinger. "Patterns of

Infection and Patterns of Evolution: How a Malaria Parasite Brought 'Monkeys and Man' Closer Together in the 1960s." *Journal of the History of Biology* 49 (2016): 359–95. Parrots and pigeons were discovered to harbour psittacosis, which caused pneumonia and systemic disease in humans: Colin Jerolmack. "How Pigeons Became Rats: The Cultural-Spatial Logic of Problem Animals." *Social Problems* 55 (2008): 72–94; Mark Honigsbaum. "'Tipping the Balance': Karl Friedrich Meyer, Latent Infections, and the Birth of Modern Ideas of DiseaseEcology." *Journal of the History of Biology* 49 (2016): 261–309. More recently, animals have been implicated in the emergence and spread of AIDS, SARS and Ebola: Nicholas Johnson (ed.) *The Role of Animals in Emerging Viral Diseases.* Amsterdam: Academic Press, 2013.

While typically, historians do not include insects and parasitic worms in their definitions of 'animal', Chapter 5 shows that parasitologists did. Looking at the histories of these creatures, as studied within the fields of tropical medicine and parasitology, offers a different perspective on animals as hosts and transmitters of infection between humans and other species of animal. Key studies which recognize the parasite as a historical actor include: Timothy Mitchell. "Can the Mosquito Speak?" In *Rule of Experts: Egypt, Technopolitics, Modernity*, 19–53. London: University of California Press, 2002; Ulli Beisel, Anne Kelly and N. Tousignant. "Knowing Insects: Hosts, Vectors and Companions of Science." *Science as Culture* 22 (2013): 1–15 and other papers in that volume; Rohan Deb Roy. "Quinine, Mosquitoes and Empire: Reassembling Malaria in British India, 1890–1910." *South Asian History and Culture* 4 (2013), 65–86.

Animals as Food

As food, animals were important to the history of medicine in two key ways. First, and more prominently, as transmitters of diseases to humans, and second as suppliers of valuable nutrition to humans. However, whether they threatened human health or benefited it, the animals themselves rarely feature in historical accounts. Instead they 'disappear' into their bodily products, or are sidelined by the microbes they disseminated. A rare exception is Jonathan Saha's "Milk to Mandalay: Dairy Consumption, Animal History and the Political Geography of Colonial Burma." *Journal of Historical Geography* 54 (2016): 1–12.

For a historical overview of animals as threats to human consumers, see Patrick Zylberman. "Making Food Safety an Issue: Internationalized Food Politics and French Public Health from the 1870s to the Present." *Medical History* 48 (2004): 1–28. Like other hosts and transmitters of zoonotic diseases, animals as food became more threatening to human health in the late nineteenth century, as greater affluence, changing tastes and the expanding meat trade provided new opportunities for them to spread disease via their meat and milk. At the same time, new tools were developed for detecting and controlling these diseases. Their application to the meat-borne parasitic disease, trichinosis, are discussed above under 'Animals aspathological specimens'. However, it is tuberculosis that has received the lion's share of the historical attention. Late-nineteenth-century debates over its spread via cow's meat and milk, and the often controversial methods adopted for its control—namely, removal of meat from the food chain, the pasteurization of milk, the tuberculin testing and slaughter of cows, and (in select countries) the BCG vaccination of cows—offer important insights into changing patterns of production and consumption, farming economies, veterinary–medical relationships, the state's responsibility for food safety, and the development of new disease-control technologies.

Key works on the history of tuberculosis include: D. Cousins and J. Roberts. "Australia's Campaign to Eradicate Bovine Tuberculosis: The Battle for Freedom and Beyond." *Tuberculosis* 81 (2001), 5–15; Keir Waddington. "The Science of Cows: Tuberculosis, Research and the State in the United Kingdom, 1890–1914." *History of Science* 39 (2001): 355–81; Anne Hardy. "Professional Advantage and Public Health: British Veterinarians and State Veterinary Services, 1865–1939." *Twentieth Century British History* 14 (2003): 1–23; B. Orland. "Cow's Milk and Human Disease: Bovine Tuberculosis and the Difficulties Involved in Combating Animal Diseases." *Food and History* 1 (2003): 179–202; Susan Jones. "Mapping a Zoonotic Disease: Anglo-American Efforts to Control Bovine Tuberculosis Before World War I." *Osiris* 19 (2004): 133–48; Keir Waddington. "To Stamp Out 'So Terrible a Malady': Bovine Tuberculosis and Tuberculin Testing in Britain, 1890–1939." *Medical History* 48 (2004): 29–48; Keir Waddington. *The Bovine Scourge: Meat, Tuberculosis and Public Health, 1850–1914.* Woodbridge: Boydell & Brewer, 2006; Delphine Berdah. "La Vaccination Des Bovides Contre La Tuberculose En France, 1921–1963: Entre Modele Epistemique et Alternative a L' Abattage." *Revue d'Etudes En Agriculture et Environnement* 91 (2009): 393–415; Gillian Colclough. "'Filthy Vessels': Milk Safety and Attempts to Restrict the Spread of Bovine Tuberculosis in Queensland." *Health and History* 12 (2010): 6–26; Alan Olmstead and Paul Rhodes. *Arresting Contagion: Science, Policy, and Conflicts over Animal Disease Control*. Cambridge: Harvard University Press, 2015; P. Robinson. "A History of Bovine Tuberculosis Eradication Policy in Northern Ireland." *Journal of Epidemiology and Infection* 143 (2015): 3182–95; Peter Atkins. *A History of Uncertainty: Bovine Tuberculosis in Britain, 1850 to the Present*. Winchester University Press: Winchester, 2016.

Cow's milk could threaten human health by the transmission of other diseases which originated in the cow, and by the contamination or adulteration of milk after it had left the cow. Several authors have described efforts to define, identify and manage these health threats, and their implications for producers, processors and consumers (but not cows): Peter Atkins. "The Pasteurisation of England: The Science, Culture and Health Implications of Milk Processing, 1900–1950." In *Food, Science, Policy and Regulation in the Twentieth Century: International and Comparative Perspectives*, edited by Jim Phillips and David F. Smith, 37–51. London: Routledge, 2000; Gareth Enticott. "Lay Immunology, Local Foods and Rural Identity: Defending Unpasteurised Milk in England." *Sociologia Ruralis* 43 (2003): 257–70; Elizabeth Cullen Dunn. "The Pasteurized State: Milk, Health and the Government of Risk." *Endeavour* 35 (2011): 107–15; Jacob Steere-Williams. "The Perfect Food and the Filth Disease: Milk-Borne Typhoid and Epidemiological Practice in Late Victorian Britain." *Journal of the History of Medicine and Allied Sciences* 65 (2014): 514–45; Jacob Steere-Williams. "Milking Science for Its Worth: The Reform of the British Milk Trade in the Late Nineteenth Century." *Agricultural History* 89 (2015): 263–88.

Similar issues are touched on in overview histories of milk: Melanie DuPuis. *Nature's Perfect Food: How Milk Became America's Drink*. New York University Press: New York, 2002; Peter Atkins. *Liquid Materialities: A History of Milk, Science and the Law*. Farnham: Ashgate, 2010; Kendra Smith-Howard. *Pure and Modern Milk: An Environmental History since 1900*. Oxford: Oxford University Press, 2016. These accounts also refer to the perceived benefits of milk consumption and efforts to promote it, particularly among children. Farmers benefited from the increased sale of this product: Peter Atkins. "Fattening Children or Fattening Farmers? School Milk in Britain, 1921–1941." *The Economic History Review* 58 (2005): 57–78; Cariin Martiin. "Swedish Milk, a Swedish Duty: Dairy Marketing in the 1920s and 1930s." *Rural History* 21 (2010): 213–32; Virginia Thorley. "Australian School Milk Schemes to 1974: For the Benefit of Whom?" *Health and History* 16 (2014): 63–86.

The outbreak of bovine spongiform encephalopathy during the 1980s and 1990s in Britain saw the appearance of an entirely new food-borne zoonosis: Patrick Van Zwanenberg and Erik Millstone. *BSE: Risk, Science and Governance.* Oxford: Oxford University Press, 2005; Kiheung Kim. *The Social Construction of Disease: From Scrapie to Prion.* London: Routledge, 2007. Its definition as a zoonoses was delayed and contested: David Miller. "Risk, Science and Policy: Definitional Struggles, Information Management, the Media and BSE." *Social Science & Medicine* 49 (1999): 1239–55; Peter Washer. "Representations of Mad Cow Disease." *Social Science & Medicine* 62 (2006): 457–66. The crisis which resulted is widely acknowledged as both a symptom of, and a driver of critical changes in, the relationships between British science, media, policy and wider publics: Gwendolyn Blue. "Food, Publics, Science." *Public Understanding of Science* 19 (2009): 147–54. It followed a series of other public controversies about food, disease and scientific uncertainty that occurred in relation to typhoid in meat, *Salmonella* in eggs and *E. coli* in meat and milk: David F. Smith. "Food Panics in History: Corned Beef, Typhoid and 'Risk Society.'" *Journal of Epidemiology and Community Health* 61 (2007): 566–70; Hugh Pennington. "*E. Coli* O157 Outbreaks in the United Kingdom: Past, Present, and Future." *Infection and Drug Resistance* 7 (2014): 211–22; A. Hardy. *Salmonella Infections, Networks of Knowledge, and Public Health in Britain, 1880–1975.* Oxford: Oxford University Press, 2014.

This atmosphere of controversy and concern has continued into the twenty-first century, with debates about the role of the poultry industry in the spread of campylobacter: Steve Hinchliffe et al. *Pathological Lives: Disease, Space and Biopolitics.* Chichester: Wiley Blackwell, 2016; the presence of horsemeat in 'beef' products: Yasmin Ibrahim and Anita Howarth. "Contamination, Deception and 'Othering': The Media Framing of the Horsemeat Scandal." *Social Identities* 23 (2017): 212–31; and the agricultural usage of antibiotics: Carol Morris,

Richard Helliwell and Sujatha Raman. "Framing the Agricultural Use of Antibiotics and Antimicrobial Resistance in UK National Newspapers and the Farming Press." *Journal of Rural Studies* 45 (2016): 43–53. These episodes highlight changing human concerns about the health and welfare of animals, as well as anxieties about the health and moral risks *for humans* of present-day systems for producing food from animals.

Animals as Points of Comparison

As noted above under 'experimental material', animals that performed as experimental subjects sometimes acted also as points of comparison with other species. However, more commonly within biomedical settings they were assumed to be homologous 'models' of humans: Cheryl Logan. "Before there Were Standards: The Role of Test Animals in the Production of Empirical Generality in Physiology." *Journal of the History of Biology* 35 (2002): 329–63. The extent to which the practices known as 'comparative pathology' actually involved animals acting as points of comparison merits further investigation. They performed this role within the observational form of comparative pathology that was practiced within the zoo (Chapter 2), and by the founder of tropical medicine, Patrick Manson: Shang-Jen Li. "Natural History of Parasitic Disease: Patrick Manson's Philosophical Method." *Isis* 93 (2002): 206–28; but accounts of the experimental form of this activity do not always make the practice of comparison explicit. For example: P.M. Teigen. "William Osler and Comparative Medicine." *Canadian Veterinary Journal* 25 (1984): 400–5; William F. Bynum. "'C'est une Malade!' Animal Models and Concepts of Human Diseases." *Journal of the History of Medicine and Allied Sciences* 45 (1990): 397–413; Lise Wilkinson. *Animals and Disease: An Introduction to the History of Comparative Medicine.* Cambridge: Cambridge University Press, 1992; Erika Jensen-Jarolim, "Definition of Comparative Medicine: History and New Identity." In *Comparative Medicine, Anatomy and Physiology*, edited by Erika Jensen-Jarolim, 1–18. Wien: Springer, 2014.

Recent analyses that explore the intersections between these two traditions offer intriguing insights into how the comparison of different animals' blood sera or their susceptibility to parasitic infection were used in the twentieth century to draw conclusions about their biological relationships: Bruno J. Strasser. "Laboratories, Museums, and the Comparative Perspective: Alan A. Boyden's Quest for Objectivity in Serological Taxonomy, 1924–1962." *Historical Studies in the Natural Sciences* 40 (2010): 149–82; Rachel Mason Dentinger. "Patterns of

Infection and Patterns of Evolution: How a Malaria Parasite Brought 'Monkeys and Man' Closer Together in the 1960s." *Journal of the History of Biology* 49 (2016): 359–95.

Animals did act as points of comparison elsewhere in medicine, notably in efforts to compare human and animal brains and minds: Robert J. Richards, *Darwin and the Emergence of Evolutionary Theories of Mind and Behavior*. Chicago: University of Chicago Press, 1987. Historians have analysed the significant impact of nineteenth-century theories of evolution, common mental descent, and degeneration on contemporaneous neurology, psychology and psychiatry. Animals, their illnesses and their pathologies are usually marginal in these accounts, though there have been important correctives: Marion Thomas. "Are Animals Just Noisy Machines? Louis Boutan and the Co-Invention of Animal and Child Psychology in the French Third Republic." *Journal of the History of Biology* 38 (2005): 425–60; Edmund Ramsden and Duncan Wilson. "The Suicidal Animal: Science and the Nature of Self-Destruction." *Past and Present* 224 (2014): 201–42.

There is an extensive, related scholarship of animals as points of comparison in the history of emotions. For example: Liz Gray. "Body, Mind and Madness: Pain in Animals in Nineteenth-Century Comparative Psychology." In *Pain and Emotion in Modern History*, edited by Rob Boddice, 148–63. Basingstoke: Palgrave Macmillan, 2014. Scholars are only just beginning to explore the twentieth-century history of comparative neurology: A.C. Palmer. "The Comparative Society for the Study of Comparative Medicine 1957–1992: An Exercise in 'One Medicine'." *Veterinary History* 17 (2014): 238–56.

Better documented is the animal as a point of comparison in work taking place post-Second World War at the intersection of ethology, primatology and sociobiology with psychiatry. Harry Harlow's studies of rhesus monkeys and their affiliations with John Bowlby's attachment theories are perhaps best known: Marga Vicedo. "The Evolution of Harry Harlow: From the Nature to the Nurture of Love." *History of Psychiatry* 21 (2010): 190–205; but see also: Richard W. Burkhardt. *Patterns of Behavior: Konrad Lorenz, Niko Tinbergen, and the Founding of Ethology*. Chicago: University of Chicago Press, 2005, especially Chapter 10; Chloe Silverman. "'Birdwatching and Baby-Watching': Niko and Elisabeth Tinbergen's Ethological Approach to Autism." *History of Psychiatry* 21 (2010): 176–89, and other contributions to the special issue "A Hundred Years of Evolutionary Psychiatry (1872–1972)." *History of Psychiatry* 21 (2010); Erika L. Milam. "Making Males Aggressive and

Females Coy: Gender across the Animal-Human Boundary." *Signs* 37 (2012): 935–59. Comparing animal brains and minds continues to resonate today: Laurel Braitman. *Animal Madness: How Anxious Dogs, Compulsive Parrots, and Elephants in Recovery Help Us Understand Ourselves.* New York: Simon & Schuster, 2014.

Animals as Shapers and Products of Environments and Ecologies

Medical historians have only infrequently addressed how, within medical contexts, animals act as shapers and products of environments. If we take the category 'animal' to include bacteria, then the gradual, piecemeal later-nineteenth-century shift from miasmatic to bacteriological theories of infection, and concurrent discussions of the evolution and spontaneous generation of disease, reveal how doctors perceived microorganisms to shape and be shaped by their surroundings: Michael Worboys. *Spreading Germs: Disease Theories and Medical Practice in Britain, 1865–1900.* Cambridge: Cambridge University Press, 2000; William F. Bynum. "The Evolution of Germs and the Evolution of Disease: Some British Debates, 1870–1900." *History and Philosophy of the Life Sciences* 24 (2002): 53–68. The same was true of parasites: John Farley, "Parasites and the Germ Theory of Disease." In *Framing Disease: Studies in Cultural History*, edited by Charles Rosenberg and Janet Golden, 33–49. New Brunswick: Rutgers University Press, 1992.

Such perceptions were sustained into the twentieth century, when ecologists and other biologists observed infection in humans and animals, giving rise to ideas of 'disease ecology', in which microorganisms were understood as part of wider systems of interaction between multiple species and changing environmental conditions: Warwick Anderson. "Natural Histories of Infectious Disease: Ecological Vision in Twentieth-Century Biomedical Science." *Osiris* 19 (2004): 39–61; Gregg Mitman. "In Search of Health: Landscape and Disease in American Environmental History." *Environmental History* 10 (2005): 184–210; Susan Jones. "Population Cycles, Disease, and Networks of Ecological Knowledge." *Journal of the History of Biology* 50(2) (2016): 357–91; see also Pierre-Olivier Méthot and Rachel Mason Dentinger. "Ecology and Infection: Studying Host-Parasite Interactions at the Interface of Biology and Medicine." *Journal of the History of Biology* 49 (2016): 231–40 and other papers in that issue.

Environmental historians have more to say about animals as shapers and products of their environments. However, their interests overlap only occasionally with those of medical historians and they sometimes depart from them in employing contemporary scientific knowledge to understand how organisms and natural environments acted in history: Libby Robin and Jane Carruthers. "Introduction: Environmental History and the History of Biology." *Journal of the History of Biology* 44 (2011): 1–14. For a critique of this approach, see Sverker Sörlin and Paul Warde. "The Problem of the Problem of Environmental History: A Re-Reading of the Field," *Environmental History* 12 (2007): 107–30. This scholarship offers one model for placing non-humans at the centre of historical narratives in ways that demonstrate their interactions with the environment around them.

For recent examples from a large body of literature, see: William Beinart. "Transhumance, Animal Diseases and Environment in the Cape, South Africa." *South African Historical Journal* 58 (2007): 17–41; Miles Alexander Powell. "People in Peril, Environments at Risk: Coolies, Tigers and Colonial Singapore's Ecology of Poverty." *Environment and History* 22 (2016): 455–82; Tiago Saraiva. *Fascist Pigs: Technoscientific Organisms and the History of Fascism*. Cambridge: MIT Press, 2016. While the animals in these accounts are often large mammals, some histories also address the lives of insects, worms and other less charismatic animals: Nick Bingham. "Bees, Butterflies, and Bacteria: Biotechnology and the Politics of Nonhuman Friendship." *Environment and Planning A* 38 (2006): 325–41; Jacob Bull. "Between Ticks and People: Responding to Nearbys and Contentments." *Emotion, Space, and Society* 12 (2014): 73–84; Franklin Ginn, Uli Beisel and Maan Barua. "Flourishing with Awkward Creatures: Togetherness, Vulnerability, Killing", *Environmental Humanities* 4 (2014): 113–23; Derek Lee Nelson. "The Ravages of Teredo: The Rise and Fall of Shipworm in US History, 1860–1940." *Environmental History* 21 (2016): 100–24. Especially relevant to the history of medicine is Jamie Lorimer's recent work on the human microbiome: "Gut Buddies: Multispecies Studies and the Microbiome." *Environmental Humanities* 8 (2016): 57–76.

Also worth mentioning is 'evolutionary history', which attempts to directly examine the entanglement of organic biological change and human history: Susan R. Schrepfer and Philip Scranton (eds).

Industrializing Organisms: Introducing Evolutionary History. New York: Routledge, 2004; Abraham H. Gibson. *Feral Animals in the American South: An Evolutionary History*. Cambridge: Cambridge University Press, 2016; Joshua Specht. "The Rise, Fall, and Rebirth of the Texas Longhorn: An Evolutionary History." *Environmental History* 21 (2016): 343–63. Most relevant to medical historians in this literature is Edmund P. Russell's inclusion of the evolution of antibiotic resistance in his programmatic *Evolutionary Biology: Uniting History and Biology to Understand Life on Earth*. Cambridge: Cambridge University Press, 2011.

Index

A. Woods et al., *Animals and the Shaping of Modern Medicine*, Medicine and Biomedical Sciences in Modern History,
https://doi.org/10.1007/978-3-319-64337-3

I

J

K

www.ingramcontent.com/pod-product-compliance
Lightning Source LLC
LaVergne TN
LVHW082119200926
848484LV00008B/1982